LIPPINCOTT MANUAL OF
MEDICAL-SURGICAL NURSING

Volume 1

LILLIAN SHOLTIS BRUNNER,
RN, MSN, ScD, FAAN
Consultant in Nursing, Schools of Nursing: Bryn Mawr Hospital and Presbyterian-University of Pennsylvania Medical Center; formerly Assistant Professor of Surgical Nursing, Yale University School of Nursing

DORIS SMITH SUDDARTH,
RN, BSNE, MSN
Consultant in Health Occupations, Job Corps Health Office, U.S. Department of Labor; formerly Coordinator of the Curriculum, Alexandria Hospital School of Nursing

CONTRIBUTORS

Herbert H. Butler, MD

Emergency Department Physician, Underwood-Memorial Hospital, Woodbury, New Jersey; Immediate Past President, New Jersey Chapter American College of Emergency Physicians

James F. Elam, PhD

Clinical Biochemist, Pathology Department, Alexandria Hospital, Alexandria, Virginia

Joseph B. Mizgerd, MD

Director, Department of Pulmonary Medicine, Washington Adventist Hospital, Takoma Park, Maryland

Alfred Munzer, MD

Associate Director, Department of Pulmonary Medicine, Washington Adventist Hospital, Takoma Park, Maryland

CONTRIBUTORS TO THE UK EDITION

Barbara Dunn, SRN, SCM, RCNT, RNT, DipN

Nurse Tutor, Nurse Education Centre, St Luke's Hospital, Guildford

Leonard Evans, BA, SRN, ONC, RCNT, RNT

Senior Tutor, Royal Orthopaedic Hospital, Birmingham

Cynthia Gilling, SRN, SCM, RNT

Assistant Director of Nurse Education, The Princess Alexandra School of Nursing, The London Hospital, London

Susan A Gowers, SRN, RCNT

Senior Nursing Officer (Capital Planning), Trent Regional Health Authority, formerly Senior Nursing Officer, Royal Marsden Hospital, London

Rosemarie Hawkins, SRN

Department of Occupational Medicine, Cardiothoracic Institute, Brompton Hospital, London

Morgan Hicks, SRN, OND, RCNT, Cert Ed, RNT

Tutor, Charing Cross Hospital School of Nursing, Charing Cross Hospital, London

Elizabeth Keighley, SRN, RSCN, RCNT, DipN

Clinical Teacher, JBCNS Course in Neuromedical/Neurosurgical Nursing, Cambridge School of Nursing, Addenbrooke's Hospital, Cambridge

Geraldine Matthison, SRN

Formerly Sister, Endocrine Unit, St Thomas's Hospital, London

Margaret Reed, SRN, DipN, Cert Ed, RNT

Tutor (Continuing and Inservice Education), Cambridge School of Nursing, Addenbrooke's Hospital, Cambridge

Lynette Stone, BA, SRN, SCM (NSW)

Nursing Officer (Outpatients), St John's Hospital for Diseases of the Skin, London

THE LIPPINCOTT MANUAL
OF MEDICAL-SURGICAL NURSING

VOLUME 1

Lillian S. Brunner and Doris S. Suddarth

Harper & Row, Publishers
London

Cambridge
Mexico City
New York
Philadelphia

San Francisco
São Paulo
Singapore
Sydney

British Library Cataloguing in Publication Data

Brunner, Lillian
    Lippincott manual of medical-surgical nursing.
    Vol. 1
    1. Nursing
    I. Title   II. Suddarth, Doris
    610.73   RT41

ISBN 0-06-318207-6

Typeset by Inforum Ltd, Portsmouth
Printed and Bound by The Bath Press, Avon

NOTE:
The publishers wish to state that, whilst every effort has been made
to ensure the accuracy and correctness of the information
contained herein, the authors of the original work from which this
adaptation is taken cannot be held responsible for any changes
made to the original text in the course of the adaptation.

CONTENTS

Volume 1

Volume 2

Volume 3

FOREWORD

In recent years, there have been many American nursing books introduced on to the British market. Although most of these are very well presented, the differences in terminology and in some nursing practices have been great disadvantages.

The *Lippincott Manual*, which is very widely used in America, has been completely adapted for the UK by trained nurses in this country, each having a specialized knowledge in a particular field.

The information is tabulated for easy reference and we believe that these three volumes of medical-surgical nursing will form a useful source of information for both learners and trained nurses. We would like to thank our professional colleagues for their willing help and advice while we were gathering this information.

The first volume of *The Lippincott Manual of Medical-Surgical Nursing* introduces the basic nursing concepts within the framework of the nursing process. Other sections in this volume refer to conditions which are encountered in every sphere of nursing, such as the elderly patient, the cancer patient and those undergoing surgery.

The second volume introduces interrelated subjects, such as the cardiovascular system, disorders of the blood and respiratory system and, in the latter part, disorders of the digestive system, metabolism and the endocrine system. Although in the past, the emphasis may have been on the medical treatment of many of these disorders, modern investigations, a greater knowledge of physiology and improved techniques mean that surgery can now cure or alleviate many conditions. A full awareness of the physiological reasons for specialized nursing care is essential to all those concerned with caring for the patient in hospital and planning rehabilitation.

The third volume is concerned with two closely related groups of subjects. The first group consists of disorders of the nervous system itself, and the special senses of hearing and sight. Some of the disorders of the musculoskeletal system are also due to problems of nervous control. The second part of this volume has sections on the kidney, urinary tract and reproductive disorders. New techniques for treating patients with these disorders have been included and, importantly, the physiological changes which occur as a result of these problems are detailed.

Together these volumes will provide a valuable source of information, so that nurses will be able to understand fully the reasons for the decisions they make when planning the total care of their patients.

Barbara Dunn, 1982

Chapter 1

TOTAL PATIENT CARE

The aim of nursing is to assist a patient in overcoming problems which have caused a disturbance in normal physical or psychological functioning.

To reach this aim, it is necessary for the nurse to acknowledge the individuality of the patient, to identify the cause and extent of the problem, and to provide nursing interventions which will alleviate or solve the problem. This must be done logically and methodically.

One framework in which this can be accomplished is by the use of the nursing process. The nursing process involves several steps which aim to provide total and on-going care.

1 *Recognition* of the unique identity of the individual patient.
2 *Assessment* of individual needs.
3 *Appraisal* of problems—physical, psychological and social.

These steps involve an interview between the nurse and the patient, or a relative, in order to gather relevant information, which must be documented. This information is gathered together in the form of a nursing history.

4 *Planning and implementing* nursing care. This must be in full accord with medical care as prescribed.
5 *Evaluating* the care which has been given.
6 *Reappraising* needs and problems.

1

OBTAINING A NURSING HISTORY

General Principles

1 The first step in caring for a patient and gaining his active co-operation, is to gather a complete and accurate nursing history.
2 Time spent in establishing a good nurse–patient relationship, as early as possible, will enable the patient to feel more relaxed, and be able to talk about the particular problems which are causing him concern.
3 Skill in interviewing will affect both the accuracy of the information which is obtained, and also the quality of the nurse–patient relationship. This point cannot be overemphasized.
4 The purpose of the interview is to encourage an exchange of information between patient and nurse. In order to do this, some basic conditions are necessary. These include:
   a. The provision of privacy for the interview, in as quiet a place as possible, with a comfortable situation for both patient and nurse.
   b. Beginning the interview with a courteous greeting and an introduction. Explain who you are and why you are there.
   c. A pleasant tone of voice, with unhurried words, and the attitude of a sensitive listener, so that the patient will feel free to express his thoughts and feelings.
   d. The patient must feel that his words are being understood.
   e. A sympathetic attitude. At times, the patient may hint at underlying problems, but may be unable to put them into words. The nurse should help the patient to overcome this difficulty by altering her method of approach and reassuring the patient about the necessity for this particular information.
   f. Guidance of the interview, so that the necessary information is obtained, but without inhibiting the patient from expressing anxieties not covered by the questions.

Types of Information Needed

Personal details, e.g., name, address, age, date of birth, general practitioner. The patient will usually be able to answer these questions fluently, and will gain confidence in doing so.

Personal and Social History

The purpose of this is:

1 To identify the patient's life style, as this may have some bearing on the present condition, and also the present and future ability of the patient to cope with the condition.
2 To have a basis for developing a plan of care which will be suitable for this particular patient, for instance, involving personal, family or financial resources.
3 To gain knowledge about living patterns, e.g., sleep, meals, exercise, so that a plan of care can be devised which will disrupt these patterns as little as possible.
4 To help the patient develop a workable plan of care at home, based on knowledge of the home conditions.
5 To discover if the patient's occupation is directly or indirectly related to the present problems.

6 To determine if the religious convictions of the patient may necessitate any modification of the normal nursing procedures or therapy, e.g. dietary requirements, refusal of blood tranfusions.

Family History

The purpose of this is:

1 To picture the patient's family health. This may reveal a hereditary or a familial tendency to a disease.
2 To supplement the social history of the patient. When enquiring about brothers and sisters, for example, information will usually be forthcoming about the closeness or estrangement of members of the family. This is often a useful point when considering resources that are available for future care.

Medical History

The purpose of this is:

1 To gain a subjective view from the patient about his interpretation of his specific problems, and also his expectations of the possible diagnosis and outcome.
2 To gain an objective view by observation of the patient, and by examination and tests which are carried out by the doctor.

Principles of Obtaining a Medical History

Obtaining a medical history, does not mean that the nurse will undertake a full physical examination of the patient.

1 It does mean that the nurse will find out from the patient the particular problems that have occurred, which necessitated medical advice and admission to hospital.
2 When talking to the patient, the nurse will use her ears, not only for listening to the actual words spoken by the patient, but also for the tone of voice, and, for instance, signs of breathlessness.
3 The nurse will use her eyes for observing signs of physical or psychological discomfort, for example, painful movements or unwillingness to make eye contact. Also, any signs of abnormalities of the skin or underlying tissues.
4 The nurse will use her sense of smell, not only to detect problems of maintaining cleanliness, but also problems of incontinence, discharges or ketotic breath.
5 Before obtaining a medical history, the nurse will have already gained information about the personal and social background of the patient. When asking about bodily disfunctions, it is important to put the questions using appropriate language for the individual patient.
6 It is vital that the nurse never 'talks down' to the patient or appears to underestimate his intelligence. It is also necessary for her to use words which are clearly understood.
7 The interview must be conducted in a relaxed, unhurried manner, and the nurse must not appear to the patient to be merely interested in filling in a complicated form. However, in order that a comprehensive and accurate history is obtained, the information must be recorded in a methodical manner. A relatively unstructured form may be used. For example:

PROBLEM CHART			NAME...................
Respiration	Mobility	Nutrition and Digestion	Communication [Physical and Psychological Problems]
Circulatory	Sleeping and Rest	Elimination	Establishing and Maintaining Relationships

Alternatively a diagram (Fig. 1.1) may be used which will call to mind the important points to be covered. The diagram method may be particularly useful when evaluating or replanning nursing care.

RECORDING THE INFORMATION

General Guidelines

1 Keep in mind the purpose of recording the information and the audience for whom it is intended. This serves to guide the form and content of the record.
2 Remember that the patient's record is a legal document. Facts must be identified and stated precisely and accurately. Bias and misinterpretation must be avoided.
3 Avoid duplication of material. This makes careful reading of the record very time consuming, and so scanning over the facts is likely, with the possibility of errors occurring.
4 The facts must be recorded clearly and in a logical sequence.
5 Avoid using abbreviations unless they are in common usage, and well known to any readers using the record.
6 Record the information as soon as it is obtained, to minimize the chance of errors or omissions.

IDENTIFYING PROBLEMS

After recording the information which has been obtained (a) subjectively from the patients themselves and (b) objectively from the observations made by the nurse, the next step is to identify the particular problems and implement the nursing care.

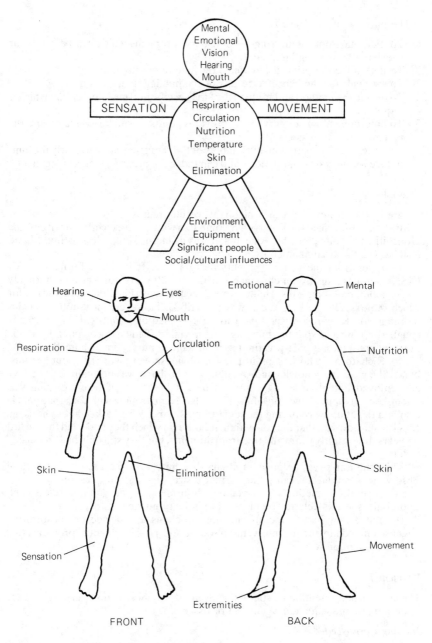

Figure 1.1.   Diagram to indicate important points to be covered in interview.

The purpose of this stage is:

1   To pick out from the nursing history, those problems which can be solved or alleviated by nursing intervention.
2   To determine the priorities in which these require attention.
3   To set goals for the expected results of the nursing intervention.
4   To decide the method and frequency of the specific nursing intervention which is required.
5   To determine at what intervals the previous points should be evaluated and the patient situation reassessed.
6   To write a care plan, so that all members of the care team can see clearly the aims of care for the particular patient, and can judge the progress that is being made.

Example

A case history is included which highlights certain points.

Mr Richardson, aged 68. Emergency admission with acute exacerbation of chronic bronchitis. On admission, Mr Richardson was cyanosed, breathless, confused and restless. He was accompanied by his wife.

The letter from the general practitioner gave the following information. 'Mr Richardson has a history of chronic bronchitis for 20 years, for which he normally takes Salbutamol 4 mg t.d.s. He developed a chest infection 2 days previously, for which Amoxycillin 250 mg q.d.s. was prescribed. However, on visiting him this morning, Mr Richardson was found to be cyanosed and confused. He normally coughed up mucoid sputum, but was now having difficulty in coughing up thick, purulent sputum. His wife was finding it difficult to nurse him at home.'

Mrs Richardson, who was about 65, was obviously very worried about her husband. She gave the following information. Her husband was normally fairly active and enjoyed doing gardening, although he got breathless if heavy digging was attempted. His appetite was only fair, and he had some trouble with constipation. He also had to get up twice during the night to pass urine. When asked about housing, Mrs Richardson said that they owned their house, in which they had lived for the last 35 years. It was fairly warm and free from draughts, but they still only had an outside toilet.

While the nurse was helping Mr Richardson into bed, she used her powers of observation and did not cause him further distress by a lot of questions.

By these three methods of obtaining information (recognition, assessment, appraisal), she was able to complete a preliminary nursing history.

The nurse now had to identify nursing problems and decide on the priority, because immediate nursing intervention was necessary. The essential problems that required attention were:

Problem 1

The patient had retention of sputum, causing airway obstruction, leading to CO_2 retention and inadequate oxygenation of tissues.

Nursing Care Needed

1   Support patient in an upright position.

2   Give oxygen 28% via Ventimask at 4 l/min.
3   Give moist inhalations as per instructions or plan.
4   Encourage patient to expectorate, and be present when physiotherapist is giving care to learn suitable technique for helping Mr Richardson.
5   Encourage him to take at least 120 ml clear fluids hourly.

Evaluation

1   Check position of patient hourly.
2   Check oxygen mask and adequacy of supply of oxygen hourly.
3   Converse with Mr Richardson to evaluate state of confusion.
4   Observe amount and type of sputum 4 hourly, and renew sputum containers as necessary.

Goal

To clear the retained sputum and to permit increased tissue perfusion with oxygen.

Problem 2

Because of poor tissue perfusion, age, state of nutrition and confusion, there is an increased tendency of development of pressure sores. Norton Scale score 11. (See Rehabilitation Concepts.)

Nursing Care Needed

1   Sit patient on sheepskin.
2   Whilst maintaining an upright position, alter weight from side to side every hour.
3   Assess reddening of skin 4 hourly.
4   Use bed cradle to allow free movement of feet and relieve pressure.

Evaluation

Review of Norton Scale twice daily.

Goal

1   To prevent the occurrence of pressure sores.
2   To improve the general condition of the patient. Dietitian to advise about suitable diet.

These two problems would need priority attention. Further factors to be considered would include:

1   Provision of nourishing diet and fluid intake to improve general health and to alleviate the problem of constipation.
2   Assessment of nocturia.
3   Possible intervention to provide inside toilet. (Grant may be available from Council.)
4   Ensure the understanding of both Mr and Mrs Richardson into the cause of this hospitalization, and the prevention of further chest infections.

The implementation of nursing care is given in detail throughout the book, either under Rehabilitation Concepts, or chapters on specific conditions.

Evaluation and Reassessment

The purpose of this is:

1 To discuss whether the observations which were made, were adequate.
2 To measure the effectiveness of the nursing care.
3 To discuss the physical and psychological reactions of the patient to the nursing care.
4 To identify whether:
    a. A goal has been reached and the problem solved.
    b. Further time should be allowed for continuation of present nursing care.
    c. Modification of existing care is needed.
    d. The existing care is inappropriate and should be radically altered.
    e. New problems have arisen which may necessitate alteration of priorities.

Total patient care, using the nursing process is an on-going method of adapting to the individual needs of each patient. In different clinical areas, the method of recording the history and the pattern of the nursing care plan may vary, but the personalized approach to the care of the patient must remain.

FURTHER READING

Books

Bower, F L (1972) The Process of Planning Nursing Care, C V Mosby
Hunt, J M and Marks-Maran, D (1980) Nursing Care Plans, HM&M
Kratz, C (editor) (1979) The Nursing Process, Baillière Tindall
Lewis, L W (1980) Fundamental Skills in Patient Care, J B Lippincott
Little, D E and Carnevalli, D L (1976) Nursing Care Planning, J B Lippincott
Matheney, R V (editor) (1978) Fundamentals of Patient-Centred Nursing, C V Mosby
Thompson, B and Bridge W (1981) Teaching Patient Care, HM&M
Yura, H and Walsh, M B (1978) The Nursing Process, Appleton Century Crofts

Articles

Castledine, G (1980) From one fellow to another: take better care, Nursing Mirror 151: 12
Crow, J (1977) The nursing process. 2. How and why to take a nursing history, Nursing Times 73: 950–957
Crow, J (1977) The nursing process. 3. A nursing history questionnaire for two patients, Nursing Times 73: 978–982, 983–994
Fleming, J (1973) The secret of total patient care, Nursing Mirror 136: 37
Henderson, V (1973) On nursing care plans and their history, Nursing Outlook 21: 378–379
Jones, C (1977) The nursing process: individualized care, Nursing Mirror 144: 13–14
Kratz, C (1977) The nursing process, Nursing Times 73: 854–855
Little, D E and Carnevalli, D L (1976) Nursing care plans: let's be practical about them, Nursing Forum 6: 61–76
Macfarlane, J (1975) What do we mean by care? Nursing Mirror 141: 47–48
Macfarlane, J (1976) A charter for caring, Journal of Advanced Nursing 1: 187–196
Nursing Times (1977) The nursing process. Report on the WHO regional office for Europe meeting to examine aspects of the nursing process, Nursing Times 73: 11
O'Hare, E (1980) The gingerbread man, Nursing Times 76: 318–321

Chapter 2

REHABILITATION CONCEPTS

Rehabilitation involves an active, dynamic programme aimed at enabling an ill or disabled person to achieve the greatest possible physical, psychological, social and economic competence.

Objective of Rehabilitation

To enable an ill or disabled person to achieve maximum functional efficiency by the use of an individualized approach to solving the particular problems which affect that person.

REHABILITATION TEAM

Rehabilitation is a creative process; it calls for a team of people working together with the patient and the relatives, and contributing the specialized services that may be required to help the patient function as well as possible. In planning and evaluating the care plan, all members of the team should contribute their opinions.

The rehabilitation team consists not only of doctors, nurses, physiotherapists and occupational therapists, but also involves social workers and possibly vocational guidance counsellors and disablement resettlement officers.

REHABILITATION NURSING FUNCTIONS

1   Identify the problems which are preventing the patient from achieving his maximum efficiency, and develop a plan of nursing care to help the patient to overcome these problems.

Virginia Henderson has listed the Components of Basic Nursing Care, which highlight the points with which the patient may need help.

a. Helping the patient with respiration.

b. Helping the patient with eating and drinking.

c. Helping the patient with elimination.

d. Helping the patient maintain a desirable posture in walking, sitting and lying; and helping him move from one position to another.

e. Helping the patient to rest and sleep.

f. Helping the patient with selecting clothing, dressing and undressing.

g. Helping the patient maintain body temperature within normal limits.

h. Helping the patient keep the body clean and well groomed and protect the skin.

i. Helping the patient to avoid dangers in the environment; and protecting others from any potential danger from the patient, such as infection or violence.

j. Helping the patient to communicate with others—to express his needs and feelings.

k. Helping the patient to practise his religion or conform to his concept of right and wrong.

l. Helping the patient with work, or with productive occupation.

m. Helping the patient with recreational activities.

n. Helping the patient to learn.

2   Provide direct nursing care that will maintain optimum physical and mental health for the patient and meet his medical treatment needs.

3   Supply nursing care which prevents the complications which may occur because of lack of mobility, and eliminate the possibility of cross infection.
4   Establish a sustained, supporting nurse–patient relationship.
5   Participate in the retraining of the patient in self-care activities.
6   Provide health care and teaching that will meet the needs of the individual patient and also the family.
7   Record and report nursing observations of the patient's condition, progress and personal needs, as well as the action taken to meet these needs.
8   Assist with patient discharge plans and ensure continuity of home care or follow-up care with the community services or outpatient department.
9   Evaluate the nursing care in terms of the overall goals.

CAUSES OF DISABILITY (Table 2.1)

Primary disability—the result of a pathological process (congenital, trauma, inflammatory, etc.)
Secondary disability—the result of either inactivity or contraindicated and injurious activity.
Disuse syndrome—disabilities due to inactivity.

PSYCHOLOGICAL IMPLICATIONS OF PROLONGED ILLNESS OR DISABILITY

Prolonged illness or disability has a tremendous impact on a patient's image of himself. There may be an actual change of body shape or function, e.g., amputation or colostomy. There will be a change of psychological and social status—from being a person able to manage the normal physical functions, to a person who is wholly or partially dependent upon someone else. A patient with illness or disability has normal needs which have to be met by different methods.

Nursing Objectives

1   To be aware of the factors influencing the patient's behaviour.
2   To help the patient to feel worthwhile.

Nursing Insight

The way in which the patient relates to others will be affected by the way in which he perceives changes in his body image.

EMOTIONAL REACTIONS OF A PATIENT TO PROLONGED ILLNESS OR NEWLY ACQUIRED DISABILITY

Period of Confusion, Disorganization and Denial

1   The patient is in a state of conflict, and has to cope with problems of forced dependence, loss of self-esteem and with feeling that personal and family integrity are threatened.

Table 2.1. Causes and Prevention of Disability

	Condition	Cause	Prevention
1	Muscle atrophy (diminution in muscle strength and size)	Lack of exercise	Exercise
2	Joint contracture (limited range of movement)	Lack of joint movement	Passive movements, splinting, positioning
3	Metabolic disturbances		
	Osteoporosis	Lack of weight bearing ability	Active movements
		Postmenopausal problems	
	Urinary tract stones	Immobilization	Mobilization
		Dehydration/concentrated urine	High fluid intake
		Urinary tract infection	High fluid intake Prompt treatment of infections. Avoid catheterization
4	Circulatory disturbances		
	Venous thrombosis	Slowing of venous return	Foot and leg exercises
		Varicose veins	Elastic stockings
		Poor positioning in operating theatre	Appropriate padding on theatre table
		Lack of motion in lower extremities	Early mobilization
	Hypostatic pneumonia	Poor position. Prolonged rest in one position	Frequent change of position. Breathing exercises. Early mobilization
	Pressure sores	Pressure. Immobility	Frequent change of position. Appropriate padding on theatre table. Assessment of patients at risk. See p. 41
5	Sphincter disturbances		
	Urinary incontinence	Lack of opportunity	Regular toilet routine
	Urinary retention	Lack of opportunity	Regular toilet routine
		Fear and embarrassment	Provision of privacy and comfort. See p. 15
	Constipation	Lack of suitable diet	Adequate fluids and roughage
		Lack of exercise	Early mobilization
		Lack of opportunity	Regular toilet routine
6	Psychological disturbance	Separation from accustomed environment. Institutional routine	Nursing care is planned to take into account patient's normal living routine
		Inactivity	Early mobilization
		Sleeplessness	Suitable environment. See p. 36
		Depression	Correct psychological preparation before hospitalization and explanation of treatment and future care

2   The patient uses mechanism of denial by refusing to accept new limitations.
   a. May have false hopes for a speedy and complete recovery.
   b. May regress and become self-centred and childlike.
   c. May attempt to remain 'normal' and nondisabled.
   Denial is the mechanism used particularly by those who have placed great value on strength, attractive appearance and social status.

Period of Depression and Grief. A Period of Reaction

1   Appears to grieve for his lost functions or altered body image.
2   Depression is also due to inactivity and sensory deprivation, because of restricted environmental stimulation.
3   Limited mobility and sensory stimulation may produce behavioural disruptions.

Period of Adaptation and Adjustment

1   Redirection of energies towards coping with physical functioning.
2   The patient revises his body image and modifies the former picture of himself. He has a reorientation of himself.
3   The patient accepts a degree of dependency.
4   He accepts the limitations imposed by the condition.
5   He begins to make realistic goals for the future.

HELPING THE PATIENT WITH RESPIRATION

Nursing Objectives

1   To assist the patient to retain a position which will allow maximum use of respiratory muscles.
2   To provide a suitable environment, this includes temperature, humidity, ventilation and lack of pollution.
3   To assist the patient in clearing his air passages by various nursing procedures.

Nursing Programme

1   Arrange for appropriate physiotherapy teaching for the patient. This may include postural drainage, breathing exercises. Arrange other nursing activities to allow the patient to get maximum benefit from physiotherapy, e.g., it is better not to arrange meal times immediately after physiotherapy, as the patient may be too tired to eat; and not to arrange physiotherapy immediately after a meal as this may cause vomiting.
2   If analgesia is required to allow the patient to breathe more freely without pain, this should be given 20–30 min before the physiotherapist arrives.
3   Perform tasks for the patient which he would normally be able to do for himself, but are now too difficult because insufficient oxygen is causing weakness and dyspnoea.
4   Arrange with the relatives to limit the amount of visitors, as too many will cause exhaustion because of the effort required by the patient for prolonged conversation.

5   Arrange for meals which do not require too much mastication, as the patient will be too tired to finish the meal, which may lead to undernourishment.
6   Any anxiety or overexcitement will increase the respiration rate, thus requiring more muscular effort. This may lead to panic by the patient who may now find difficulty with speaking and making his fears known to the nurse. She must anticipate the need for reassurance, and give practical help to restore quiet, rhythmic breathing.
7   Adequate fluid intake is essential because:
    a. A patient with respiratory difficulties may use mouth breathing, resulting in a dry, coated mouth.
    b. It is essential to prevent constipation occurring, which will result in straining to defaecate, causing anxiety and dyspnoea.

In order to allow the patient to regain as much independence as possible, ordinary daily tasks, such as dressing and preparing meals, should be simplified into easy steps so that he can perform these with maximum self-reliance. For instance, front fastening clothes will need less exertion to put on than ones which have to be pulled over the head. Kitchens and living rooms should have shelves and cupboards which contain the equipment that is constantly used, at a suitable height, so that bending or stretching are avoided.

Before the patient goes home, consideration must be given to the provision of suitable heating and ventilation, and possibly financial assistance may be needed to help pay for this.

Detailed treatment for specialized respiratory disorders will be found in Volume 2, Chapter 3.

HELPING THE PATIENT WITH EATING AND DRINKING

Nursing Objectives

1   To identify the particular problems, physical or psychological, which are causing concern to the patient.
2   To enable the patient to overcome his problem, as far as possible by his own efforts.
3   To enable the patient to ingest the correct type and amount of nourishment.
4   To maintain the dignity of the patient.

Nursing Programme

1   Whenever possible, the patient should be given a choice of food, and should be encouraged to state his preferences.
    a. There is wide variation in likes and dislikes for different types of food.
    b. There may be cultural or religious restrictions on various foods or times for meals.
    c. There may be physical difficulties with mastication and swallowing.
2   An interest in the choice of food is often an indication of the improvement of the physical or psychological state of the patient.

3   Although a choice should be given, in some cases guidance may be necessary, to encourage the patient to choose a well-balanced meal. However, in some cases, a strict dietary regime is necessary.

4   The nurse must remember her role as an educator, and explanation of the reasons for the necessity of certain foods must be given.

5   Meal times should be pleasurable times, and a social occasion. The environment should be pleasant and have a relaxed atmosphere.

   a. If possible, the dining area should be away from the ward, so that patients can relax in the day room, away from the ward activities.

   b. Any dressings or treatments should be completed well before meal times, so that no uncomfortable or distressing procedures are carried on, which could cause anxiety to the patient.

   c. Patients should be encouraged to meet together at meal times.

   d. Each patient must be made as comfortable as possible. This includes using toilet facilities before meals, and also the provision of suitable chairs or supporting pillows to give an upright position.

6   Any patient with a disability should be given help in the most appropriate way, without causing embarrassment. For example, a patient with Parkinson's disease or multiple sclerosis may feel conspicuous if food or fluids are spilt, and they may tend to withdraw from social contact. Special drinking cups, and cutlery with large handles may help to overcome some of the difficulties, but the attitude of the nurse in accepting the occasional mess and the tactful manner in clearing up is the main thing in encouraging the patient to continue making an effort to feed himself.

7   Mouth care and also the provision of drinks with meals is essential.

8   Whenever possible, flexible meal times should be provided to fit in as nearly as practicable with the patient's own eating habits. Some patients may not normally have a main meal at mid-day, but have the main meal in the evening, or vice versa. On admission to hospital the change in routine may cause considerable upset and loss of appetite.

9   In many cases, there is no reason why relatives cannot bring in some special delicacy which may tempt the appetite of the patient, and which has been prepared in a way which he will enjoy.

10   If the patient chooses the menu on the previous day, latitude must be given for change of mind, perhaps because of the change in condition, and provision made for alternative meals, without making the patient feel a nuisance.

HELPING THE PATIENT WITH ELIMINATION

Problems with Micturition

Nursing Objectives

1   To enable the patient to empty his bladder at suitable intervals.
2   To prevent urinary tract infection, and to preserve renal function.
3   To help the patient to maintain his dignity and be socially acceptable.

Nursing Programme

1   Make a plan of definite times for the patient to try to empty his bladder.
2   Whenever possible, the patient should be encouraged to go out to the toilet, so that privacy is ensured. If this is not possible, a commode may be provided and the bed well screened from other patients.
3   Give sufficient oral fluids at regular intervals. Wait for 30 min, then ask the patient to attempt to pass urine. The patient may apply pressure on the lower abdominal area.
4   The interval should be 2 hourly to begin with, and this may be increased to 3 hourly during the day time. The patient may be woken during the night if this is thought to be desirable for the particular patient.
5   Frequent testing of the urine is necessary, especially for bacterial infection, which must be treated.
6   The patient should be encouraged to dress in his own clothes. If necessary, incontinence appliances or garments may be provided, as reassurance, until the patient has confidence in his ability to control micturition.
7   It is essential that the patient is able to get to the toilet easily, without delay, and also that any garments can be removed without difficulty; for instance, a patient with rheumatoid arthritis affecting the hands may have a particular problem, and the delay in removing garments may cause incontinence.
8   Encouragement and maintenance of dignity are essential.
9   Encourage the patient to make decisions concerning his future care, and to perform as many self-help tasks as possible. Boredom and apathy must be avoided at all costs.
10 Stimulate an interest in the environment, which must be made as interesting as possible.

Problems with Defaecation

Nursing Objectives

1   To develop regular bowel habits, if possible by natural methods.
2   To prevent faecal incontinence, impaction or irregularity.

Nursing Programme

1   Establish a specific and definite time for bowel movement.
    a. Note must be taken of the patient's normal bowel habits, as wide variations can occur in individuals.
    b. Attempts should be made within 15 min of a meal, usually breakfast, as this maximizes the stimulation of peristalsis, and the gastrocolic and duodenocolic reflexes.
2   Promote good dietary habits.
    a. Adequate fluid intake.
    b. Addition of bran to the diet. This is probably most acceptable in the form of breakfast cereals.
    c. Provision of raw and cooked vegetables, and plenty of fruit. It is essential to check the state of the patient's teeth or dentures to ensure adequate mastication.
3   In cases of diarrhoea, a rectal examination should be done, to eliminate the possibility of faecal impaction causing spurious diarrhoea.

4   Encourage as much mobility and muscular exercise as the patient can manage.
5   The use of suppositories may be necessary at first, as this will stimulate the anorectal reflex.
6   Make sure the patient is in a comfortable position, either on a commode or in the toilet. The provision of a footstool may help the patient to make the best use of his muscles, as this position most nearly approximates the physiological position for defaecation.
7   The temporary use of aperient drugs may be necessary, but these should not be used routinely.
8   The provision of privacy, an odour free atmosphere and absolute cleanliness are essential. Also the facilities for personal hygiene.

For care of the patient with neurological disturbances of bladder and bowels, see Chap 1, Vol. 3.

HELPING THE PATIENT WITH MOBILITY

1   One of the main fears of a disabled person, is the fear of being unable to move or to be unable to control a movement. This produces a feeling of total dependence on others.
2   Deformities and complications of illness or injury can often be prevented by frequent changes of position, proper positioning in bed or chair and exercise.

Purposes for Changing Positions

1   To prevent contractures.
2   To prevent pressure sores by relieving pressure and stimulating the circulation.
3   To promote lung expansion and drainage of respiratory secretions.

Principles of Body Alignment

Dorsal or Supine Position

1   The head is in line with the spine, both laterally and antero-posteriorly.
2   The trunk is positioned so that flexion of the hips is minimized.
3   The arms are slightly flexed with the hands resting on the bed.
4   The legs are extended.
5   The heels may be suspended in a space between the mattress and footboard.
6   The toes are pointing upwards.

Side-lying or Lateral Position

1   The head is in line with the spine.
2   The uppermost hip joint is slightly forward and supported by a pillow in a position of slight abduction.
3   A pillow supports the arm, which is flexed at both the elbow and shoulder joints.

Prone Position

1   The head is turned laterally and is in alignment with the rest of the body.
2   The arms are abducted and externally rotated at the shoulder joint; the elbows are flexed.

3   A small flat support may sometimes be needed to be placed under the pelvis, extending from the level of the umbilicus to the upper third of the thigh.
4   The lower extremities remain in a neutral position.
5   The toes are suspended over the edge of the mattress.

Therapeutic Exercises

Exercise involves the function of muscles, nerves, bones and joints as well as the cardiovascular and respiratory systems. The return of function depends on the strength of the musculature that controls the joint.

Objectives

1   To develop and retrain deficient muscles.
2   To restore as much normal movement as possible.
3   To maintain and build muscle strength.
4   To maintain joint function.
5   To prevent deformity.
6   To retrain for muscular co-ordination.
7   To stimulate circulation.
8   To build up tolerance and endurance.

Types of Exercises

1   Passive.
2   Active assisted.
3   Active.
4   Resisted.
5   Isometric or static.

Passive

An exercise carried out by the therapist or the nurse without assistance from the patient.

1   Purposes:
   a. To retain as much joint range of movement as possible.
   b. To maintain circulation.
2   Action:
   a. Stabilize the proximal joint and support the distal part.
   b. Move the joint smoothly, slowly and gently through its full range of movement.
   c. Avoid producing excessive pain.

Active Assisted

An exercise carried out by the patient with assistance from the therapist or the nurse.

1   Purpose: To encourage normal muscle action.
2   Action:
   a. Support the distal part and encourage the patient to take the joint actively through its range of movement.

b. Give only the amount of assistance necessary to accomplish the action.

c. Short periods of activity should be followed by adequate rest periods.

Active

An exercise accomplished by the patient without assistance.

1   Purpose: To maintain and increase muscle strength.
2   Action:
    a. When possible, active exercise should be done against gravity.
    b. The joint is moved through its full range of movement without assistance from nurse or therapist.
    c. The patient should not substitute another joint movement for the one intended.

Resisted

An active exercise carried out by the patient working against resistance produced by either manual or mechanical means.

1   Purpose: To provide resistance in order to increase muscle power.
2   Action:
    a. The patient moves the joint through its full range of movement while the therapist provides slight resistance at first and then progressively increases resistance.
    b. Sandbags and weights can be used and are supplied at the distal part of the involved joint.
    c. The movements should be done smoothly.

Isometric or Static

Alternately contracting and relaxing a muscle while keeping the part in a fixed position. This exercise is performed by the patient.

1   Purpose: To maintain strength when a joint is immobilized or when it should not be put through a range of movement.
2   Action:
    a. The patient contracts or tightens the muscle as much as possible without moving the joint.
    b. He holds for several seconds, then 'lets go' and relaxes.

Range of Movement Exercises

Range of movement is the movement of a joint through its full range in all appropriate planes. It may be passive, active or resisted.

Objectives

1   To maintain function and prevent deterioration.
2   To maintain or increase the maximal movement of a joint.

Underlying Principles

1   Range of movement testing is done by the doctor or physiotherapist to determine the movement that exists at the joint areas. Testing sets realistic and positive goals.
2   The patient's range of movement is affected by his physical condition, the disease process and his genetic make-up.
3   Each joint in the body has a normal range of movement.
4   Joints may lose their normal range of movement, stiffen, and produce a permanent disability.
5   Range of movement exercises are individually planned since there is a wide variety in the degree of movement which patients of different body builds and age groups are capable.
6   Range of movement exercises should be carried out whenever there is physical inactivity, provided the patient's clinical condition allows such activity.

Techniques of Range of Movement

1   Place the patient in a supine position with his arms to the side and the knees extended.
2   Hold the extremity either side of the joint, e.g., elbow, wrist or knee, and move the joint slowly, smoothly and gently through its range. This is repeated about three times.
3   Avoid moving a joint beyond its free range of movement; avoid forcing movement. The movement should be stopped at the point of pain.
4   When spasticity is present, move the joint slowly to the point of resistance.
5   Refer to Fig. 2.1 for joint movement, and Fig. 2.2 for a pictorial review of range of movement exercises.

Definitions

Abduction—movement away from the midline of the body.
Adduction—movement towards the midline of the body.
Flexion—bending of a joint so that the angle of the joint diminishes.
Extension—the return movement from flexion; the joint angle is increased.
Inversion—movement that turns the sole of the foot inwards.
Eversion—movement that turns the sole of the foot outwards.
Dorsiflexion—flexing or bending the ankle towards the leg.
Plantar flexion—flexing or bending the ankle in the direction of the sole.
Pronation—rotating the forearm so that the palm of the hand is downwards.
Supination—rotating the forearm so that the palm of the hand is upwards.
Rotation—turning or movement of a part around its axis.
   Internal rotation—turning inwards towards the centre.
   External rotation—turning outwards, away from the centre.

Preparation for Transfer of Patient

Objective

To develop the ability to raise and move the body in different positions.

SHOULDER

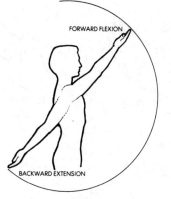
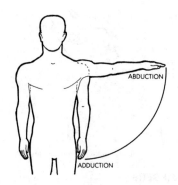

ELBOW

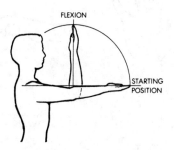

FOREARM

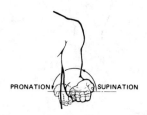

WRIST

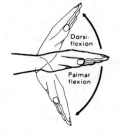
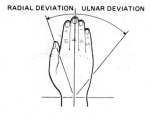

Figure 2.1   Range of movement exercises.

THUMB

ADDUCTION　　　　　ABDUCTION　　　　　OPPOSITION

FINGERS

ADDUCTION

ABDUCTION

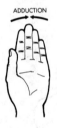

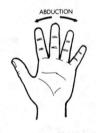

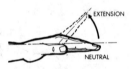

EXTENSION

NEUTRAL

ANKLE　　　　　　　　**FOOT**

DORSI-FLEXION　　　PLANTAR FLEXION

EVERSION　　　　　INVERSION

THE FOOT

Figure 2.1 (cont.)

TOES

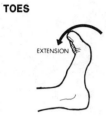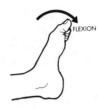

HIP

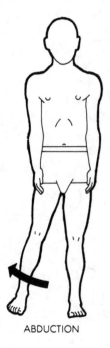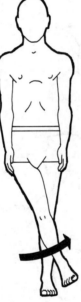

ABDUCTION   ADDUCTION   INTERNAL ROTATION   EXTERNAL ROTATION

Figure 2.1 (cont.)

KNEE

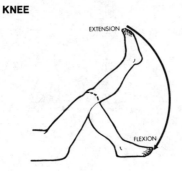

CERVICAL SPINE

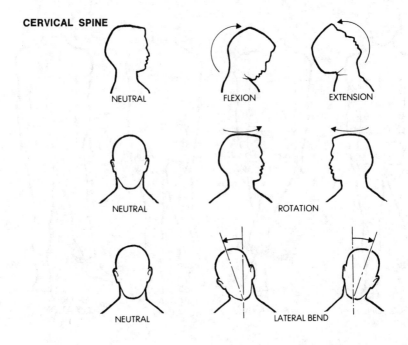

Figure 2.1 (cont.)

SHOULDER: Flexion

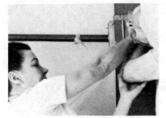

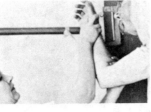

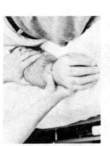

1. Start by placing one hand above the patient's elbow. Hold the patient's hand with your other hand.

2. Lift his arm up from the side of his body.

3. Move the arm slowly and gently toward his head as far as possible without causing pain.

4. If the headboard prevents full forward flexion, bend the arm at the elbow.

5. Lift arm again before returning to side or neutral position. Repeat the exercise.

SHOULDER: Abduction and Adduction

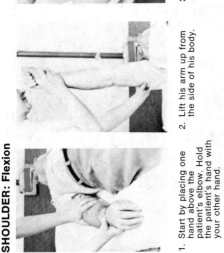

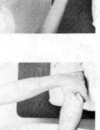

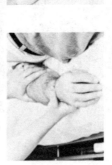

1. Place one hand above the patient's elbow. Hold his hand with your other hand.

2. Keeping his arm straight, move it sideways away from his body.

3. Bend and move the arm slowly around toward the patient's head. Move his arm back as far as possible without pain.

4. Return the arm to the side or neutral position. Repeat the exercise.

Figure 2.2. Range of motion.

* From Nursing '72, April, 1972.

SHOULDER: Internal and External Rotation

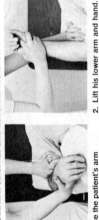

1. Place the patient's arm pointed away from his body, elbow bent. Hold his upper arm against the mattress.

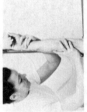

2. Lift his lower arm and hand.

3. Move his lower arm and hand slowly and gently back toward his head as far as possible without causing pain.

4. Return his arm to the starting position. Repeat exercise.

SHOULDER: Cross Adduction

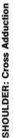
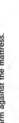

1. Place one hand on the patient's arm above his elbow. Hold his hand with your other hand.

2. Lift his arm.

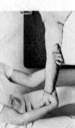

3. With arm at shoulder height move arm across the body as far as possible toward the other shoulder.

4. Return the arm to the starting position. Repeat the exercise.

FOREARM: Supination and Pronation

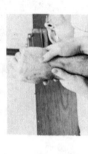

1. Starting position: Note the position of the patient's hand and the nurse's hands.

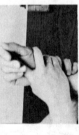

2. Twist the palm of the patient's hand toward his face.

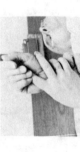

3. Then, twist the palm of his hand back toward his feet. Repeat.

Figure 2.2 (cont.)

WRIST AND FINGER: Extension and Flexion

1. Hold the patient's wrist with one hand and his hand with your other hand.

2. Bend his hand backward while keeping his fingers straight.

3. Straighten the hand.

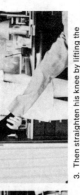

4. Bend his hand forward, closing his fingers to make a fist. Open his hand and repeat the exercise.

THUMB: Flexion and Extension

1. Hold the patient's fingers straight within one of your hands. Bend the patient's thumb into the palm of his hand with your other hand.

2. Pull his thumb back so that it points away from his palm. Repeat the exercise.

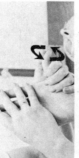

3. Move his thumb around in a circle. (circumduction)

KNEE AND HIP: Flexion and Extension

1. Place one of your hands under the patient's knee. Place your other hand on the heel of his foot.

2. Lift his leg and bend it at the knee. Move his leg slowly back toward his head as far as it will go without hurting him.

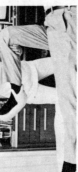
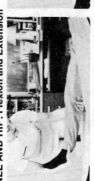

3. Then straighten his knee by lifting the foot upward. Lower his leg to the starting position and repeat the exercise.

Figure 2.2 (cont.)

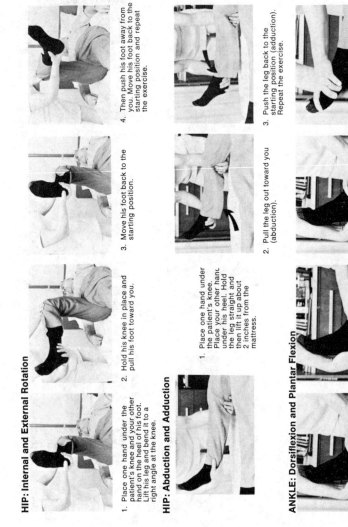

HIP: Internal and External Rotation

1. Place one hand under the patient's knee and your other hand on the heel of his foot. Lift his leg and bend it to a right angle at the knee.

2. Hold his knee in place and pull his foot toward you.

3. Move his foot back to the starting position.

4. Then push his foot away from you. Move his foot back to the starting position and repeat the exercise.

HIP: Abduction and Adduction

1. Place one hand under the patient's knee. Place your other hand under his heel. Hold the leg straight and then lift it up about 2 inches from the mattress.

2. Pull the leg out toward you (abduction).

3. Push the leg back to the starting position (adduction). Repeat the exercise.

ANKLE: Dorsiflexion and Plantar Flexion

1. Hold the patient's heel with your hand, letting the sole of his foot rest against your arm.

2. Press your arm against the bottom of the foot, moving it back toward the leg (dorsiflexion). At the same time, pull on the heel.

3. Move your arm back to the starting position.

4. Move your hand up to the top of the foot, below the toes. Push down on the foot to point the toes and at the same time, push up against the heel (plantar flexion).

Figure 2.2 (cont.)

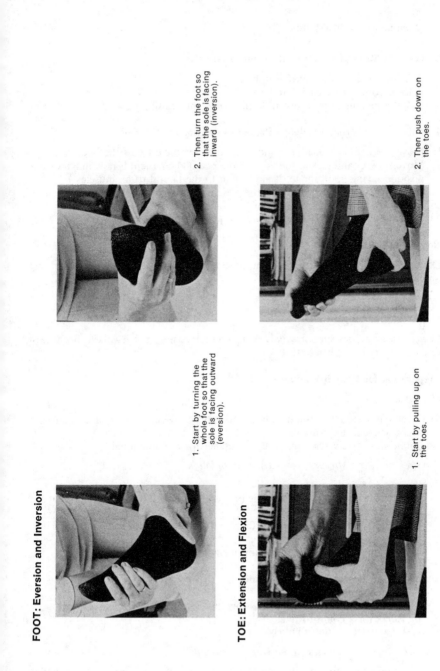

FOOT: Eversion and Inversion

1. Start by turning the whole foot so that the sole is facing outward (eversion).

2. Then turn the foot so that the sole is facing inward (inversion).

TOE: Extension and Flexion

1. Start by pulling up on the toes.

2. Then push down on the toes.

Figure 2.2 (cont.)

Exercises to Strengthen Arm and Shoulder Muscles

1   Ask the patient to sit upright in bed.
2   Place a book under each hand.
3   Ask the patient to push down on the book, thus raising his body weight.

Technique for Moving a Helpless Patient to the Edge of the Bed

1   Move the patient's head and shoulders towards the edge of the bed.
2   Move his feet and legs to the edge of the bed. (The patient is now in a crescent position giving good range of movement to the lateral trunk muscles.)
3   Place both your arms well under the patient's hips. (Before the next manoeuvre tighten or set the muscles of your back and abdomen.)
4   Straighten your back while moving the patient towards you.

Nonweight-bearing Transfers

Done by double lower-extremity amputees, or paraplegics who are not wearing braces (Fig. 2.3).

Crutch Walking

Crutches are artificial supports that assist patients who need aid in walking because of disease, injury or a birth defect.

Preparation for Crutch Walking

Objectives

To develop power in the shoulder girdle and upper extremities that bear the patient's weight when crutch walking.
To obtain the correct type and size of crutches for the individual.

To Strengthen the Muscles Needed for Ambulation

1   For quadriceps contraction.
    a. With the patient's leg flat on the bed, ask the patient to dorsiflex the foot and raise the heel off the bed.
       The next points will vary according to the capabilities of each patient. These are average times.
    b. Maintain the muscle contracture for a count of five.
    c. Relax for a count of five.
    d. Repeat this exercise 10–15 times hourly.
2   For gluteal contraction.
    a. Contract or pinch the buttocks together for a count of five.
    b. Relax for a count of five.
    c. Repeat 10–15 times hourly.

To Strengthen the Muscles of the Upper Extremities

1   Ask the patient to flex and extend arms slowly whilst holding traction weights. Gradually increase the poundage of the weights.

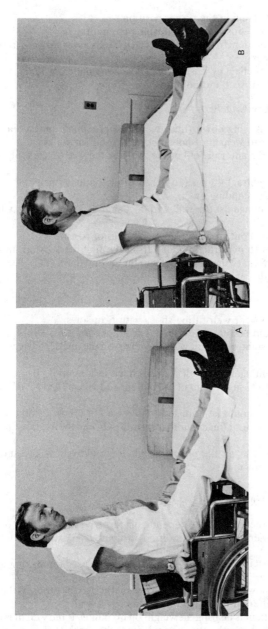

Figure 2.3. Vertical transfer of a paraplegic patient. a. Place the wheelchair facing the bed as close to the bed as possible. Lock brakes. Instruct the patient to push up on his hands and arms and slide his body forward onto the bed. b. This is a nonweight-bearing transfer in which the patient learns to transfer on the same level. Later this type of nonweight-bearing transfer can be done to a higher and lower level by the push-up method.

2   Do push-ups while lying in the prone position.
3   Squeeze rubber ball—this increases grasping strength.
4   Raise head and shoulders from the bed, stretch hands as far forward as possible.
5   Sit up on bed or chair.
    a. Raise body from chair by pushing hands against the chair seat.
    b. Raise body out of seat and hold position. Relax.

To Measure for Axillary Crutches

1   When the patient is lying down (this gives an approximate measurement).
    a. Ask the patient to wear the shoes normally used for walking.
    b. Measure from the anterior fold of the axilla to the sole of the foot, then add 5 cm (2 in).
    c. Alternatively, subtract 40 cm (16 in) from the patient's height.
2   When the patient is standing erect.
    a. Stand the patient against the wall with feet slightly apart and away from the wall.
    b. Mark 5 cm (2 in) out from the side to the tip of the toe.
    c. Measure 15 cm (6 in) straight ahead from the first mark. Mark this point.
    d. Measure from 5 cm (2 in) below axilla to the second mark. This measurement is the crutch length.

Crutch Stance

1   Ask the patient to wear well-fitting shoes with firm soles.
2   The crutches should be fitted with large rubber suction tips.
3   Ask the patient to stand by a chair with his weight on the unaffected leg to achieve balance.
4   Position the patient against a wall with his head in a neutral position.
5   Place crutches 5 cm (2 in) in front of the patient and 10 cm (4 in) to the side (Fig. 2.4).
    a. The hand piece should be adjusted to allow a 30° elbow flexion.
    b. There should be a four finger width insertion between the axillary fold and the arm piece.
    c. A foam rubber pad on the underarm piece should relieve pressure on the upper arm and thoracic cage.

Teaching the Crutch Gait

1   The selection of the crutch gait depends on the type and severity of the disability and the patient's physical condition, arm and trunk strength and/or body balance.
2   Teach the patient at least two gaits—a faster gait to be used for making speed and a slower one for use in crowded places.
3   Show the patient how to change gait from one method to the other, as this relieves fatigue since a different combination of muscles is used.
4   Make sure the patient is bearing his weight on his hands. If the weight is borne on the axilla, the pressure of the crutch can damage the brachial plexus and produce crutch paralysis.

Crutch Gaits

Four-Point Gait (four-point alternate crutch gait)

Crutch–foot sequence (Fig. 2.5): (1) right crutch, (2) left foot, (3) left crutch, (4) right foot.

1   This is a slow but stable gait; the patient's weight is constantly being shifted.
2   Four-point gait can be used only by patients who can move each leg separately and bear a considerable amount of weight on each of them.

Two-Point Gait (two-point alternate crutch gait)

Crutch–foot sequence (Fig. 2.6): (1) right crutch and left foot, (2) left crutch and right foot simultaneously.

1   This is a faster gait but requires more balance since there are only two points of contact with the floor.

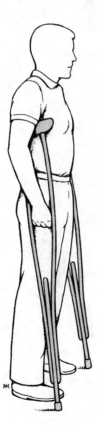

Figure 2.4.   Crutch stance.

Four–Point Gait

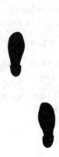
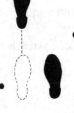

| Right crutch forward | Advance left foot | Left crutch forward | Advance right foot |

Figure 2.5. Four-point gait.

Two–Point Gait

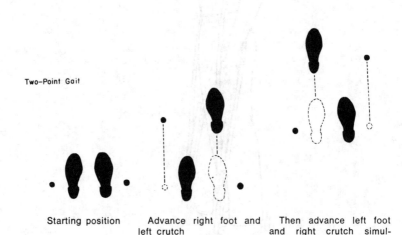
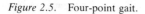

| Starting position | Advance right foot and left crutch | Then advance left foot and right crutch simultaneously. |

Figure 2.6. Two-point gait.

Three-Point Gait

Crutch–foot sequence (Fig. 2.7): (1) both crutches and the weaker lower extremity simultaneously, (2) then the stronger lower extremity.

1   This is a fairly rapid gait but requires more strength and balance.
2   The patient's arms must be strong enough to support his entire body weight.

Tripod Crutch Gait

Tripod Alternate Crutch Gait

Crutch–foot sequence: (1) right crutch, (2) left crutch, (3) swing body and legs forward.

Tripod Simultaneous Crutch Gait

Crutch–foot sequence (Fig. 2.8): (1) both crutches, (2) swing body and legs forward.

1   The patient constantly maintains a tripod position.
2   At the start, both crutches are held fairly widespread out front while both feet are held together in the back.
3   These gaits are slow and laboured.

Swinging Crutch Gaits

Swinging-to Gait

Crutch–foot sequence: (1) both crutches forward, (2) then lift and swing body *to* crutches, (3) place crutches in front of body and continue.

Swinging-through Gait

Crutch–foot sequence: (1) both crutches forward, (2) lift and swing body *beyond* crutches, (3) place crutches in front of body and continue.

1   In the swinging crutch gaits, both legs are lifted off the ground simultaneously and swung forward while the patient pushes up on the crutches.

CANE USE

Purposes

A cane is used for balance and support.

1   To assist the patient to walk with greater balance and support and less fatigue.
2   To compensate for deficiencies of function normally performed by the neuromuscular skeletal system.
3   To relieve pressure on weight-bearing joints.
4   To provide forces to push or pull the body forward or to restrain the forward motion of the patient while walking.

Underlying Principles

1   A firm wooden stick fitted with a 1.5 in rubber suction tip to provide traction while walking, provides good stability for the patient. An adjustable, aluminium stick is available, but is very expensive.

Three–Point Gait

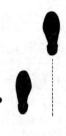

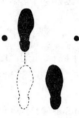
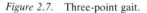

Starting position   Advance both of   Balance weight on   Then advance
                          the crutches and the   both crutches   good foot
                          weak foot

Figure 2.7.   Three-point gait.

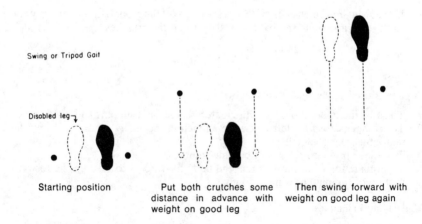

Swing or Tripod Gait

Disabled leg

Starting position   Put both crutches some   Then swing forward with
                          distance in advance with   weight on good leg again
                          weight on good leg

Figure 2.8.   Tripod sumulatneous crutch gait.

2 The stick handle should be level with the greater trochanter when the patient is wearing his normal walking shoes.
3 The patient's elbow should be flexed 25–30° when the stick is the correct length.

Technique for Walking with a Stick

Teach the patient as follows.
1 Hold the stick in the hand opposite to the affected extremity, i.e., the stick should be held on the good side.
2 Move the cane at the same time that the affected leg is moved (Fig. 2.9).
3 Keep the stick fairly close to the body to prevent leaning.
4 When climbing stairs:
   a. Step up with unaffected leg, with both stick and affected leg on lower step.
   b. Then place stick and affected leg on higher step.
   c. Reverse this procedure for descending steps. The unaffected, or stronger, leg goes up first and comes down last.

HELPING THE PATIENT TO REST AND SLEEP

Nursing Objectives

1 To identify and overcome the particular problems which are preventing adequate rest and sleep.
2 To enable the patient to establish a routine which will allow for mental and physical relaxation as well as actual sleeping time.
3 To substitute physiological methods and habits for drug use.
4 To promote a positive attitude to relaxation.

Nursing Programme

1 Establish a good nurse–patient relationship. This will encourage the patient to express his anxieties and fears, and enable the nurse to give full explanations of procedures and plans of care, both immediate and in the future. Encourage the patient to make suggestions for his future rehabilitation.
2 Provide an environment which will prove interesting for the patient. Boredom and apathy must be prevented at all costs.
3 Pain must be relieved by the appropriate means for the individual patient. Fear and anxiety increase pain, and should be eliminated. Analgesic drugs should be available for patients who will obviously need them, e.g., postoperatively. Patients with a terminal illness must have a realistic programme provided so that pain is prevented and not allowed to become uncomfortable or even unbearable before relief is provided. Specialist advice in conjunction with the pain clinic must be available. See Care of Patient with Cancer (p. 277).
4 Plan for definite periods of relaxation during the day, when no interruptions for nursing procedures, doctor's rounds or visitors will occur.
5 During rest and sleeping times, ensure quietness, dimmed lights, adequate warmth and ventilation.
6 Check that discomfort is not caused by full bladder or bowels, and provide a suitable warm or cold drink.

7   Give encouragement to the patient about the progress made during the day to induce a relaxed frame of mind.
8   For anxious or very ill patients, the presence of a nurse or relative sitting quietly by the bed will provide a feeling of confidence and companionship which is conducive to relaxation.
9   Check the patient's previous sleeping habits, and try to provide a plan of care that does not interfere or vary too much from this.

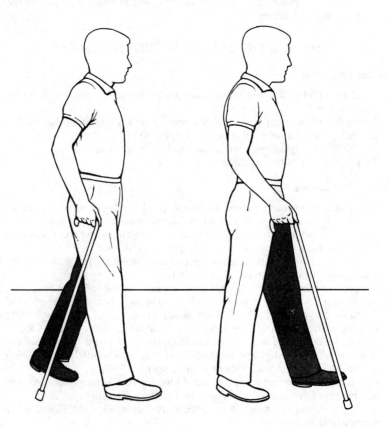

Figure 2.9.   Walking with a cane.

HELPING THE PATIENT WITH SELECTING CLOTHING, WITH DRESSING AND UNDRESSING

Nursing Objectives

1 To help the patient to obtain clothes which:
   a. Express his own personal preference.
   b. Are easy for that individual to put on or take off.
   c. Are in keeping with the environment.
   d. Are fresh and clean.
2 To teach the patient and relatives the best way of putting on garments and removing them, and the use of any special aids which can help.

Nursing Programme

1 Identify the particular problems which the patient may have in selecting clothing.
   a. The patient may have a psychological state in which he as lost interest in his own appearance. This may be an actual psychiatric disorder, but is also present as the result of many physical illnesses, particularly if the patient is very weak.
   b. The patient may have been unable to obtain the type of clothes of his choice because of lack of mobility and being unable to go shopping. Reliance may have been put on relatives or friends who may not have understood the special preferences of the patient, or, as often happens, clothes may have been given as Christmas or birthday presents, which are not really to the taste of the patient.
   c. The patient may be unable to, or have great difficulty in, obtaining clothing which is suitable for a particular disability, e.g., garments with front or extra large openings.
   d. Financial difficulties which have prevented the patient from buying new clothes.
2 Always encourage the patient to choose the clothes which he wishes to wear that day. If the patient has his own clothes, provision must be made for these to be kept in a suitable cupboard, and hung up if possible. If hospital clothes are worn, there should be a sufficient variety of size, colour and style so that individuality is retained.
3 Ensure that laundering facilities are available for personal clothes if the relatives are unable to take these home for washing.
4 Obtain advice from the occupational therapy department for special problems.
5 Encourage the patient to be as independent as possible. Although dressing may take a considerable time, it will give the patient a feeling of achievement.
6 When new clothes are being bought, either a special shopping expedition should be arranged, or else the patient should have access to several mail order catalogues or fashion magazines, and must have an option of returning clothes if they are not suitable.
7 No patient must be left without suitable underwear, even though there may be a problem with incontinence. This is degrading and unnecessary.

HELPING THE PATIENT TO MAINTAIN BODY TEMPERATURE WITHIN NORMAL LIMITS

Nursing Objectives

1   To provide an environment with a stable temperature and satisfactory humidity.
2   To provide specialized nursing procedures for those patients in whom the physiological control of body temperature has been affected, either producing hypothermia or hyperthermia.
3   To maintain a satisfactory condition of the skin, so that the normal mechanisms of heat regulation can function efficiently.
4   To provide suitable personal and bed clothing for the climatic conditions.

Nursing Programme

1   Ensure a constant temperature within the whole area in which the patient will be moving around. This includes bathrooms and sleeping areas as well as day rooms. It is important to consider the provision of adequate heating in the home, well before the time of discharge of the patient, particularly in vulnerable patients, e.g., very young or old, and those with limited mobility. The constant temperature must be maintained throughout the whole of the 24-hour span.
2   Financial grants may be provided for elderly patients at home in order to provide adequate heating. See Care of the Ageing Person (p. 51).
3   To identify patients with a problem in maintaining body temperature, e.g., those with an infection, those with cerebral lesions which may affect the heat regulating centre, those with metabolic disturbances, hypo- or hyperthyroidism.
4   Close observation is needed for a patient suffering from a rigor—with the provision of light, but warm, coverings during the shivering stage; the provision of a fan during the hot stage, and tepid sponging of the skin of the patient to allow reduction of temperature by evaporation.
5   Provide clothing of suitable materials. Cotton is the best material for patients with a raised temperature. Several layers of nonconstricting, light material are suitable for those in need of warmth.
6   Adequate fluid intake is essential for a patient with pyrexia.
7   Hot food and drinks with a sufficient energy content are essential for those with a temperature below normal.

REMEMBER: A sudden rise in temperature or a drop to subnormal temperature may indicate a deterioration in the condition of the patient, and must be reported to the doctor.

HELPING THE PATIENT TO KEEP HIS BODY CLEAN AND WELL GROOMED AND TO PROTECT THE SKIN

Nursing Objectives

1   To assist the patient in maintaining a high standard of personal hygiene.
2   To protect the integrity of the skin in patients at risk.
3   To encourage the patient to take an interest in care of the hair, face and nails.

Nursing Programme

1 Provide facilities for cleanliness of the skin. This may necessitate:
   a. A complete bed bath for a helpless, or very ill, patient.
   b. Provision of a bowl of water and the necessary toilet requisites, placing the patient in a well-supported position, and encouraging the patient to wash and dry his face and hands, and perhaps arms and chest as well, if this can be done without causing undue fatigue or strain.
   c. Assisting the patient with a bath or shower, using mechanical lifts or bath appliances as necessary.
   d. Supervising the patient attending to his own personal hygiene and only providing assistance when needed.
2 Providing aids for those with a disability of hands or arms, or those with limited movement.
3 Remember that the nurse is also a teacher, and some patients with a low standard of personal hygiene need tactful guidance and encouragement. *However*, apparent lack of cleanliness may be due to physical or psychological incapacity, and may be a cause of distress to the patient.
4 The hair must be thoroughly brushed and combed. Women should be encouraged to take an interest in the styling of their hair and a hairdresser should make frequent visits. It is important for the nurse to ascertain if any patient is unwilling to ask for a visit from the hairdresser because of financial difficulties, and to tactfully arrange for this through hospital funds. If the patient's own hairdresser wishes to come, this should be encouraged.
5 The nurse should be able to shampoo the patient's hair either in bed or in the bathroom as frequently as needed.
6 All men should be encouraged to shave themselves. If this is not possible, a barber or the nurse should perform this.
7 Mouth cleanliness is essential. This can usually be accomplished by the patients themselves using a normal shaped toothbrush and paste, but a large handle may be needed for those who have difficulty in holding thin articles.
8 Although the aim of rehabilitation is to achieve as much independence as possible, many patients may find cutting and care of finger and toe nails is beyond their capability, and a chiropodist should visit.
9 Advice and practical help must be available for a patient who needs special cosmetics, e.g., for covering scar tissue, or for provision of wigs or prostheses.

PREVENTION AND TREATMENT OF PRESSURE SORES (DECUBITUS ULCERS)

Pressure sores are localized areas of necrosis occurring in the skin and subcutaneous tissues as a result of pressure.

Altered Physiology

Pressure; tissue anoxia and ischaemia; necrosis of tissue cells; sloughing and ulceration; infection; sepsis; involvement of underlying tissues; rapidly irreversible condition.

Two types of lesions can occur: (a) Superficial lesions which are visible immediately; (b) Lesions which occur in deeper tissues due to prolonged pressure, which may not be visible for 24–48 hours after the pressure occurs, e.g., bad positioning on an operating table, with only a thin layer of padding.

Causes

Pressure

Pressure exerted on skin and subcutaneous tissues by bony prominences and by the object on which the body rests (mattress, stretcher, plaster bed, etc.) interferes with the blood supply of the tissues and if it is prolonged will cause tissue death.

Contributing Factors

1 Immobilization and lack of normal movement, particularly if associated with neurological, circulatory and orthopaedic conditions.
2 Sensory and motor deficits.
   a. Sensory loss produces lack of awareness of pain and pressure.
   b. Motor paralysis with associated muscular atrophy causes lack of movement and reduction in padding between overlying skin and underlying bone.
3 Poor nutrition—negative nitrogen, phosphorous, sulphur and calcium balance will produce wasting of tissue, osteoporosis and loss of weight.
   a. Anaemia.
   b. Hypoproteinaemia.
   c. Vitamin deficiencies particularly ascorbic acid.
4 Oedema which interferes with supply of nutrients to the cells.
5 Friction, moisture and heat irritate the skin, making it less resistant to injury.
6 Infection destroys tissue.
7 Shearing force—caused by gravitational forces that pull the patient's body down towards the foot of the bed, and by resisting forces creating friction on the skin surface.
   a. Pulling tissues so that surface tissues and blood vessels are stretched and injured.
   b. It happens when a patient is pulled up in the bed instead of being lifted clear of the sheets; is allowed to slump down in a chair or bed; moves in bed by digging heels and elbows into the mattress.
8 Changes in the skin (especially in the elderly, because of reduced production of sebum).

Sites

1 Weight bearing bony prominences which are covered only by skin and small amounts of subcutaneous fat. Most (75%) pressure sores occur at such sites (Fig. 2.10).
2 Other bony promontories—knees, malleoli, heels and elbows.

Signs and Symptoms

1 Redness.
2 Dusky, cyanotic blue-grey area indicating capillary occlusion and subcutaneous weakening.

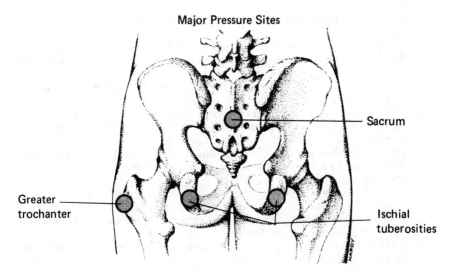

Figure 2.10. Pressure areas.

3 Blistering.
4 Break in the skin progressing to tissue necrosis.

Preventative Measures

1 Identify patients at particular risk. This can conveniently be undertaken using the Doreen Norton Risk Scoring System (Table 2.2). Any patient who scores 12 or less needs very specialized care. The frequency with which the score should be assessed varies with individual patients, but all nurses should be alert to the fact that a significant change in the condition of the patient means a reassessment of the score.
2 Relieve pressure.
   a. By encouraging the patient to keep active.
   b. Turn the patient regularly, at 1, 2 or 4 hourly intervals to allow the blood to flow back into the tissues which are affected by pressure.

Table 2.2.   Pressure Sore Risk Assessment Scoring System (Doreen Norton)

A Physical Condition		B Mental Condition		C Activity		D Mobility		E Incontinent	
Good	4	Alert	4	Ambulant	4	Full	4	Not	4
Fair	3	Apathetic	3	Walk/help	3	Slightly limited	3	Occasionally	3
Poor	2	Confused	2	Chairbound	2	Very limited	2	Usually/urine	2
Very bad	1	Stuporous	1	Bedfast	1	Immobile	1	Doubly	1

    c. If possible position the patient on all four sides in sequence, laterally, dorsal and prone.

3   Use pillows or pads to relieve pressure around particular areas, e.g., heels. Sheepskins, natural or synthetic, can be placed under the patients buttocks, and sheepskin bootees can be used to prevent friction on heels.

4   Use a bedcradle to lift the weight of the bedclothes off the limbs so that there is no impediment to free movement.

5   Avoid placing the patient on a poorly-ventilated mattress that is covered with plastic or impermeable material. If this is unavoidable, a thick cotton under-blanket should be used.

6   Draw sheets should not be used as a routine, only when absolutely necessary. This applies to cotton draw sheets as well as plastic sheets.

7   Maintain meticulous skin hygiene.
    a. Wash skin with mild soap, rinse and *blot* dry with a soft towel.
    b. Keep local areas dry, clean and free from excretions.
    c. If the skin is very dry, or if the patient is doubly incontinent, the use of a barrier cream may be necessary.

8   If the patient is bedbound, use active and passive exercises to avoid movement, and to improve muscular, skin and vascular tone.

9   Mobilize the patient as soon as possible. If actual ambulation is not possible, a change of position from a bed to a chair will help.

10   Use alternating pressure mattresses or chairs, which helps to improve the circulation as well as relieving pressure.

11   Inspect the skin frequently for signs of pressure.
    a. A patient with paraplegia must be taught to inspect his skin, using a mirror.
    b. Keep the patient's weight off reddened areas until it has completely cleared.

12   Relieve pressure over the ischial area for patients sitting in wheel chairs for any length of time. Teach paraplegic patients to do push-ups every hour for intermittent relief of pressure over ischial tuberosities.

13   Inspect any areas where friction may occur from the edge of plaster casts, splints and bandages.

14   Improve the nutritional state of the patient. Sufficient protein and vitamin C intake are essential.

15   A check on the general health of the patient, to exclude anaemia, and diabetes as well as cardiovascular disorders.

Principles of Treatment of a Pressure Sore

1   Completely remove pressure from the area. This may mean putting pressure on other vulnerable sites, and vigorous preventative measures must be taken to avoid the skin breaking down in these places.

2   Clean the ulcer daily. This is essential if sepsis or necrotic tissue are present.

3   Topical applications may be needed for specific reasons, e.g., a streptokinase gel to remove a persistent slough. There are very many preparations which can be used according to the age, condition and skin type of the patient. However, the first aim of the nurse must be to relieve pressure.

4   The use of ultraviolet light may be beneficial.

5   Ensure good nutrition. Extra protein and vitamin intake may be needed.

HELPING THE PATIENT TO AVOID DANGERS
IN THE ENVIRONMENT

Nursing Objectives

1 To encourage the patient to be involved in self-care without causing himself any injury.
2 To alert the patient to dangers inherent in a disabled person, e.g., through lack of mobility.
3 To provide a safe environment without restricting the initiative of the patient.

Nursing Programme

1 Ensure freedom from potential hazards.
   a. At floor level, e.g., trailing flexes, slip mats, spilt food or water.
   b. Unguarded fires, wheelchairs without fixed castors or brakes.
   c. Overhanging shelves, dazzling lights, inconvenient steps.
2 Clothing must not restrict free movement.
3 No trailing belts or ties as these can cause falls.
4 Shoes must be well fitting. It is important to avoid the wearing of slippers, as they will not provide a firm footing.
5 All drugs must be clearly labelled, with the name and the time they are to be taken. Various methods may be employed to clarify that drugs are taken at the correct time, e.g., colour coding, the use of bubble packs so that actual times can be written on them. Avoidance of unnecessary medication.
6 Safety in the bathroom. There should be aids for the patient to get in and out of the bath, and also a nonslip mat in the bottom of the bath.
7 Safety in the kitchen. There should be easy access to shelves and cupboards. The cooking hob must be at a suitable level. If gas is used, a self-igniting device should be provided. A suitable storage cupboard for food as well as a refrigerator. This is essential because people who have a disability may not be able to get to the shops very frequently, and may have to buy food to last for several days at a time. This must be stored in a cool, airy place, free from contamination.
8 Any dressings or infected material must be able to be disposed of safely and easily for the patient.
9 A review of the situation, both from the physical and psychological aspect, at regular intervals is essential.
10 Any mechanical equipment used to help the patient must be regularly serviced.

HELPING THE PATIENT TO COMMUNICATE WITH OTHERS

Nursing Objectives

1 To form a channel of communication between the patient and the nurse, preferably by verbal, or if necessary, by nonverbal means.
2 To encourage the patient to communicate willingly with staff, other patients and his relatives.
3 To combat apathy and provide a stimulating environment.
4 To monitor the amount of nurse–patient interaction.

Nursing Programme

1   Identify the particular physical or psychological problems which are causing blockages of communication.
2   An unsuspected or unacknowledged degree of deafness may be present. An appointment with the audiometry department should be made, and a suitable hearing aid provided. It is important that the hearing aid must be kept in good repair and that batteries are readily available. Also, that both patient and relatives understand its use.
3   A patient with aphasia, perhaps due to a cerebrovascular accident, is suffering considerable frustration because of the lack of ability to communicate.
   a. Specialist treatment from the speech therapist is essential.
   b. Nonverbal means of communication must be sought, these may include picture cards or word boards.
4   All nurses working in a ward must be aware of the amount of time which is spent communicating with each patient. In some cases, this may amount to less than 1 hour a day actually giving personal attention to a patient. Ways of improving this situation must be sought.
5   Even though a patient may be unable or unwilling to communicate with others, it is necessary for someone to talk to them as a sensible human being. On discharge from hospital, care must be taken that the patient will have outside contacts, and will not be isolated.
6   Note must be taken of anybody who withdraws from communicating with others. This may be a sign of deterioration of his physical and psychological state which may need medical intervention.
7   Encourage the patient to be with other people, e.g., clubs, outings, church attendance.

   Communication acknowledges the existence of another person. Failure or refusal to communicate turns the person into a thing, an inanimate object.

HELPING THE PATIENT TO PRACTISE HIS RELIGION OR TO CONFORM TO HIS CONCEPT OF RIGHT AND WRONG

Nursing Objectives

1   To allow the patient to practise his religion without interference.
2   To encourage the patient to actively participate in making balanced decisions about treatment.
3   To respect the right of the patient to decline a particular form of treatment if it is against his religious principles, and, whenever possible, to provide alternative care.

Nursing Programme

1   Identify a patient who has a particular religious belief which may demand modification of the normal medical or nursing provisions.
2   Acknowledge the uniqueness of the individual by involving him in all decisions affecting present and future treatment. Many ethical issues may arise, and these must be treated with sympathy and understanding.

3 Arrange for the hospital chaplain, clergyman or spiritual adviser to visit the patient if he wishes to see them. Provide a quiet place of privacy for them. Make it possible for the patient to receive the sacraments which are part of his religious life. All this should be done without making the patient feel that he is causing trouble or disorganization of hospital routine.
4 The nurse should make herself aware of the main principles of various religions, the demands made by these on the life of a person, and, if the patient wishes, be able to discuss these with him, with tolerance and understanding.
5 The nurse must not deliberately set out to impose her own beliefs on a patient.
6 When possible, a patient should be involved as a part of his own religious group or community, visits to his own church should be arranged if possible and visits from other church members should be encouraged.

HELPING THE PATIENT WITH WORK OR PRODUCTIVE OCCUPATION

Nursing Objectives

1 To enable the patient to achieve a feeling of independence by accomplishing some form of gainful employment.
2 To help the patient to fulfil the more basic physiological and psychological needs in order to reach higher levels of self-fulfilment. These have been described by Maslow (Fig. 2.11.)

Nursing Programme

1 Co-operate with the occupational therapy department and physiotherapy in assessing the physical or psychological handicaps which are hindering the patient from obtaining gainful employment.
2 Discuss with the patient the type of work which he has previously done, and his wishes for the future. Encourage him to make full use of special abilities.

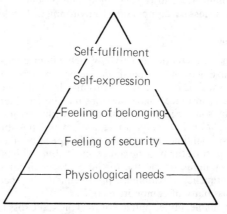

Figure 2.11.   Maslow's hierarchy of needs.

3   Special prostheses should be provided, for instance, for upper or lower limb amputees.
4   For patients who are severely disabled, e.g., tetraplegic, an electronic machine may be provided which can enable them to operate various machinery and use a typewriter. This is known as Patient Operated Selector Mechanism (POSSUM). This could enable a patient to use his thoughts and ideas in some form of work.
5   Some form of mobility may be needed. Each individual must be assessed carefully to see which is the most suitable form of transport, e.g., hand-controlled wheel chairs, battery controlled chairs, or a car adapted for a special disability. A Disability Mobility Allowance may be available. Also, there may be concessions on hire purchase of a car, motor insurance, as well as concessionary fares on most public transport.

Useful addresses include:

The Disablement Income Group, Atlee House, Tonynbee Hall, 28 Commercial Street, London EC1

Disabled Drivers Association, Ashwellthorpe Hall, Ashwellthorpe, Norwich NR16 1EX

The Royal Association for Disability and Rehabilitation, 23/25 Mortimer Street, London W1N 8AB

The Disability Alliance, 5 Netherhall Gardens, London NW3 5RN
6   One of the most important people who can help, is the disablement resettlement officer, who can provide information about retraining schemes and sheltered workshops. Many people, however, are able to find a productive activity of their own.

HELPING THE PATIENT WITH RECREATIONAL ACTIVITIES

Nursing Objectives

1   To encourage the patient to participate in some activity which will provide enjoyment, without necessarily yielding an end product.
2   To provide the necessary equipment or environment for this activity.

Nursing Programme

1   Identify the type of recreational activity which will give most enjoyment to the patient. The nurse may wish to persuade the patient to undertake some activity which she thinks will be beneficial, but this may be quite against the inclinations of the patient. For instance, Bingo sessions may be considered an ideal recreational activity by some people, and fill others with horror.
2   If physical recreation is needed, there are several possibilities. Many sports centres have a special time set aside for handicapped people so that help can be given with transporting them to the centre and helping with the special sport. This may include swimming, or the use of the gymnasium for various ball games. There are 450 branches of Riding for the Disabled, also special archery groups. There is the possibility of competitive sport.
3   Libraries are available, either public libraries or Red Cross Libraries which may provide mobile facilities.

4 Further study may be a form of recreation. The Open University provides many courses and excellent tutorial contacts for those people who cannot attend the normal tutorial sessions, and may require special help, e.g., with writing down the assignments.
5 Social clubs of all kinds are available. It is often possible for the patient to join a club which provides a specialist interest, e.g., music societies, archaeological societies, chess clubs. Most of these are only too willing to provide help with transport to the club meetings.
6 If the patient is housebound, a visiting occupational therapist may help to provide materials for recreational activities. Amateur radio may enable a disabled person to literally keep in contact with the rest of the world.

HELPING THE PATIENT TO LEARN

Nursing Objectives

1 To enable the patient to learn the best way of coping with his particular problem.
2 To enable the patient to be aware of the medical background of his problem, as far as possible for each individual, and to encourage him to ask questions about possible treatments or future plans.
3 To teach the patient any necessary modifications of his former life style which may be needed.

Nursing Programme

1 All nurses must be aware of their function as teachers. They must also be aware that much of the teaching must be done by indirect methods or by example.
2 Work out objectives for the patient to reach within a certain time, and break these down into manageable steps, e.g., objective: the patient will learn to dress himself will be broken down into various parts, such as the patient will learn to put on his shoes using a long-handled shoe horn. The patient must gain a feeling of satisfaction by achieving each step.
3 The nurse may well have a specific teaching function in the field of preventative medicine, for instance, hygiene. Also, in teaching a patient about the administration of his drugs, the dangers of missing doses and the possible side-effects which would require medical assistance. The safe storage of the drugs must be taught. The technique of giving injections will have to be taught to many diabetic patients.
4 Repeat each teaching session as often as required until the patient has gained confidence in his own ability to control the situation. Adjust the level of teaching to match the intellectual ability of the patient. Never assume that the patient has a knowledge of medical matters, but never talk down to the patient.

FURTHER READING

Books

Adams, A et al. (1980) Assessing Vital Functions Accurately, Nursing Skillbooks, Intermed Communications

Altschul, A (1972) Patient–Nurse Interaction, Churchill Livingstone
Burnes, E M, Isaacs, B and Gracie, T (1975) Geriatric Nursing, Heinemann Medical
Campbell, A V (1975) Moral Dilemmas in Medicine, Churchill Livingstone
Downie, P A and Kennedy, P (1978) Lifting, Handling and Helping Patients, Faber
    & Faber
Henderson, V (1977) Basic Principles of Nursing Care, International Council of
    Nurses
Lewis, L W (1980) Fundamental Skills in Patient Care, J B Lippincott
Matheney, R V (1972) Fundamentals of Patient-Centred Nursing, C V Mosby
Redman, B K (1972) The Process of Patient Teaching in Nursing, C V Mosby
Saunders, C (1977) Care of the Dying, Nursing Times Reprint, Macmillan Journals
Shopland, A et al. (1979) Refer to Occupational Therapy, Churchill Livingstone
Stockwell, F (1972) The Unpopular Patient, Rcn Research Publications
Tarling, C (1980) Hoists and Their Uses, Heinemann Medical
Watson, J (1979) Medical/Surgical Nursing and Related Physiology, W B Saunders

Articles

Agate, J (1977) Pressure sores, mechanical and medical factors, Nursing Mirror 144:
    i–iii
Bateman, J M (1979) Rudiments of nursing care. 1. Helping the patient with eating
    and drinking, Nursing Times 75: 957–959
Evans, P M and Massey, R (1979) Rudiments of nursing care. 4. Helping the patient
    with respiration, Nursing Times 75: 1106–1107
Hall, E M (1979) Rudiments of nursing care. 3. Helping the patient with productive
    occupations, Nursing Times 75: 1061–1062
Lowthian, P T (1977) A review of pressure sore prophylaxis, Nursing Mirror 144:
    vii–xi
Mackenzie Stuart, A (1979) Financial aid for the disabled, Nursing 5: 226–227
Miller, V (1979) Rudiments of nursing care. 2. Helping the patient learn, Nursing
    Times 75: 1016–1017
Robinson, W (1978) Aids for the disabled, Nursing Mirror 147: Supplement
Rumbold, G C (1979) Rudiments of nursing care. 6. Protecting the patient and other,
    Nursing Times 75: 1191–1192
Swann, F (1979) Rudiments of nursing care. 5. Helping the patient to communicate
    with others, Nursing Times 75: 1148–1149
Woodbine, A (1979) Pressure sores—a review of the problem, Nursing Times 75:
    1087–1088

Chapter 3

THE AGEING PERSON

Definitions

Gerontology is the study of older persons and the ageing process.
  Social gerontology is the study of the ageing process and its impact on the individual and his society.
  Geriatrics is medical treatment of older persons.

BODILY CHANGES ASSOCIATED WITH AGEING

General Principles

1 Ageing occurs at all levels of bodily function—cellular, organic and systemic. Almost every organ loses functional capacity.
2 There is a reduction of reserve capacity due to actual loss of individual cells in various organ tissues of the body. The ageing body lacks reserve power.
3 Ageing proceeds at different rates in different systems in the same individual.
4 In general, adjustment to physiological changes is made by reducing the level of activity.

Changes in Homoeostasis

Homoeostasis is the ability of the body to restore equilibrium.

1   Decrease in functional capacity and efficiency of co-ordinating systems within the body.
    Progressively limited capacity to respond to stress.
2   Diminution of functional reserve—person more vulnerable to disease, death more likely; more time required for body to return to normal after illness.
3   Temperature regulation less efficient, causing increased risk of hypothermia.

Changes in the Nervous System

1   Progressive loss of brain cells and their fibres, brain compensates for this.
2   Progressive atrophy of the convolutions (gyri) of the brain surface and consequent widening and deepening of the spaces (sulci) between the convolutions.
3   Decrease in blood flow to the brain.
4   Loss of postural reflexes causing unsteadiness of gait.
5   Slower reaction time; more time required for decision making.
6   Gradual failing of memory (particularly short-term memory).
7   Personality changes—appear to be related to blood supply to brain as well as to changes in nervous system.

Changes in Skin and Subcutaneous Tissues

1   Epidermis thins generally, although it may thicken in some areas.
2   Dermis becomes relatively dehydrated and loses strength and elasticity; skin is prone to excessive dryness and itching.
3   Blood flow to peripheral areas of body decreases.
4   Loss of subcutaneous fat gives characteristic appearance to skin—folds, lines, wrinkles, slackness.
5   Focal pigmentary discolorations occur.
6   Ecchymoses may appear—due to greater fragility of the dermal and subcutaneous vessels.
7   Sweating decreases.
8   Thickening and hardening of nails.

Changes in Musculoskeletal System

1   Lessening of muscular strength, endurance and agility.
2   Postural changes—from structural changes in ligaments, joints and bones. Ligaments calcify and ossify; joints stiffen from erosion of cartilaginous joint surfaces; ossification and degenerative changes occur in synovium (lining of joint cavities).
3   Increase in curvature of spine.
4   Bone changes—bones become porous and lighter and lose much of their density (see Osteoporosis).

Changes in the Special Senses

1   Vision—decrease in visual acuity and in ability to accommodate to light; falling off of lateral vision, receding clarity.

Clinical problems include presbyopia (impaired vision due to ageing), senile cataract, glaucoma.

2 Hearing—loss of some hearing ability; inability to hear higher pitches; greater difficulty in hearing normal ranges of sound.

3 Voice—lower volume; slower rate of speech.

4 Smell and taste—dulling of sense of smell; decrease in number of taste buds.

5 Less acute sensations of touch; slowing of reflexes.

Changes in the Cardiovascular System

Heart

1 Effectiveness of pumping action of heart is reduced.

2 Cardiac output and stroke volume decreases.

3 With diminishing cardiac reserve the heart reacts poorly to stress.

4 Fat deposits around heart may increase; thickening and loss of flexibility of valves due to sclerosis and fibrosis.

5 Blood flow through the coronary arteries may be lessened.

Vascular

1 Progressive chemical and anatomic changes in arteries, with an increase in cholesterol, other lipids and calcium.

2 Elastic fibres progressively straighten, fray, split and fragment.

3 As aorta becomes less elastic and there is increasing resistance to blood flow, systolic hypertension may develop.

4 Increased tendency to varicose veins.

Changes in the Respiratory System

1 Elasticity of lungs and chest wall decreases—partly due to an alteration in the structure of collagen. Calcification of cartilage of rib cage.

2 Less oxygen diffusion—due to increase in collagen and scar tissue in lung and to decrease in blood flow to the lung.

3 Reduction in amount of blood flow to lungs—contributes to arrhythmias.

4 Decline in total lung capacity and concurrent increase in residual volume—producing decrease in function.

Changes in the Gastrointestinal System

1 Gastrointestinal function impeded by loss of teeth, impaired swallowing mechanism and diminishing gastric and enzyme secretions.

2 Tooth decay is increased because of decreased saliva.

3 Less absorption of nutrients and minerals.

4 Reduced motility of stomach.

5 Decreasing peristalsis—due to generalized weakness of muscle activity; constipation is a common complaint.

Changes in the Urinary System

1 Decrease in kidney function and adaptability.

2 Reduction of blood flow to kidneys—due to decrease in cardiac output and increase in peripheral resistance.
3 Diminished filtration rate and tubular function.
4 Structural changes in kidneys. Loss of glomeruli may be 50%.

Metabolic Changes

1 Production of gonadal hormones is reduced; cortisol secretions decrease.
2 Decline in production of thyroid-stimulating hormone of pituitary and of thyroid hormones secreted by thyroid gland.
3 Glucose tolerance curve tends towards that of the diabetic. Reduced production of insulin.
4 Decline in ability to adapt or respond to stress.
5 Liver enzymes less efficient.

Changes in the Reproductive System

1 Sexual desires and capabilities, though modified, may remain in late life.
2 Cessation of sexual activity is due in part to decline of physical health in one or both partners or to death of partner.

PSYCHOSOCIAL INFLUENCE OF AGEING ON HEALTH

Psychosocial Aspects

Both physical and mental health are inter-related with psychosocial aspects of ageing.

1 Decrease in self-esteem due to loss of:
   a. Earning power. Although many people will have paid into voluntary pension schemes as well as the compulsory contribution into the national pension scheme, and so will be receiving a definite weekly amount, this often does not keep up with the rise in inflation. It is difficult for an elderly person to find a small, part-time job, and there is the possibility of the retirement pension being decreased if earnings exceed a certain amount. If Supplementary Benefit has to be provided, this may give a feeling of inadequacy, and that this is accepting charity.
   b. Status and work role. An elderly person may feel that the regard and respect which they received was due to their role at work and not due to themselves. This may cause them to withdraw and disengage from the mainstream of life.
   c. Social roles and resources because of loss of contact with work colleagues.
   d. Family and friends through death or moving away.
2 Lack of meaningful activity.
3 Negative stereotype or prejudices of society against the aged.
4 Loss of cognitive functioning (thinking, perceiving, remembering) may be caused by lack of interest or concentration.
      Decline in mental and physical capabilities—poor short-term memory, loss of speed and agility.
      Sensory disabilities—these make individuals suspicious and distrustful of others.

Physical Disabilities Affecting Adaptation

1 Perceptual impairment.
2 Hearing losses—lead to depression and suspiciousness.
3 Lack of sexual desire and capacity.
4 Loss of speed and psychomotor response—inability to travel.
5 Subjective awareness of ageing.
6 Cultural devaluation.
7 Slowing down of psychological processes.
8 Personality defects exaggerated. Eccentric and hysterical trends become more obvious.

Adaptive Techniques Employed by the Aged

1 Disengagement—mutual withdrawal between individual and society; can produce chronic depression.
2 Activity.
3 Paranoid retreat.
4 Integration—person accepts ageing and ages gracefully.
5 Adherence to specific routine with resistance to change (helps failing memory).

DISEASE ASPECTS OF AGEING

General Effects

1 Manifestations of disease are modified by old age.
2 More than one disease may be present—over 40% of ageing persons have more than one illness.
3 Elderly persons respond to treatment more slowly and to a lesser degree.
4 There is less resistance to stress—one major illness lowers resistance and allows other illnesses to appear.
5 Illnesses tend to cluster during closing years of the very old person's life—chain reaction of one degenerative process leading to another and finally to death.

Specific Aspects

1 Most common diseases are those of circulatory system and atherosclerosis.
     Arterial disease causes cardiac, renal and neurologic problems.
2 Elderly persons are more vulnerable to acute infections of respiratory tract—increasing numbers have chronic lung disease.
3 They are prone to gastrointestinal diseases, particularly functional diseases.
4 Incidence of cancer increases—may be of many years' duration.
5 There are changes in arterial walls (arteriosclerosis), in joint spaces (arthritis) and in functioning of certain endocrine glands (diabetes).
6 Hypothalamic temperature regulation less efficient—increased risk of hypothermia.
7 Loss of muscle tone, effecting limbs, bladder and bowels.

Mental Illness

1   Older persons constitute the largest single group of patients in mental hospitals.
 a. Many problems that produce stress in old age arise from conflicts that have not been adequately resolved throughout life—extrinsic or intrinsic.
 b. Psychiatric symptoms in the elderly may also be caused by metabolic, toxic, infectious, cardiac, respiratory or drug-induced disorders.
2   Patient may exhibit delusions, hallucinations and other signs of brain decompensation.
3   Anxiety and depression are common emotional problems.
4   Suicide in aged is allied to physical disease, social isolation and grief; more prevalent among men.

MEDICAL AND NURSING MANAGEMENT OF THE AGED

Health Maintenance and Preventative Care

Objective

To maintain a state of physical, mental and social well-being, and to enable the individual to retain a state of independence in physical and psychological functioning.

1   Encourage forward planning for retirement in consultation with partner or family. This should include:
 a. Planning for retirement income. In addition to the state pension, contributory or noncontributory schemes are provided by many firms, or private insurance schemes are available.
 b. Planning for retirement housing. Full consideration must be given to this. A smaller house in the same area, which is easy to maintain, has adequate heating facilities, and is within easy reach of a shopping area. It is unwise for elderly people to move to some apparently 'ideal' location in the country or at the sea, where they have no relatives or friends, and where the demands on the social services may already be excessive.
 c. Attendance at preretirement courses (which cover the above and much more).
 d. Planning for retirement activities and hobbies.
2   Encourage a positive approach to health.
 a. Special over 60s clinics for well people run by the local health authority by general practitioners in health centres. These may include special screening programmes for such conditions as diabetes mellitus, hypertension, chest conditions and myxoedema. Some primary care teams are developing screening and assessment programmes independently.
 b. Health visitors who are attached to a general practice can identify all the old people registered with the doctor and provide information and help for those who have no need to visit the surgery, as well as those who attend for medical advice.
 c. Because a person is old, it is not inevitable that they suffer from ill health. Any disorders should be treated.

3   Provide information about the high risk of accidents due to falls. These may be due to locomotor disabilities, environmental risks, poor lighting and poor eyesight, as well as pathological conditions. Help should be available to give advice about particular danger areas in any house and special equipment which can be provided to minimize these hazards. Working areas should be arranged so that bending down and stretching above head height are avoided. In the house ensure that there is easy access to toilet and baths.

To prevent falls:

a. Efforts must be made to ensure a steady gait.

b. Encourage the wearing of proper shoes rather than slippers.

c. Good foot care and chiropody services are essential.

d. Hands should be kept free for holding onto rails or supports rather than carrying articles.

4   Recreational activities should be encouraged. These may be run by a day centre, or by various social or welfare organizations. Occupational facilities at home should be discussed. Help with gardening can be very important for men, who often have difficulty in adjusting to retirement.

5   Statutory and voluntary services should be used. These include:

a. The primary health care team, i.e., general practitioner, who will be the key person in treating overt and latent physical and mental ill health; health visitor who gives health education advice and information about available services and benefits, and also identifies present and future problems; the community nurse who carries out care, possibly only helping with bathing or carrying out the complete care of a helpless patient. The community nurse identifies problems and initiates other services, e.g., home helps, Meals on Wheels. The community doctor acts as co-ordinator.

b. Chiropodist, optician and dental care.

c. Home helps—an hourly charge is made for this according to patient's income.

d. Meals on Wheels is a statutory service, but this may be supported financially and with voluntary support by Age Concern, WRVS, schools, etc. British Red Cross helps with transport, social clubs and visiting. Youth groups help with home decorating and gardening. Lunch clubs may be held in an old people's day centre, or in a residential home or in a village hall.

e. Day centres may be run by the social services department or by voluntary organizations. These provide meals at reduced prices, occupational and rec-reational facilities. Volunteers may help with transport.

f. Day hospitals, which are usually run by the hospital, where, as well as the facilities which are available at the day centre, there is also medical assessment, bathing facilities, medical and nursing care and physiotherapy and occupational therapy. Transport facilities are provided by the ambulance service.

g. Good neighbour schemes. Thse are run by many different groups, e.g., churches, Women's Institutes, young wives groups, and they have many different functions, the main one is to make contact with an elderly person who needs some sort of support, e.g., someone to talk to, help with shopping. An emergency call system, e.g., a card in the window, may be available. In any post office, there is a list of voluntary services available. Many areas have a branch of Age Concern, which organizes a great deal of help through various resources.

6   Financial help is available through social security. It must be explained that this is

not charity but an entitlement. Rent or rate rebates, via the local authority, pay-as-you-go schemes for heating costs or additional supplementary benefit for heating costs.

7   For elderly people who need continuous care in their own homes, a constant attendance allowance may be payable.

   a. Outings and holidays—some social service departments arrange subsidized or free holidays for the elderly, and various organizations have schemes (see appendix).

   b. Travel concessions may vary in different areas, e.g., in greater London free bus travel is available. In other areas, a special card can be purchased, which entitles the holder to half-price fares. British Rail also reduce fares for the elderly. It is important that elderly people keep in touch with their friends and relations, so full advantage should be taken of these concessions.

Nutritional Considerations for the Aged

1   Nutritional requirements of the elderly are similar to those of adults, except that energy intake should be reduced.

   a. Energy needs diminish with age, both metabolic rate and activity decrease, so that energy requirements of the aged are reduced.

   b. The energy intake is adjusted on an individual basis to maintain normal weight.

   c. Protein requirements are not reduced but protein utilization may be less efficient in old age.

   d. Calcium intake should be as great as that of a younger person—high incidence of osteoporosis in older women.

   e. Older persons usually have inadequate intake of calcium, ascorbic acid and riboflavin due to insufficiency of milk, fruit and vegetables in the diet.

2   Nutritional deficiencies are frequently encountered in the elderly.

   a. Vitamin C and K deficiencies—ecchymoses due to capillary fragility.

   b. Vitamin A deficiency—fissuring of skin around mouth.

   c. Vitamin B deficiency—glossitis, angular stomatitis, megaloblastic anaemia —B_{12} and folic acid deficiency.

   d. Vitamin D deficiency—osteomalacia.

   e. Mineral deficiencies—demineralization of bone.

3   Factors affecting nutritional habits of the elderly.

   a. Food habits of a lifetime.

   b. Social factors (eating alone).

   c. Food fads.

   d. Poor dental health; ill-fitting dentures.

   e. Shopping problems.

   f. Reduced income and financial problems; high cost of many protein foods.

   g. Lack of motivation for meal planning and food preparation.

   h. Decreased appeal of food—loss of taste buds; less acute sense of smell.

   i. Difficulty with preparation of food because of stiff hands and lack of mobility.

   j. Mental deterioration and memory loss—meals may be omitted.

4   Fluid intake should be at least 1.5 l daily. It is essential that this is not decreased because of the fear of incontinence. This will aggravate the problem.

Drug Therapy and the Aged

Factors Altering Drug Response in the Elderly

1 Diminished production of liver enzymes that break down substances, including drugs; majority of drugs are metabolized and detoxified by the liver.
2 Increase in circulation time (due to reduced cardiac efficiency) may have cumulative effect.
3 Diminished kidney function—lower rate of elimination leads to drug accumulation and toxicity.
4 Decrease in amount of gastric acid inhibits absorption of acid-requiring drugs.
5 Diminished ability to maintain homoeostatic balance.

Nursing Implications

1 Be aware that drug effect is more pronounced in old persons. The potential for adverse reactions and interactions is greater.
 a. Old people may not be able to handle multiple medications or may omit to take them.
 b. They appear to be more sensitive to digoxin, diuretics, aspirin, warfarin sodium, etc.
2 Obtain a medical and drug history.
 a. Check nutritional status.
 b. Ask what over-the-counter medications the patient is taking (laxatives, antacids, aspirin); these may affect the interaction of prescribed drugs.
3 Usually the doctor will hold the dosage to lowest effective amount; doses may be given further apart.
 a. Reinforce verbal instructions with written instructions to the patient, family and primary care team.
 b. Write what the drug is used for—e.g. 'to stop indigestion after meals'.
 c. Explain possible side effects.
 d. Be sure the drug name and instructions for taking it are typed in large letters on the label, and that containers can be opened easily.
 e. Arrange drug schedule to coincide with a regular activity (arising, eating, retiring)—helps patient to remember to take drug.
 f. Arrange some sort of check-off system.
4 Carry out periodic drug review.
 a. Ask patient to bring medication with him on next visit to doctor or clinic.
 b. Assess for patient compliance, response to therapy, possible side effects, drug interactions.

Nursing Approach to the 'Confused' Old Person

1 Changes in mental status may be the first sign of illness in the elderly.
 a. Expect an underlying physical cause in any patient who has *sudden* changes in intellectual functioning.
 b. Confusion and disorientation may be first sign of infection, pneumonia, cardiac failure, coronary occlusion, electrolyte imbalance, stroke, dehydration, anaemia, malignancy.

2 Ageing is not synonymous with senility—senile dementia is a *degenerative* disease of the elderly.
3 A new environment may bring on confused behaviour without physiological causes.
   a. Be optimistic over this turn of events; act on the assumption that this behaviour is temporary.
   b. Accept the person as he is now, without judgement or criticism.
   c. Pay attention to what the patient is saying—often a person who is considered confused is only transiently so and much of what he is saying makes sense.
   d. Call the person by name each time a contact is made; touch the patient when you speak to him.
      (1) Talk directly to him.
      (2) Answer questions in simple, short sentences.
   e. Tell the person who you are, and why you are there.
   f. Keep the patient oriented with respect to time and place.
      (1) Remind him of time, dates and place each morning and whenever necessary.
      (2) Keep a calendar and clock, both with easily readable numbers, within his range of vision.
      (3) Keep the room well lighted to reduce confusion and fear.
   g. Have the patient's personal belongings where he can see and use them.
   h. Maintain a calm environment. Remove unduly stressful stimuli.
   i. Arrange for visits from others to counteract isolation.
      (1) Have family sit by bed so patient can see and touch them.
      (2) Utilize services of a volunteer if no family is available.
   j. Attempt to alleviate the patient's anxiety.
      (1) Hold the patient's hand—many aged persons have no one to touch them.
      (2) Use warm baths, warm milk, back massage and understanding and compassion.
   k. See that the patient wears his glasses, and that they are clean, also hearing aid, dentures or other prostheses.
   NOTE: Be sure he is drinking enough fluids.
4 Avoid endorsing confused behaviour.
   a. Do not agree with confused statements.
   b. Avoid letting the patient 'ramble'. Direct him back to reality.
   c. Be consistent. Each member of the health care team should know the nursing objective and use the same approach.
5 Plan the patient's daily activities and adhere to the plan to promote security.

Foot Care of the Elderly

1 Care of the feet in the elderly and chronically ill patient is a vital part of nursing.
2 Systemic diseases such as diabetes mellitus, arterial insufficiency and the arthritides often are compounded by loss of sensation, abnormal gait patterns and impaired vision; thus the assessment made by the nurse is of prime importance, and may be diagnostic.

Care of the Elderly in Long-term Accommodation

Long-term accommodation may be run by the local health authority or privately.

1 Private homes may be:
   a. Rest homes for the elderly who need hotel type accommodation but not nursing care. Residents must be mobile and continent. Help with bathing is usually available, but night attendance is not always possible.
   b. Nursing homes for people who need nursing care. They are supervised by a trained nurse 24 hours a day.
2 Local authority accommodation may be:
   a. Sheltered accommodation (statutory service), individual flats, bungalows or bedsitters with washing and cooking facilities, with a warden in charge. There may be communal dining room facilities for some meals and a lounge for social gatherings. A call system is often installed.
   b. Part III accommodation (old people's homes, statutory service). Residents must be continent and mobile, i.e., able to transfer and be wheelchair independent. Care attendants are employed to help with general tasks, bathing, dressing, etc. A community nurse usually visits if nursing care is required for a time.
   c. Health authority geriatric ward or unit—all types of problems will be nursed—acute (diagnostic and fast rehabilitation) and long term (slow rehabilitation and total care). Physical and psychological care is provided. Social admissions may be taken on a short-term basis to give relatives a break.

With the health and local authority accommodation, a deduction is made from the state pension. A small portion of the pension is always given to the patient for their own personal use. With private homes, the patient is responsible for the whole cost. If, through rising prices, a long-term resident is unable to meet the increased fees financial help may be available. Any elderly person who remains in a National Health Service (NHS) hospital for longer than 6 weeks, has his state pension reduced until he is discharged.

NOTE: It is essential that the team approach to the care of the elderly is carried out, so the expertise of various members of the team may contribute to the physical, psychological and social side of care.

Nursing Patients in a Geriatric Ward

Essential Guidelines

Patients may be in a long-term geriatric ward for many years, and this is their *home*. All efforts must be made to make the ward as homelike as possible. A plan of care for each patient must be formulated, and the care which is received by each patient must be evaluated frequently and regularly (case conferences). *Positive, individualized patient care is essential*.

The geriatric ward should be:

1 Purpose built, or efficiently adapted for the particular needs of the geriatric patient, and heated to the temperature required by the elderly rather than the staff.
2 Within easy access for visiting, taking into account that the patients' friends and relatives may belong to the same age group.

3   Have a good outlook, be preferably on a ground floor, so that the patient feels a contact with the outside world.
4   Have clearly identifiable toilet facilities within easy reach of sleeping and day room areas. Commodes should always be used in preference to bed pans.
5   Facilities for a degree of privacy, and also maintenance of dignity during toilet and nursing procedures.
6   TV and radio should be used positively and not as background noise.
7   Be free from hazards, e.g., slippery floors.
8   Avoid restrictive equipment—cot sides, fixed chair fronts, restrainers.

See Rehabilitation Concepts for more detail.
Nursing Care must be:

1   Geared to the particular needs of the geriatric patient. Routine must be flexible and adjusted to the needs of the individual patient, e.g., there may be considerable variation in sleeping patterns. It is not necessary for all patients to be woken up or put to bed at the same time.
2   Carried out by staff who are sympathetic to the needs of the elderly, who have skills needed for these patients, who are open minded and aware of current research and ideas, and willing to implement new procedures if they are in the interests of their patients.
3   Planned so that a full range of medical and surgical investigations and care must be available, but it is essential that the terminal stage of old age must be peaceful, dignified, free from pain or discomfort, and that overvigorous methods of treatment are very carefully considered, before causing the patient added stress. Positive planning for the latter stages of any illness are essential and the very best medical and nursing care is required at this stage. See Rehabilitation Concepts for care of bladder, bowels and help with dressing.
4   Planned to add life to years and not years to life.

Nursing Care of Elderly Patients in Their Own Homes

The full resources of the health service and the social services should be used to enable elderly persons to remain in their own home or with relatives if they wish. It is essential that these resources are known to them, and include financial help, home help services, Meals on Wheels, as well as all the resources available through the primary care team, such as equipment.

Essential Guidelines

1   Members of the care team are entering the house at the invitation of the patient and their approach to the patient and the relatives should reflect this fact. They should therefore try to preserve an empathic and nonjudgemental approach.
2   Team management of the care of the elderly is necessary, and regular case conferences by members of the primary health care team should examine all aspects of care. Many teams may designate one member to be the prime carer. This person may make an assessment visit and then act as co-ordinator for the various services. This person may be the health visitor initially, but in the course of time, if the elderly person's physical condition deteriorates, it may be more appropriate for the district nursing sister to assume this role.

3   Adaptations to the house should be carried out where necessary, to provide extra safety measures, and also increase the mobility of the patient. Facilities for the safe and easy storage and preparation of food must be available.

4   The method of heating the house should be carefully considered, because of the danger of hypothermia, the risk of fire, and also from the financial problem.

5   If relatives are living with the patient, they should be given full support and encouragement. Holiday admissions to a geriatric unit should be available and may provide a welcome break for both the patient and the relatives. It is essential that both the patient and the relatives have an area of privacy at home, where they can have visitors, and where the various members of the family can have their own hobbies without constant interference. As already mentioned, planning for retirement and old age should take place with information from various sources, and after consultation with the family.

6   If the elderly person is living on their own, some method of summoning help must be available, e.g., card in the window, alarm bell or light. Neighbours should be aware of the fact of this person being on their own.

7   If adequate help can be given, many elderly people can safely remain in their own homes, in familiar surroundings with the maximum degree of independence.

GUIDELINES: Trimming the Toenails (Fig. 3.1)

The nails of elderly persons usually grow very slowly, but they have a tendency to become thickened and deformed from trauma to the nail matrix, vascular insufficiency and nutritional changes.

Equipment

Foot care tray containing:
One pair nail clippers: 11 cm (4·5 in)   Towel
Orange sticks   Sterile Telfa or nonadherent dressing
Antiseptic   Sterile cotton-tipped applicators
Sterile Kling or adherent gauze   Emery boards
Band-Aids

Procedure

Nursing Action	Reason
Preparatory Phase	
1 Explain the procedure to the patient.	1 Proper explanation of any procedure reduces apprehension and ensures patient co-operation.
2 Soak the feet in tepid water for 5 min. An antibacterial skin cleanser (pHisoHex®) may be added to the soak.	2 Soaking softens the nail plate, loosens subungual debris, decreases the possibility of bacterial infection and relaxes the patient.
3 Dry the feet by blotting instead of wiping.	3 The use of friction may injure delicate, atrophic and ischaemic skin.

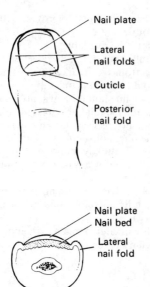

Nail plate

Lateral
nail folds

Cuticle

Posterior
nail fold

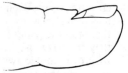

Nail after cutting

Nail plate
Nail bed

Lateral
nail fold

Figure 3.1.   a. Anterior and cross section of toenail. b. After the nail is cut, the nail plate should be long enough so that it rests freely and without pressure on the nail bed.

Performance Phase

1   Sit facing the patient. Place his feet on a foot rest or improvised foot rest (hassock).

2   Observe the nails, skin temperature, texture and colour. Look for breaks in the skin, infection, redness and oedema.

3   Locate the nail and differentiate the nail from the nail bed. A cotton bud can be used for this.

4   Apply antiseptic to areas around toenails before debriding or cutting nail plates.

5   Thin the nail plate by rubbing the emery board across the nail surface if necessary.

3   The growth pattern of some nail plates is altered so that it is frequently difficult to differentiate nail plate from nail bed.

4   This is a precaution which reduces the chance of secondary bacterial infection.

5   The nails may be so thick that thinning is required before cutting is possible.

Nursing Action	Reason
6 Using only the tip of the nail clippers, start at one corner and take small bites across the entire nail plate, following the contour of the nail plate. Little or no force should be necessary.	6 The nail should be cut so that it rests freely and without pressure on the nail bed (Fig. 3.1). It should be cut even with the end of the toe.
7 Smooth the nail edges with an emery board.	7 This prevents irregular nail edges from irritating adjacent toes and from tearing hose.
8 Use an orange stick to carefully debride around and under the nail plate.	8 Debriding removes subungual debris which may be causing discomfort.
9 Apply antiseptic to nail plates and toes that have been treated.	9 This action helps prevent infection.

Nursing Alert: Avoid cutting nails if force is required, if a toe is exuding purulent material or is gangrenous, or if a subungual neoplasm is suspected. The toenails of a patient with diabetes mellitus should only be cut by a qualified chiropodist.

A toe nail (Fig 3.2) should not be treated by a nurse. A qualified chiropodist will deal with this problem.

Skin Care of the Elderly

The skin of the elderly tends to become dry and thin. Care must be taken to avoid (a) pressure on any area for a prolonged time, (b) friction from shoes, walking aids, chairs and (c) dampness, which predisposes to skin lesions.

Skin lesions are common and should be treated as a long-standing infection can occur, and malignant changes missed. Seborrhoeic warts, pruritis and rodent ulcers are common. Squamous cell epithelioma may occur on lips, ears and penis. Extremes of temperatures can cause skin problems. Warm clothing should be worn, bedsocks are better at night-time than hot water bottles. The skin in the pretibial area is

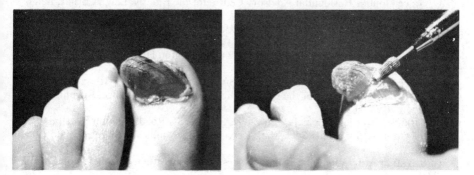

Figure 3.2. Ram's horn nail.

vulnerable, and in the ankle area particularly if varicose veins are present. Such people should avoid sitting with their legs directly in front of a fire for a long time or with their legs crossed as this impairs circulation. Frequent movement should be encouraged to promote good circulation in the legs.

Eye Care of the Elderly

Visual acuity should be checked every 2 years. This is essential for safety but also for orientation and social communication. Misunderstandings can occur if an elderly person apparently ignores neighbours or friends, or is unable to read notices. The possibility of cataract or glaucoma must be remembered. Discharging eyes may be a problem, and these should be gently swabbed, and the appropriate eye drops instilled. See Chap. 3, Vol. 3, Eye Disorders.

APPENDIX. ADVISORY SERVICES AND USEFUL ADDRESSES

Age Concern, Bernard Sunley House, 60 Pitcairn Road, Mitcham, Surrey CR4 3LL.

British Association for the Services to the Elderly, 86 York Street, London W1.

British Deaf Association, 38 Victoria Place, Carlisle, Cumbria CA1 1HU.

British Society for Research on Ageing, Department of Medicine, Leeds University, Leeds LS1 3EX.

Chest, Heart and Stroke Association, Tavistock House, North, Tavistock Square, London WC1H 9JE.

Citizen's Advice Bureaux, local branches in most towns. Addresses found in the post office.

Distressed Gentlefolk's Aid Association, Vicarage Gate House, Vicarage Gate, London W8 4AQ.

Elderly Invalid's Fund and Old People's Advisory Service, 10 Fleet Street, London EC4Y 1BB.

Friends of the Elderly and Gentlefolk's Help, 42 Ebury Street, London SW1 0LZ.

Grace Gould's Residential Advisory Centre for the Elderly, Leigh Corner, Leigh Hill Road, Cobham, Surrey KT11 2HW.

Health Education Council, 78 New Oxford Street, London WC1A IAH.

Help the Aged, 8–10 Denman Street, London W1A 2AP.

Information Service for the Disabled, 346 Kensington High Street, London W14 8NS.

Marie Curie Foundation, 124 Sloane Street, London SW1X 9BB.

National Corporation for the Care of Old People, Nuffield Lodge, Regents Park, London NW1 4RS.

Parkinson's Disease Society of the UK, 81 Queen's Road, London SW19 8NR.

Salvation Army Men's Social Services, 110–112 Middlesex Street, London E1 7HZ.

Salvation Army Women's Social Services, 280 Mare Street, Hackney, London E8 1HE.

Women's Royal Voluntary Service, 17 Old Park Lane, London W1Y 4AJ.

SUMMARY OF THE PRINCIPLES UNDERLYING THE NURSING MANAGEMENT OF THE ELDERLY PATIENT

1 Nursing care must be individualized, taking into consideration the patient's past experiences, needs and invidual goals.

2 Realistic and attainable goals, which are understood by the patient, are set to help him gain a sense of accomplishment and purpose.
   a. Engage in mutual goal-setting when possible.
   b. Keep communicating to the patient the planned goals of his care.
   c. Support his belief in his own inner resources.

3 The patient should be an active participant in his own plan of care.
   a. Learn something about him before the initial encounter; find out the strengths of the patient.
   b. Consult his preferences.
   c. Concentrate on what the patient can do, and praise frequently to encourage further effort.
   d. Ask his opinions.
   e. Encourage him to make choices and decisions.
   f. Avoid making decisions for him; this promotes low self-esteem, dependency and depression.
   g. Support him during his periods of anxiety.
   h. Urge him to remain active.

4 Nursing activities should be done *with* the patient rather than *for* him.

5 Necessary modifications and compromises imposed by the physiological limits of ageing must be made in the medical and nursing management of the patient.

6 The individuality of the patient should be encouraged—to preserve his identity and sense of control.
   a. Encourage him to have and use personal possessions that help bridge the gap between past and present.
   b. Give the patient *time* to express his feelings.
   c. Help him retain the social graces.
   d. Help him cope with thoughts of death.

7 Elderly persons should be kept in the mainstream of life to prevent physical, emotional and mental deterioration.
   a. Stimulate mental acuity.
   b. Share your world with the patient.
   c. Remember his preferences; accept his idiosyncracies.
   d. Provide opportunities for him to do some tasks of daily living (water plants; washing up).
   e. Provide meaningful diversional activity.
   f. Give him something to look forward to.

8 The patient's potentialities should be utilized.
   a. Select activities that are in keeping with lifelong interests.
   b. Do not attempt to alter lifelong character and behaviour patterns.
   c. Give the patient time to listen, to learn and to adapt.

FURTHER READING

Books

Chartered Society of Physiotherapy (1980) Handling the Handicapped, Woodhead-Faulkner

Coni, N et al. (1978) Lecture Notes on Geriatrics, Blackwell Scientific Publications

Darnborough, A and Kinrade, D (1978) Directory for the Disabled, Woodhead-Faulkner

Eliopoulos, C (1979) Geriatric Nursing, Harper and Row

Eliott, J R (1975) Living in Hospital—The Social Needs of People in Long Term Care, King Edwards Hospital Fund

Foott, S (1977) Handicapped at Home, Design Centre Book

Goldsmith, S (1976) Designing for the Disabled, RIBA Publications

Hale, G (1979) The Source Book for the Disabled, Paddington Press

Meredith Davis, B (1979) Community Health, Preventive Medicine and Social Services, Ballière Tindall

Todd, H (1980) Old Age—A Register of Social Research, Centre for Policy on Ageing

Wells, T J (1980) Problems in Geriatric Nursing Care, Churchill Livingstone

Articles

Barrowclough, F (1977) The elderly in institutions, Nursing Mirror, 145 (24): 27–28

Barrowclough, F (1978) All nurses must share in the care of the old, Nursing Mirror, 148 (1): 13–16

Barrowclough, F (1979) Ward accidents. Danger. Why old people fall, Nursing Mirror, 148 (24): 28–29

Burton, M et al. (1981) A behavioural approach to nursing the elderly, Nursing Times, 77 (6): 247–248

Whitely, M W et al. (1981) Elderly clients and the withdrawal of night hypnotics, Nursing Times, 77 (12): 35–36

Chapter 4

CARE OF THE SURGICAL PATIENT

TYPES OF SURGERY

Optional

Surgery is scheduled completely at the preference of the patient, e.g., cosmetic surgery.

Elective

The approximate time for surgery is at the convenience of the patient; failure to have surgery is not catastrophic, e.g. superficial cyst

Required

The condition requires surgery within a few weeks, e.g. eye cataract.

Urgent

Surgical problem requires attention within 24–48 hours, e.g. cancer.

Emergency

Requires immediate surgical attention without delay, e.g., intestinal obstruction.

REGIONS AND INCISIONS OF THE ABDOMEN

See Fig. 4.1.

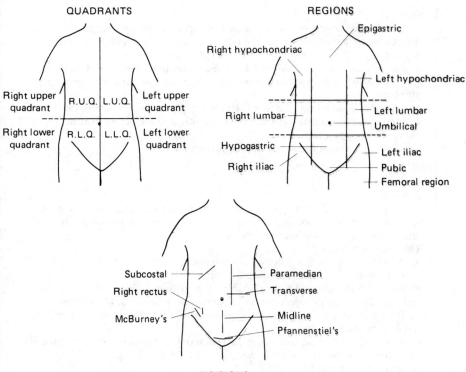

Figure 4.1.   Regions and incisions of the abdomen.

INITIAL ASSESSMENT AND EARLY PHYSICAL PREPARATION OF THE SURGICAL PATIENT

General Physical Examination and Diagnosis

1 Observe the patient for skin lesions, rashes, pressure sores and other abnormalities.
2 Engage the patient in conversation to determine his reaction to and concerns about hospitalization and the forthcoming operation.
3 Prepare him for various diagnostic tests by telling him why and how they are done and how he may contribute to the success of the test.
4 Record his reactions to tests as well as the outcome of such tests.

Specific Conditions and Their Effect on Surgery

Obesity

1   Danger:
   a. Increases difficulty involved in technical aspects of performing surgery (e.g., sutures are difficult to tie because of fatty secretions); the breakdown of wounds is greater.
   b. Postoperatively, more difficult to turn and ventilate the patient when he is lying on his side. This leads to hypoventilation, pneumonia and other pulmonary problems.
   c. Increases demands on the heart, leading to cardiovascular embarrassment.
   d. Increases possibility of renal, biliary, hepatic and endocrine disorders.
2   Therapeutic approach:
   Encourage weight reduction if time permits.

Fluid, Electrolyte and Nutritional State

1   Danger:
   Dehydration and malnutrition have adverse effects in terms of a general anaesthetic, the shock of surgery and postoperative recovery—can disturb fluid and electrolyte balance and lead to shock.
2   Therapeutic approach:
   a. Administer fluids (parenteral) as prescribed.
   b. Keep a detailed input and output record.
   c. Provide high calorie diet to alleviate malnutrition; supplement with protein and vitamin C—helps repair tissue and serves as a deterrent to infection.
   d. Recommend repair of dental caries and proper mouth hygiene to prevent respiratory tract infection.
   e. Assist with administration (and surveillance) of blood transfusion, protein hydrolysates or blood plasma if there is a protein deficiency.
   f. Assist with hyperalimentation.

Ageing

1   Danger:
   a. Recognize that physical, psychological and pathological reactions to injury are not as obvious and are slower in appearing.
   b. Be aware that the cumulative effect of medications is greater in the older person than it is in younger people.
   c. Note that such medications as morphine, scopolamine and barbiturates in the usual dosages may cause confusion and disorientation.
2   Therapeutic approach:
   a. Consider using lesser doses for desired effect.
   b. Anticipate problems from long-standing chronic disorders such as anaemia, obesity, diabetes, hypoproteinaemia.
   c. Adjust nutritional intake to conform to higher protein and vitamin needs.
   d. When possible cater to set patterns in older patients (sleeping and eating patterns, use of alcohol and laxatives).

Presence of Disease

1   *Cardiovascular:*
   a. Increased diligence is required when surgical problem is complicated by a cardiovascular problem.
   b. Avoid overloading the body with fluids (oral, parenteral, blood) because of possible congestive failure and pulmonary oedema.
   c. Prevent prolonged immobilization, which results in stasis of circulation.
   d. Encourage change of position but avoid sudden exertion.
   e. Note evidence of hypoxia and initiate therapy.

2   *Diabetes:*
   a. Be aware that hypoglycaemia due to inadequate carbohydrate intake or insulin overdosage is life-threatening in uncontrolled diabetes.
   b. Recognize the signs and symptoms of ketoacidosis and glycosuria, which can threaten an otherwise smooth surgical experience.
   c. Reassure the diabetic patient that when his disease is controlled, the surgical risk is no greater than it is for the nondiabetic person.

3   *Alcoholism:*
   a. Anticipate the additional problem of malnutrition in the presurgical alcoholic patient.
   b. Recognize that the acutely intoxicated person is susceptible to injury and may receive serious injuries without being aware of them.
   c. Be prepared to perform gastric lavage on the intoxicated patient if surgery cannot be postponed; this may lessen the chance of vomiting and aspiration during anaesthesia induction.
   d. Note that risk due to surgery is greater for the individual who is a chronic alcoholic.
   e. Anticipate the acute withdrawl syndrome (delirium tremens).

4   *Pulmonary and upper respiratory disease:*
   a. Surgery may be contraindicated in the patient who has an upper respiratory infection because an acute upper respiratory infection may be the forerunner of more serious illness, such as pneumonia.
   b. Patients with chronic pulmonary problems such as emphysema, bronchiectasis, etc., should be treated for several days preoperatively with bronchodilators, aerosol medications, postural drainage, conscientious mouth care.

5   *Concurrent or prior pharmacotherapy:*
   a. Hazards exist when certain medications are given concomitantly with others; therefore, an awareness of prior drug therapy is essential. (Example: interaction of some drugs with anaesthetics can lead to arterial hypotension and circulatory collapse).
   b. Notify anaesthetist if the patient is taking any of the following drugs:
      (1) Certain antibiotics*—may, when combined with a curariform muscle relaxant, interrupt nerve transmission, causing respiratory paralysis and apnoea.
      (2) Antidepressants, particularly monoamine oxidase inhibitors (MAOIs), increase hypotensive effects of anaesthesia.
      (3) Phenothiazines increase hypotensive action of anaesthetics.

* Neomycin, streptomycin, polymyxin A and B, colistin and kanamycin.

(4) Diuretics, particularly thiazides, cause electrolyte imbalance and respiratory depression during anaesthesia.

CONSENT FOR OPERATION

A consent form is signed by the patient, granting permission to have the operation performed as described by the surgeon. This is a medicolegal requirement and the patient's signature must be witnessed by the doctor.

Prior to signing the consent form, the patient should:

1   Be told in clear and simple terms by the surgeon what is to be done (drawings or audiovisual aids may help).
2   Be aware of the risks, possible complications, disfigurement and removal of parts.
3   Have a general idea of what to expect in the early and late postoperative periods.
4   Have a general idea of the time involved from surgery to recovery.
5   Have an opportunity to ask any questions.
6   Sign a separate form for each operation.

Purposes

1   To protect the patient against unauthorized procedures.
2   To protect the surgeon and hospital against legal action by a patient who claims that an unauthorized procedure was performed.

Circumstances Requiring Consent

1   For entrance into a body cavity, e.g., bronchoscopy, cystoscopy.
2   For general anaesthetic.

Obtaining Consent

1   *Written* permission is best and is legally acceptable.
2   Signature is obtained with the patient's complete understanding of what is to occur; it is obtained before he receives sedation and is secured without pressure or duress.
3   The form is witnessed by a doctor. It is the doctor's ultimate responsibility.
4   In emergency, permission via telephone or telegram is acceptable.
5   For a minor (or one who is unconscious or irresponsible), permission is required from a responsible member of the family—parent or legal guardian.
6   For a married minor, permission from the husband or wife is acceptable.
7   If the patient is unable to write, an 'X' to indicate his sign is acceptable if there are two signed witnesses to his mark.
8   If no parent or guardian is available, the duty administrator may be authorized to give the consent.
9   In Great Britain, 16 years is taken as the age of consent.

PREOPERATIVE PATIENT CARE

Preoperative patient care includes the giving of information to the patient who is scheduled to have an operation; such instruction may be offered by talking, discussion, use of audiovisual aids and demonstration. It is designed to help the patient understand what he is about to experience so that he can participate intelligently in more effective recovery from surgery and anaesthesia.

Value to the Patient

1   Recuperation is more rapid.
2   There is less need for medications for pain and discomfort.
3   Complications are lessened.
4   Hospitalization is shortened.

Approach to Patient Care

Obtain Nursing History and Plan Care

1   Determine what patient already knows. This can be accomplished by reading the patient's notes, by interviewing the patient and by communicating with his family and other members of the health team.
2   Encourage active participation of patients in their care and recovery.
3   Provision should be made for the patient to ask questions and express his concerns; every effort is made to answer all questions truthfully and in agreement with the medical plan of therapy.

Constantly Assess Needs of Patient as Teaching Progresses

1   Begin at his level of understanding and proceed from there.
2   Correct misinformation—provide opportunity for him to express himself.
3   Provide general information and be alert for patient needs as communication takes place. Assess his ability to absorb, his interest and his curiosity or lack of it.
   a. Explain details of preoperative preparation.
   b. Offer general information on his specific surgery. (Doctor is the resource person.)
   c. Tell when surgery is scheduled (if known) and how long it will take; explain that afterwards he will go to the Recovery Room.
   d. Let him know that his family will be kept informed and that they will be told where to wait and when they can see him; note visiting hours.
   e. Describe the Recovery Room; anticipated equipment to expect: drains, tubes, monitors.
   f. Explain the importance of his participation in his postoperative recovery. Tell him you will demonstrate to him some of the activities he will be doing postoperatively.
   g. Utilize other resource persons; doctors, therapists, chaplain, interpreters and so forth.
   h. Document in outline form what has been taught and patient's reaction.

Utilize Audiovisual Aids if Available

1   Videotapes with sound or film strips with narration are effective in giving basic information to a single patient or group of patients.
2   Booklets and brochures, if available, are helpful.
3   Demonstrate any equipment which will be specific for the particular patient. Examples:

Drainage equipment   Ostomy bag
Side rails   Monitoring equipment

NOTE: The extent of preoperative patient teaching is determined on an individual basis; determinants are the patient's previous knowledge, his desire to learn and willingness to use this new knowledge, his psychoemotional and physical condition, the amount of time available and the quality of teaching.

Preparation for Postoperative Activities (usually carried out by physiotherapist)

Activities which the patient will practise and do postoperatively include the following:

Diaphragmatic Breathing

This is a mode of breathing in which the dome of the diaphragm is flattened during inspiration resulting in enlargement of the upper abdomen as air rushes into the chest. During expiration, abdominal muscles contract.
   For the patient:

1   Assume bed position similar to that most likely to be used postoperatively (semiprone).
2   Place both hands over lower rib cage; make a loose fist and rest the flat surface of the fingernails against the chest (to feel chest movement).
3   Exhale gently and fully; ribs will sink downwards and inwards towards midline.
4   Inhale deeply through mouth and nose; permit abdomen to rise as lungs fill with air.
5   Hold this breath through a count of five.
6   Exhale and let *all* air out through mouth and nose.
7   Repeat 15 times with a brief rest following each group of five.
8   Practise this twice each day preoperatively.

Coughing

To promote the removal of chest secretions.

1   Interlace the fingers and place the hands over the proposed incision site; this will act as a splint during coughing.
2   Lean forward slightly while sitting in bed.
3   Breathe, using the diaphragm as described under diaphragmatic breathing.
4   Inhale fully with the mouth slightly open.
5   Let out three or four sharp 'hacks'.
6   Then, with mouth open, take in a deep breath and quickly give one or two strong coughs.
7   Secretions should be readily cleared from the chest; splinting the incision will reduce pain and will not harm the incision.

Turning

Circulation is stimulated, deeper breathing encouraged and pressure areas are relieved when the patient is encouraged to move from his back to the side-lying position.

1   The patient may require assistance to move onto his side; pillows have to be readjusted.
2   Place the uppermost leg in a more flexed position than that of the lower leg and place a pillow comfortably between the legs.
3   Patient is turned from one side to his back and onto other side every 2 hours.

Leg Exercises

To improve circulation.

1   While lying on the back, bend the knee and raise the foot—hold it a few seconds, extend the leg and lower it to the bed.
2   Repeat above for about five times with one leg and then do it with the other. Repeat the set five times every 3–5 hours.
3   While lying on the side, exercise the legs by pretending to pedal a bicycle.
4   As a foot exercise, trace a complete circle with the great toe.

PREOPERATIVE PROPHYLAXIS TO PREVENT POSTOPERATIVE VENOUS THROMBOSIS

Low dose heparin is sometimes given prophylactically to haemostatically competent patients over the age of 40 who are to undergo major elective abdominal or thoracic surgical procedures, and has been seen to result in an 80% reduction in postoperative pulmonary emboli.

Preoperative Screening

1   Administer no aspirin or other platelet antiaggregating drugs for 5 days prior to an operation.
2   Administer no coumarin therapy at time of operation.
3   Haematocrit, prothrombin time, partial thromboplastin time and platelet count should be within normal range prior to operation.

Dose and Duration of Prophylaxis

1   Administer 5000 International Units (I.U.) of heparin 2 hours before operation.
2   Repeat above dosage every 12 hours until discharge from hospital.

Limitations and Contraindications

1   Haemorrhagic disorders; acute or potential bleeding sites, e.g., haemophilia, postoperative oozing of blood, subacute bacterial endocarditis, severe hypertension, recent cerebrovascular accident.
2   The regime is ineffective during active thrombus formation.

Monitoring of Heparin Therapy

1   No laboratory test (whole blood clotting time, partial thromboplastin time, thrombin time, antithrombin III assay) is necessary during therapy to determine drug dosage or to prevent haemorrhage.
2   With this regime, there may be a *slight increase in minor wound haematoma*. Report this immediately.
3   This regime is followed at the discretion of the doctor.

PREPARATION OF SPECIFIC OPERATIVE AREAS

Head surgery. Obtain specific instructions from surgeon concerning the extent of shaving. *Other surgery*. See Fig. 4.2.

GUIDELINES: Preparing the Patient's Skin for Surgery

Purpose

To cleanse the skin and reduce the number of organisms on the skin so as to eliminate as far as possible the transference of such organisms into the incision site.

Pharmacophysiologic Emphasis

1   Human skin normally harbours transient and resident bacterial flora, some of which are pathogenic.
2   Skin cannot be sterilized without destroying skin cells.
3   Friction enhances the action of detergent antiseptics.
4   No existing antiseptic produces instant skin disinfection.

Equipment

Bowl of water
Soap
Gauze squares
Orange stick, protected with cotton wool to clean umbilicus if required
Razor and blades
Scissors for cutting long hair if required.

Procedure

Preparatory Phase

1   Explain to the patient the purpose of the activity.
2   Instruct the patient to assume the most comfortable and satisfactory position for the required skin preparation.
3   Expose only the area to be shaved.

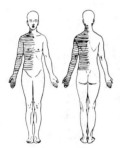

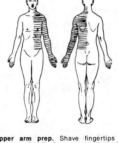

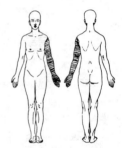

Shoulder prep. Shave fingertips to hairline, midline chest to midline spine on operative side and to iliac crest, including axillae.

Upper arm prep. Shave fingertips to neckline (hairline), on operative side from midline chest to midline spine on operative side from axilla to iliac crest. Trim and clean fingernails. Use brush on hand and nails.

Hand prep. Shave fingertips to shoulder. Trim and clean fingernails. Use brush on hand and nails.

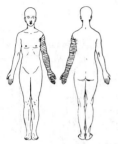

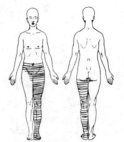

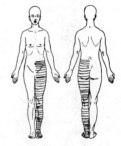

Forearm and elbow prep. Shave from fingernails to shoulder including axilla. Trim and clean fingernails. Use brush on hand and nails.

Saphenous vein ligation prep. Shave from umbilicus to toes of affected leg, or both legs. Include pubis and perineal area. Prep entire leg posteriorly.

Thigh prep. Shave from toes to 3 inches above the umbilicus, midline front and back. Complete pubic shave. Clean and trim toenails. Use brush on foot and nails.

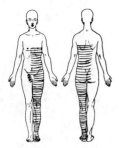

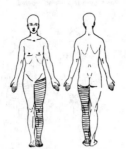

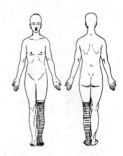

Hip prep. Shave toes to nipple line to at least 3 inches beyond midline back and front. Complete pubic shave. Clean and trim toenails. Use brush on foot and nails. Hip fractures—all preps done in the operating room.

Knee and lower leg prep. Shave entire leg, toes to groin. Clean and trim toenails. Use brush on foot and nails.

Ankle and foot prep. Shave entire leg, toes to 3 inches above the knee. Clean and trim toenails. Use brush on foot and nails.

Figure 4.2. Preoperative preparation of the patient. (From (1977) Manual on Control of Infection in Surgical Patients, J B Lippincott.

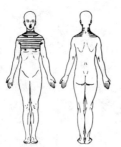

Thyroid prep. Shave from chin line to nipples, including axillary region. Extend to back of neck and upper shoulder as sketched.

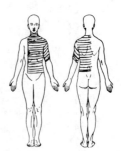

Thoracotomy prep. Shave from chin line to iliac crest, from nipple on unaffected side to at least 2 inches beyond the midline in back. Include axilla and entire arm to elbow.

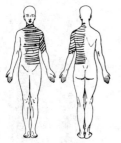

Mastectomy prep. Shave from upper neck to iliac crest, from nipple line on unaffected side to midline of back (affected side). Prep axilla and entire arm to elbow on affected side.

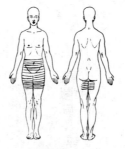

Lower abdominal prep (as for hernia, femoral vein ligation, femoral embolectomy). Shave from 2 inches above the umbilicus to mid-thigh, including the pubic area. Femoral ligation—shave to midline of thigh posteriorly. Hernia and embolectomy—shave to costal margin and down to knee as ordered.

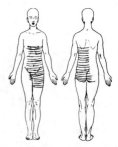

Flank prep (as for renal procedures, adrenalectomy, sympathectomy). Shave from nipple line to pubis and 3 inches beyond the midline in back. Shave pubic area. Shave upper thigh on the affected side.

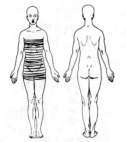

Abdominal prep. Shave from 3 inches above the nipple line to upper thighs, including pubis.

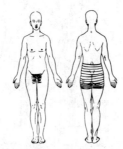

Perineal prep (as for hemorrhoidectomy, fistula-in-ano). Shave pubis, perineum, and perianal area. Shave from the waist in back to at least 3 inches below the groin.

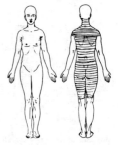

Spine prep. Shave entire back including shoulders and neck to hairline and down to knees and to both sides, including axillae.

Figure 4.2 (cont.)

Nursing Action	Reason

Performance Phase

1 Wet and lather the area well.

1 Oils, soils and organisms are removed from skin surface.

2 Cut long hairs with scissors.

2 Much easier and quicker than with a razor.

3 Provide extra attention to areas where there are folds of skin, e.g., axillae, pubic area, umbilicus. Draw loose skin taut. Use cotton-tipped applicators where necessary.

3 Greater numbers of organisms are harboured in folds of skin; removal requires extra effort.

4 If the operative area includes calloused areas or the nails, use a brush.

4 Facilitates cleansing in out-of-the-way areas.

5 With free hand, apply smooth traction in opposite direction; with other hand shave the lathered hair using firm steady strokes.

5 Traction provides a smoother surface and allows the hairs to assume a more upright position; this facilitates cutting.

6 Use a disposable or sterilized razor and a sharp new blade.

6 Avoids risk of infectious hepatitis from contaminated razor.

7 Avoid nicking the skin; report any skin abrasions.

7 An opening in the skin increases the hazard of infection.

Follow-up Phase

1 Remove all equipment and dispose of expendable materials according to local policy.
2 Unless contraindicated, it is desirable for the nonemergency patient to have a bath prior to surgery using a bacteriostatic soap.
3 Remind the patient of the necessity for keeping the prepared area clean for surgery.

IMMEDIATE PRESURGICAL PREPARATION OF THE PATIENT

Physical and Psychological Attention to the Patient

1 Provide patient with a gown to be worn to the operating room.
2 Remove hairpins; braid women's long hair; cover hair with a cap.
3 Remove dentures or plates (unless anaesthetist requests that they be left in to reduce respiratory tract obstruction); inspect mouth for foreign material such as chewing gum.
4 Remove jewellery, identify properly and place in the hospital safe; if wedding ring cannot be removed, completely cover it with adhesive surgical tape.
5 Remove contact lenses; have patient place them in properly marked receptacle (left and right), identify properly and deposit in the hospital safe.
6 Have patient micturate immediately before leaving for the operating room; measure amount and note time of micturition; record.
7 Continue to support the patient emotionally and correct any misconceptions he may have.

Premedications

Prescribed to meet individual needs.

Purposes

1 To facilitate the administration of any anaesthetic and to relax the patient.
2 To minimize respiratory tract and oral secretions and changes in heart rate and to reduce anxiety.

NOTE: Administer preanaesthetic medication precisely at the time it is ordered. If given too early, the maximum potency will have passed before it is needed; if given too late, the action will not have begun before anaesthesia is started.

Medications

1 Be ready to administer medication as soon as call is received.
2 Proceed with remaining preparation activities.
3 Indicate on the chart or preoperative check list the time when medication was administered.

Transporting Patient to the Operating Room

1 Adhere to the principle of maintaining the comfort and safety of the patient.
2 Accompany operating room attendants to patient's bedside for introduction and proper identification.
3 Assist in transferring patient from bed to stretcher, if necessary.
4 Complete chart and preoperative check list; include laboratory reports and x-rays as required in the operating room.
5 Recognize importance of co-ordinating team effort to ensure arrival of the patient in the operating room at the proper time.

The Patient's Family

1 Direct patient's family, if necessary, to the proper waiting room where magazines, television and tea may be available.
2 Acquaint the family with the fact that a long interval of waiting does not mean the patient is in the operating room all the while; anaesthesia preparation and induction take time and after surgery the patient is taken to the Recovery Room.
3 Tell the family what to expect postoperatively when they see the patient—tubes, monitoring equipment, and blood transfusion, suctioning and oxygen equipment.

IMMEDIATE POSTSURGICAL NURSING CARE

Objective

To assist the patient in recovering from the operation and from the effects of the anaesthetic agent as quickly, safely and comfortably as possible.

Nursing Alert: This phase of nursing care is geared to *recognizing* **the significance of signs and** *anticipating* **and** *preventing* **postoperative difficulties.**
    Carefully *observe* **the patient coming out of general anaesthesia until:**

1   Vital signs (blood pressure, pulse and respiration) are stable for at least 30 min and are within *his* normal range.
2   He is breathing easily.
3   Reflexes have returned to normal.
4   He is conscious, responsive and oriented to time and place.

For the patient who had regional anaesthesia, observe carefully until:
1   Sensation has been recovered.
2   Reflexes have returned.
3   Vital signs have stabilized for at least 30 min.

Immediate Nursing Assessment

Upon receiving a patient in the Recovery Room from the anaesthetist and circulating nurse, the following determinations are made:

1   Observe the patient's respiration and note his skin colour.
2   Verify the patient's identity, the operative procedure and the surgeon who performed the procedure.
3   Request a briefing on problems encountered in the operating room and those that may arise in the recovery period.
4   Determine vital signs.
5   Examine the operative site and check dressings for drainage.
6   Perform safety checks to verify that padded side rails are in place and restraints properly applied for infusions, transfusions, etc.

Nursing Management

Ensure the Maintenance of a Patent Airway

1   Place the patient in the lateral position with neck extended—this permits the best possible expansion of the lungs.
2   Allow metal, rubber or plastic airway to remain in place until the patient begins to waken and is trying to eject the airway.
   a. The airway keeps the passage open and prevents the tongue from falling backwards and obstructing the air passages.
   b. Leaving the airway in after the pharyngeal reflex has returned may cause the patient to retch or vomit.

NOTE: Many seriously ill patients return from the operating room with a tracheal tube in place; this may be left in place for hours or days and requires special management.

3   When patient is partially awake and the airway is removed, he may show signs of retching, nausea or vomiting; place him in the lateral position with the upper arm supported on a pillow. Reassure patient that operation is over and give psychological support.
   a. This will promote chest expansion.
   b. Turn the patient every hour or two to facilitate breathing and ventilation.
4   Aspirate excessive secretions when they are heard in the nasopharynx and oropharynx.

a. Using a Y-connecting tube with catheter, turn suction machine on, insert catheter into pharynx 15–20 cm (6–8 in), then close Y-tube outlet with finger to activate suction; withdraw slowly while rotating catheter.

b. If secretions are lower in the tracheobronchial tree, intratracheal suctioning may be necessary.

5   Encourage patient to take deep breaths to aerate lungs fully and prevent hypostatic pneumonia.

6   Administer humidified oxygen if required.

a. Heat and moisture are normally lost during exhalation.

b. Dehydrated patients may require oxygen and humidity because of higher incidence of irritated respiratory passages in these patients.

c. Secretions can be kept soft to facilitate removal.

7   Mechanical ventilation to maintain adequate pulmonary ventilation may be required.

Call the anaesthetist if he is not present.

Assess Status of Circulatory System

1   Take vital signs (blood pressure, pulse and respiration) frequently, as clinical condition indicates, until patient is well stabilized. Then check every 4 hours thereafter.

a. Know patient's preoperative blood pressure in order to make significant comparisons.

b. Report immediately a falling systolic pressure.

c. Variations in blood pressure and cardiac arrhythmias are reportable.

d. Respirations over 30 should be reported.

2   Recognize the variety of factors which may alter circulating blood volume.

a. Reactions to anaesthesia and medications.

b. Blood loss and organ manipulation during surgery.

c. Moving the patient from one position on the operating table to another on the stretcher.

3   Monitor temperature hourly. Over 37.7°C (100°F) or under 36.1°C (97°F) is reportable.

4   Recognize early symptoms of shock or haemorrhage.

a. Rapid, thready pulse and a falling blood pressure may indicate haemorrhage, leading to a decrease in blood volume.

b. Oxygen therapy may be prescribed to increase oxygen availability from the circulating blood.

c. Place patient in shock position with feet elevated (unless contraindicated).

d. See p. 139 for more detailed consideration of shock.

Promote Comfort and Maintain Safety

1   Provide a therapeutic environment with proper temperature and humidity; remove unnecessary blanket which might cause loss of body fluid through excessive perspiration.

2   Place side rails in protecting position until patient is fully awake.

3   Protect limb into which intravenous fluids are running so that needle will not become accidentally dislodged.

4   Turn patient frequently and maintain good body alignment.

5   Avoid nerve damage and muscle strain by properly supporting and padding pressure areas.

Continue Constant Surveillance of the Patient Until He is Completely Out of Anaesthesia

1   Be aware of the fact that the patient cannot complain of injury such as the pricking of an open safety pin, a clamp that is exerting pressure, a burn from a hot-water bottle.
2   Examine dressings for unexpected drainage or bleeding.
3   Check dressings for constriction.
4   Observe drainage tubes and catheters for proper connection and patency.
5   Note proper functioning of monitoring and suctioning devices, oxygen therapy equipment, etc.
6   Observe the patient for bladder distension.
7   Inspect skin and tissue surrounding intravenous needles to detect fluid entering the tissue.
8   Evaluate periodically the patient's status of orientation—how he responds to being addressed by his name or performs simple movements upon receiving a command.
9   Determine return of motor control following spinal anaesthesia—indicated by how the patient responds to a pinprick or a request to move a part.

Recognize Stress Factors that may Affect the Patient in the Recovery Room and Attempt to Minimize These Factors

1   Know that the ability to hear returns more quickly than other senses as the patient emerges from anaesthesia.
2   Avoid saying anything in the patient's presence that may disturb him; he may appear to be sleeping but still consciously hears what is being said.
3   Explain procedures and activities at his level of understanding.
4   Minimize his exposure to emergency treatment of nearby patients by drawing curtains and lowering voice and noise levels.
5   Treat him as a person who needs as much attention as the equipment and monitoring devices.
6   Respect his feeling of sensory deprivation and simultaneous bombardment of sensory stimuli; make any necessary adjustments to minimize this problem.
7   Make every effort to demonstrate concern for and understanding of this patient—anticipate his needs and feelings.

POSTOPERATIVE BASIC MONITORING

Nursing Alert: The most advanced electronic monitoring system cannot substitute for conscientious clinical surveillance.

Central Venous and Pulmonary Artery Catheters

Definitions

1   *Central Venous Pressure (CVP)* is measured via a catheter in the superior vena cava; it reflects right atrial pressure (see Volume 2, Chapter 1, Conditions of the Cardiovascular System).

2   *Pulmonary Artery (PA)* and *Capillary Wedge Pressure (PCWP)*.
   a. Swan Ganz catheter is positioned in pulmonary artery to measure pulmonary artery pressure.
   b. When balloon is inflated, with catheter advanced to a wedge position, the pressure transmitted measures pressure changes in left atrium. (In absence of valvular heart disease, this PCWP also reflects left ventricular end-diastolic filling pressure.)

Indications for Pulmonary Artery Catheters (PAP)

PAP indicates how efficiently the right ventricle is clearing the venous return presented to the right side of the heart at the time of measurement.

1   Increased pulmonary vascular resistance—chronic obstructive pulmonary disease (COPD).
2   Coronary artery disease requiring complicated intravenous fluid regimen.
3   Cardiac surgery and trauma.
4   Decreased left ventricular function secondary to anoxia, acidosis or electrolyte imbalance.
5   Decompensated cirrhosis, severe pancreatitis, generalized peritonitis and severe multisystem trauma.
6   Massive transfusions.
7   High CVP in the presence of underperfusion of peripheral tissues.

Complications Associated with Central Venous and Pulmonary Artery Catheters

1   CVP Catheters
   a. Infection, loss of catheter, thromboembolic complications.
   b. Complications specific to insertion site.
   c. Air embolism
   d. Perforation of right ventricle.
2   PA Catheters
   a. Pulmonary artery perforation.
   b. Pulmonary ischaemic lesions.
   c. Catheters kinking and intracardiac knotting.
   d. Heart murmurs.

Guides to the Safe Use of CVP Catheters (Volume 2, Chapter 1, Conditions of the Cardiovascular System, p.13).

POSTANAESTHETIC RECOVERY SCORING GUIDE

Many hospitals use a scoring system to determine the patient's general condition and his readiness to be released from the Recovery Room. As the patient progresses through the recovery period, his physical signs are observed and evaluated by means of an objective scoring guide.

Objective

To provide the recovery room staff with a guideline to the patient's condition following surgery and anaesthesia. This evaluation system is a modification of the Apgar score.

Physical Signs and Criteria for Their Assessment

Activity

Muscle activity is assessed by observing the ability of the patient to move his extremities spontaneously or on command.

Score: 2—able to move all extremities.
         1—able to move two extremities.
         0—not able to control any extremity.

Respiration

Respiratory efficiency evaluated in a form that permits accurate and objective assessment without complicated physical tests.

Score: 2—able to breathe deeply and cough.
         1—limited respiratory effort (dyspnoea or splinting).
         0—no spontaneous respiratory effort.

Circulation

Use changes in arterial blood pressure from preanaesthetic level.

Score: 2—systolic arterial pressure between plus or minus 20% of preanaesthetic level.
         1—systolic arterial pressure between plus or minus 20–50% of preanaesthetic level.
         0—systolic arterial pressure between plus or minus 50% or more of the preanaesthetic level.

Consciousness

Determination of the patient's level of consciousness.

Score: 2—full alertness seen in patient's ability to answer questions and acknowledge his/her location.
         1—aroused when called by name.
         0—failure to elicit a response upon auditory stimulation.

Physical stimulation should not be considered reliable since even a decerebrated patient might react to it.

Colour

This is an objective sign that is easy to recognize.

Score: 2—normal skin colour and appearance.
         1—any alteration in skin colour: pale, dusky, blotchy, jaundiced, etc.
         0—frank cyanosis.

Implications of Score

1   The patient's score is taken at stated intervals, such as every 15 or 30 min, and totalled on the official scorecard (Fig. 4.3).
2   Patients with a total score of less than 7 must remain in the Recovery Room until improved or transferred to an intensive care area.
3   This guide permits a more objective evaluation of the patient's physical condition in the recovery area (Fig. 4.3).

POST-ANESTHESIA RECOVERY ROOM
SCORING CARD

Patient: Smith, Raymond
Room: B 1083
Date: 3/7/78

Final Score: 10
Physician: Dr. J. Evans
Nurse: Mrs Peggy Fay, R.N.

Physical Signs / TIME	ACTIVITY Score	ACTIVITY Comment	RESPIRATION Score	RESPIRATION Comment	CIRCULATION Score	CIRCULATION Comment	CONSCIOUSNESS Score	CONSCIOUSNESS Comment	COLOR Score	COLOR Comment	TOTAL SCORE
Admission A.M. 11:15 / P.M.	1	Spinal anesth	1	chest & abdom. pain	1		1	Semi-conscious	1		5
½ Hour A.M. 11:45 / P.M.	1		1		2		1		1	slight pallor	6
½ Hour A.M. / P.M.											
Dismissal A.M. 12:15 / P.M.	2		2		2		2	alert verbally responsive	2	color improved	10
FINAL SCORE A.M. / P.M.	2		2		2		2		2		10

Figure 4.3.   Recovery Room scoring card.

THE PATIENT RECEIVING INTRAVENOUS THERAPY

Objectives

1 To maintain or replace the body's normal levels of water, electrolytes, vitamins, proteins, calories and nitrogen in the patient who cannot maintain an adequate intake by mouth.
2 To restore acid-base balance.
3 To replenish blood volume.
4 To provide a route for the administration of drugs.

Physiological Assimilation of Intravenous Solutions

Principles

1 Blood cells (erythrocytes, etc.) are surrounded by a semipermeable membrane.
2 Osmotic pressure is the pressure demonstrated when a solvent moves through the semipermeable membrane from weaker to stronger concentrations.
3 Osmotic characteristics of different solutions are often determined by the way they affect red blood cells.

Types of Fluids

1 *Isotonic*—a solution which has the same osmotic pressure externally as that found across the semipermeable membrane within the cell.
   a. Normal saline 0·9%
   b. Dextrose 5% in water.
   c. Ringers lactate.
   d. Balanced isotonic.
2 *Hypotonic*—a solution which has less osmotic pressure than that of blood serum; this causes the cells to expand or swell.
      Sodium chloride 0·45%.
3 *Hypertonic*—a solution which has higher osmotic pressure than that of blood serum; this causes the cells to shrink.
   a. Dextrose 5% in saline.
   b. Dextroxe 10% in saline.
   c. Dextrose 10% in water.
   d. Dextrose 5% in half-strength saline.
   e. Dextrose 20% in water.

Composition of Fluids

1 Saline solution—fluids and electrolytes (Na^+, Cl^-).
2 Dextrose—fluid and calories.
3 Ringers lactate—fluid, electrolytes (Na^+, K^+, Cl^-, Ca^{2+}, lactate).
4 Balanced isotonic—fluid, electrolytes, some calories (Na^+, K^+, Mg^{2+}, Cl^-, HCO_3-, gluconate).
5 Blood-related fluids (i.e. transfusion).
   a. Whole blood.
      (1) Approximately 45% cellular—red cells, white cells, blood platelets.
      (2) Approximately 55% plasma.
      (a) 90% water.

(b) 7% protein (albumin, globulin, fibrinogen).
(c) 2% lipids, vitamins, carbohydrates, inorganic salts.
(3) Whole blood is used to replace blood lost in acute haemorrhage.
b. Packed cells—red blood cells obtained by centrifuging whole blood and drawing off the plasma.
Packed cells are used in treatment of anaemia or for the patient in whom there is a risk of circulatory overload (congestive heart failure).
c. Fresh frozen plasma.
(1) To restore blood volume in shock.
(2) To correct hypoproteinaemia.
6   Plasma expanders: albumin, dextran, haemacel and human plasma protein fraction.
To improve circulating blood volume.
7   Parenteral hyperalimentation nutrients.

Nursing Assessment

Diagnosis and Need for Fluid Therapy

Know the major and minor medical problems of the patient as indicated in the doctor's diagnosis and the nurse's assessment of the patient.

1   Can the patient's illness affect his fluid balance?
2   What medication or treatment is he receiving that can affect fluid components? How?
3   What is the relation of his fluid intake to fluid output?
4   Does he have dietary restrictions?
5   Is he taking adequate fluids by mouth?
6   What is the doctor's plan of treatment?

Evidence of Fluid Imbalance in the Patient

1   Determine body temperature—febrile conditions suggest loss of body fluids through perspiration.
2   Is he thirsty? Possible dehydration.
3   Observe for dry, warm skin, cracked lips—signs of dehydration.
4   Check skin for elasticity—lightly pull up a pinch-fold of skin, release it. Does it rapidly resume its normal position?
5   Note colour and amount of urine—concentrated scanty urine indicates lack of fluids.
6   Compare present weight with admission weight—it may indicate fluid change.

Inspection of Prescribed Fluid and Equipment to be Used for the Infusion

1   Observe fluid for discoloration, foreign particles, cloudiness, film—if present, do not use.
2   Fluid in a bag:
Gently squeeze and observe for leakage.
3   Fluid in a glass bottle:
a. Hold flask up to light.
b. Slowly rotate flask in upright position and then on its side; carefully inspect for a flash of light that could indicate a crack.

4   Check intravenous tubing for discoloration or defects; if noted, secure new equipment.
5   Follow instructions for assembling equipment, using aseptic technique when inserting drip chamber spike into flask; flush equipment with 20–30 ml of fluid from receptacle before using.
(See Guidelines, p. 100.)

Nursing Alert: In the UK a nurse, student or qualified, is not covered by insurance to perform a venepuncture or administer intravenous fluids. These procedures are carried out by a doctor. However, some hospital authorities may allow doctors to delegate these procedures to a qualified nurse who has received instruction, but it still remains the doctor's responsibility. Nurses should check local hospital policy.

Criteria for Selecting a Suitable Vein for Venepuncture

1   Use distal branches of a large vein rather than the best sites—these are then available for emergencies.

Nursing Alert: Select lowest good vein on hand or arm initially for venepuncture or infusion. If, with subsequent venepunctures, this site is difficult to enter, move up higher on the arm. Conversely, if the antecubital fossa area is used first, and if later there is difficulty entering at this site, none of the lower veins can be used.

2   Convenient veins include the following:
   a. Back of the hand—basilic or cephalic vein (See Fig. 4.4a).
      (1) The advantage of this site is that it permits arm movement.
      (2) If later a vein problem develops at this site, another vein higher up the arm may be used.
   b. Forearm—basilic or cephalic vein (Fig. 4.4.b).
   c. Inner aspect of elbow, antecubital fossa—median basilic and median cephalic for relatively short-term infusion.
      (1) These veins are large and easily accessible.
      (2) Note, however, that this site precludes arm movement.
      (3) Choose site below elbow crease for patient's comfort.
3   Otherwise, select other available veins.
   a. Thigh—great saphenous and femoral veins.
   b. Ankle—great saphenous.
   c. Foot—venous plexus of dorsum, dorsal venous arch, medial marginal vein.

Nursing Alert: Avoid leg veins if there are marked degrees of varicosity at or above proposed site of injection. Otherwise, injected solutions may stagnate along varicosed vessels.

Methods of Distending a Vein

1   Apply manual compression above site where needle is to be inserted (Fig. 4.5).
2   Have patient periodically clench his fist (if arm is used).
3   Massage area in direction of venous flow.
4   Apply sphygmomanometer cuff (keep pressure just below systolic pressure).
5   Fasten soft rubber tubing with a haemostat.
6   Tie soft rubber tubing as a slip knot.

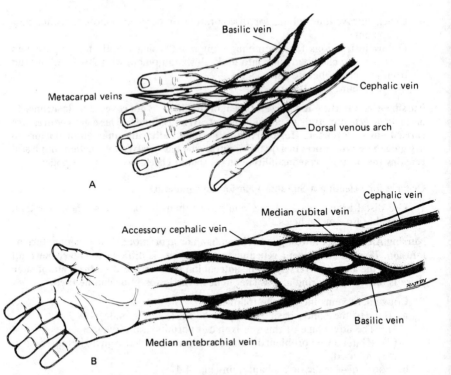

Figure 4.4.   a. Superficial veins, dorsal aspect of hand. b. Superficial veins, forearm.

7   Lightly slap vein site; this is to be done gently so that the vein is not injured.
8   Allow extremity to be dependent for a few minutes.

NOTE: Should the above measures fail, it may be necessary to perform a 'cut-down'—this is a surgical procedure exposing the vein for venepuncture; the incision site is treated as a surgical wound.

Stabilizing Extremity with a Padded Armboard

1   This is done if the patient is restless, disoriented, elderly or a child and if motion could result in infiltration into tissues or phlebitis.
2   Various kinds of armboards are available; an armboard should be padded.

Nursing Alert: If hand and arm are to be immobilized, place in normal functional position. *Contractures may occur if hand is immobilized in flat position.*

For hand: Dorsiflexion of wrist about 20–25°.
(Fig. 4.6)   Flexion of metacarpophalangeal joint about 45–50°.
Palm slightly cupped with finger flexion increasing from index to little finger.
Thumb should be extended in relaxed position and not flexed under fingers.

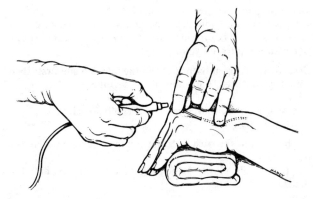

Figure 4.5.   Finger palpation of dorsal venous arch.

3   Prevent compression of nerves or blood vessels; check pulse and ask patient if pressure is too great.

Cleansing Infusion Site

1   Use a good surgical soap to thoroughly cleanse the infusion site. Dirt, dead skin, blood, mucus and oil are to be removed so that action of antiseptic is not hindered.
2   Rinse the area with an alcohol swab.
3   Apply an iodine-base antiseptic; 1 or 2% iodine in water or in 70% alcohol is effective. After 30 s, iodine can be washed off with alcohol.
   a. In patients sensitive to iodine, iodophors may be used. Do not wash off an iodophor since it provides sustained release of free iodine which may enhance the germicidal action.

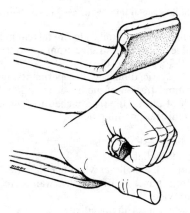

Figure 4.6.   Immobilization of hand and arm during infusion.

   b. If iodine preparations are not available, 70% alcohol is an alternative if it is applied vigorously for 1 min after the area has been cleansed.

4 Wait until area is dry before inserting needle; this is done to prevent carrying antiseptic solution into the vein.

Nursing Alert: In applying antiseptic, swab the infusion site first; then, covering an ever-widening circular area, move out to the periphery.

Providing Local Anaesthesia for Infants or Usually Sensitive Patients (performed by doctor)

1 Raise a wheal in the skin just over the vein by injecting 0·5 ml procaine hydrochloride 1·0% solution.
2 Advance the needle close to the wall of the vein so that this area is also anaesthetized.

Equipment

Needle or Catheter

Infusion may be administered through a needle (short-term) or through a catheter (long-term).

1 *Needle* (Fig. 4.7)
   a. *Metal cannula*, usually 18-, 19- or 20-gauge needle which is 2.5–4 cm long (1 or 1.5 in). This traditional intravenous needle has largely been replaced by the synthetic catheter which lends itself better to long-term use, administration of intravenous antibiotics and other medications.

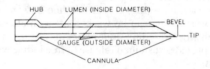

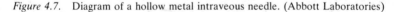

Figure 4.7.   Diagram of a hollow metal intraveous needle. (Abbott Laboratories)

   b. *Winged (scalp vein) needle*—similar to metal cannula; however, hub is replaced by two flexible wings. Sizes range from 16 to 23 gauge and length is approximately 2 cm (0·75 in). Two types:
   (1) Short length of plastic tubing with a permanently attached resealable injection site for administration of medications and/or fluids.
   (2) Variable length of plastic tubing attached to female Luer adapter—this accommodates administration equipment.
   Advantages:
   (1) Short-bevel reduces risk of:
     (a) Trauma to endothelial wall.
     (b) Extravasation or haematoma when needle enters vein.
     (c) Infiltration from puncture of opposite wall of vein.
   (2) Plastic wings provide:
     (a) A firm grip when inserting needle.
     (b) Better fixation against the skin.

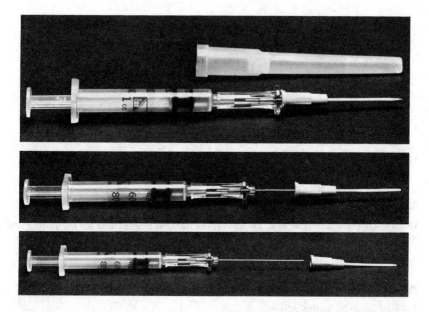

Figure 4.8. a. A catheter-threaded needle. The needle's protective sheath (above the needle in the photo) has been removed. b. After the needle and catheter have been introduced into the vein, the needle and syringe are carefully withdrawn, leaving the catheter in place in the vein. c. After the needle is withdrawn completely, the tubing from the intravenous solution is connected to the catheter. (Lewis, L W (1976) Fundamental Skills in Patient Care, J B Lippincott, p. 356.)

2 *Catheter*—radiopaque; made of synthetic polyvinylchloride (PVC), Teflon or Silastic.
   a. *Plastic needle*—catheter is mounted on needle. When puncture is made, needle and syringe are withdrawn, leaving catheter in place in the vein; tubing from intravenous receptacle is connected to the catheter (Fig. 4.8). (See Guidelines, p. 104.)
   b. *Intracath*—catheter is inserted through needle. Venepuncture is made and plastic catheter is then pushed through needle into vein to the desired length. There is less risk of infiltration with this method than with metal needle. (See Guidelines, p. 104.)
   c. *Inlying catheter* requires a cutdown procedure and is useful in keeping a vein open in patient who has obscured or collapsed vessels.

Bevel

To facilitate entering a vein with least injury to skin, the bevel should face:

1 Upwards—when entering a vein lumen which is larger than the needle (Fig. 4.9a).
2 Downwards—when entering a small vein with lumen which approaches the size of the needle (Fig. 4.9b).

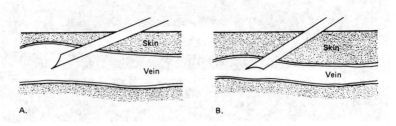

Figure 4.9.   Position of needle in vein.

Rate of Flow of Fluid in Infusion Therapy

Doctor will prescribe flow rate. However, the nurse is responsible for regulating and maintaining the proper rate.

Patient Determining Factors

1   Surface area of the patient.
     The larger the person, the more fluid he requires and the faster he utilizes it.
2   Patient condition.
     If patient has cardiovascular or renal problems, the rate may be restricted.
3   Age of patient.
     Administer fluid more slowly to elderly patient to prevent increase in venous pressure.
4   Tolerance to solutions.
     Example—Test protein sensitivity by administering protein hydrolysates slowly.
5   Fluid composition for this particular patient.
     When drugs are administered via infusion, the effect desired often depends on speed of administration.

Factors Affecting Rate of Flow

1   Pressure gradient—the difference between two levels in a fluid system.
2   Friction—the interaction between fluid molecules and surfaces of inner wall of tubing.
3   Diameter and length of tubing.
4   Height of column of fluid.
5   Size of opening through which fluid leaves receptacle.
6   Fluid viscosity—the thicker the fluid, the slower the flow.
7   Vein trauma, clots, plugging of vents, etc.
8   If there is any question regarding rate of fluid administration, check with doctor.

Calculation of Flow Rate

Speed regulation of an intravenous infusion is most important. Small drop giving sets have guidance on the speed flow printed on the packet, but normal size drop giving sets have to be calculated.

Remember if the patient moves it can alter the rate of flow.

Normally there are 15 drops per ml.

Method $$\frac{ml \ per \ bottle}{hours \ to \ be \ given} \quad \times \quad \frac{no. \ of \ drops \ per \ ml \ (15)}{no. \ of \ minutes \ per \ hour \ (60)}$$

For example: The doctor prescribes 500 ml of fluid to be given over a 4-hour period. This would mean:–

$$\frac{500}{4} \ \times \ \frac{15}{60} \ = 31.2 \quad \text{(approximately 30 drops per minute)}$$

GUIDELINES: Venepuncture

Venepuncture is the puncturing of a vein with a needle (steel or plastic) attached to a syringe. This procedure is usually performed by a doctor and the nurse may be asked to assist.

Purpose

1   To obtain blood samples for analysis, cross matching.
2   To administer fluids, blood, medications.
3   To perform tests requiring a needle in a vein.

Equipment

Tourniquet, usually rubber tubing or flat latex rubber, approximately 37·5 cm (15 in). (Blood pressure cuff is effective because it can be pumped to the desired 100 mmHg)
Sterile gauze squares or cotton ball with iodine-base antiseptic or alcoholic swab
Sterile syringe: 10 or 20 ml depending on amount of blood desired
No. 18 needle–with disposable needles, the likelihood of a burr is practically non-existent. If there is any question, draw needle through sterile gauze—a burr will pick up threads. A needle with a burr should be discarded
Shaving equipment if necessary.

Procedure

Doctor's/Nursing Action	Reason

Preparatory Phase

1   Wash hands thoroughly.

2   Explain procedure to patient.

    2   Most patients have had experience of venepuncture.

3   Select site: shave area if necessary.
     The back of the hand, the back of the arm, or the antecubital vein is used (in order of preference).
     Vein selection is determined by size, elasticity and distance below skin. (Shave hair if necessary.)
     Vein should be distinct, easily observable, and palpable; it should be large enough for a needle to enter.

4   Ascertain if there is satisfactory distension of the vein.

    4   This is done by observation or by drawing the skin tight over the vein.

5   Make decision about whether to use a tourniquet or not.

    5   Pulling the skin taut over the vein usually makes the vein prominent enough.

6   If tourniquet is used, do not apply too tightly—venous flow should be stopped but arterial flow should continue (radial pulse should be palpable).

    6   Improperly applied tourniquet may cause blood stasis and may result in blood chemistry alterations. This is why some prefer to apply a blood pressure cuff to 100 mmHg.

7   Scrub area with iodine-base antiseptic or alcohol swab. Allow to dry.

    7   To reduce number of skin micro-organisms.

8   If vein is prominent, it is not necessary to request patient to make a fist.

    8   Fist-making may increase ammonia concentration in the blood.

Performance Phase

1   Insert the needle, bevel up, through the skin, parallel to the vein.

    1   Usually a single sliding stroke can be used to enter skin and vessel.

2   If vessel rolls, it may be necessary to penetrate the skin first at a 30° angle and then apply a second thrust parallel to the skin to enter the vessel.

    2   Satisfactory penetration is evidenced by appearance of blood coming back into syringe.

3   Direct needle into vein; this usually means a slight change in direction to avoid going through the other side of the vessel.

    3   If tourniquet was used, remove at this time to prevent extravasation of blood.

4   For blood sampling: Draw desired amount of blood into syringe.

    4   Blood should flow easily; if suction is required, reposition needle to avoid haemolysis.

Doctor's/Nursing Action	**Reason**

Follow-up Phase

1 Place cotton swab over vein at site of puncture and withdraw needle.	1 Instruct patient to hold cotton ball in place with slight pressure for 2–3 min. If oozing continues, apply a strip of adhesive tape over a fresh sterile cotton ball.
2 Slowly inject blood specimen into proper receptacle, label and see that specimen is delivered to proper laboratory.	2 Record venepuncture and purpose of blood specimen.

GUIDELINES: Arterial Puncture

An *arterial puncture* is the entering of an artery for the purpose of drawing blood for blood gas determination or for other laboratory study.

NOTE: see Nursing Alert, p. 91, the same applies to arterial puncture.

Equipment

Iodine-base antiseptic
Lignocaine (0·5%) 0·5 ml in a 1·0 ml syringe
Heparinized syringe with No. 25g needle (radial puncture)
Heparinized syringe with No. 22g needle (femoral or brachial puncture)

Procedure

Doctor's/Nursing Action	**Reason**
1 Wash hands carefully.	1 To minimize possibility of infection.
2 Check arm for colour, temperature and pulses for adequacy of circulation.	2 Particularly note brachial, radial and ulnar pulses. If there is any question regarding circulation check with doctor.
3 If patient's concern is not allevi- aesthetic will be injected first so	3 Inform patient that a local an- ated, hyperventilation could pro-

Doctor's/Nursing Action	Reason
that the drawing of blood will cause little discomfort.	duce atypical blood values.
4 Have patient in a comfortable position.	4 Sitting in a chair or semirecumbent position in bed is acceptable.
5 Cleanse puncture site; then follow with iodine-base antiseptic.	5 Be sure site is free of soil, dead skin or debris which would interfere with action of antiseptic.
6 Dorsiflex patient's wrist slightly— determine strongest pulse.	6 To determine best puncture site.
7 Puncture artery, entering at a 45° angle over strongest pulse area.	7 Holding needle with bevel up, pierce skin and artery using same technique as for venous puncture (p. 98).
8 Note 'flashback', keep needle steady, and withdraw required sample; remove needle.	8 This indicates entrance into artery.
9 Apply constant pressure over puncture site for at least 5 or 6 min.	9 Time can be increased if there is a coagulation problem; pressure is applied until bleeding stops.
10 Hold syringe and needle in a vertical position and eject all air; cap needle with needle cover.	10 Air would alter gaseous content of blood.
11 Apply firm pressure for 5 min or longer if necessary. Special care is required for patients with bleeding disorders. Inform doctor if haematoma occurs.	
12 Transport syringe and needle with blood specimen to laboratory immediately.	12 If the analysis will not take place within 5 min, entire syringe is placed in ice water to preserve condition of blood.

GUIDELINES: Administering an Intravenous Infusion Using the Cubital Fossa

NOTE: See Nursing Alert, p. 91.

Procedure

Doctor's/Nursing Action	Reason
Preparatory Phase	

1 Place patient in bed in semirecumbent position.
  Inform him of the procedure and its purpose.
	1 This is comfortable for the patient and permits arm to assume a flexed comfortable position.
	  To secure his understanding and co-operation.

Doctor's/Nursing Action	Reason
2 Remove sleeve of patient's garment.	2 To permit removal of gown or pyjama top if necessary while infusion is in progress (without cutting sleeve).
3 Position (but do not tighten) tourniquet under lower end of upper arm (5 cm (2 in) above joint).	3 To immobilize arm while needle or catheter is in vein; this will prevent dislodging of needle and injury to vein.
4 Place padded splint under arm; fix arm to splint by bandaging firmly (see p. 93).	4 Padding will prevent constriction of nerves or blood vessels.
5 Connect intravenous materials; hang fluid receptacle after checking label for proper solution.	5 Intravenous fluids are considered medications; labelling must be verified.
6 Allow fluid to flow through the system; tighten the clamp; lay sterile needle on sterile surface until arm is prepared.	6 To eliminate air bubbles which could cause air emboli in the circulatory system.

Performance Phase

1 Tighten tourniquet.
    Ends of tubing should be opposite or away from infusion site.
	1 To distend veins (for better visualization) by preventing blood flow back to heart.
	    To prevent contamination of injection area by tubing ends.

2 Request patient to open and close his fist. Palpate and note suitable vein for injection.	2 Contracting muscles of lower arm forces blood into veins, which distends them further.
3 Cleanse skin thoroughly, using an antiseptic (at room temperature) on a cotton ball; apply friction in a circular pattern outwards from injection site.	3 To remove skin pathogens and sebum which might otherwise be drawn into the subcutaneous tissue or vein as the needle is advanced. Avoid application of cold antiseptic solution particularly if patient has very small veins; cold application would further constrict the vessels.
4 Use thumb to apply tension on tissue and vein about 5 cm (2 in) distal to injection site.	4 To aid in anchoring the vein as the needle is introduced.
5 Hold the needle at a 45° angle alongside the wall of the vein in the direction of and near the intended site of injection; pierce skin.	5 This angle permits greatest ease and accuracy in entering the vein.
6 Decrease angle of needle until it is nearly parallel with the skin and slightly to one side of the vein;	

Doctor's/Nursing Action	Reason
apply pressure in same direction as puncture and enter the vein.	
7 If there is a backflow of blood through the needle, the vein has been entered; advance the needle slowly about 2·5 cm (1 in) while lifting the vein.	7 To prevent the needle from becoming dislodged and puncturing the posterior wall of the vein.
8 Release tourniquet.	8 To permit infusion solution to enter circulatory system.
9 Release clamp on infusion tubing and relax skin tension.	9 To allow flow of solution and to prevent blood from clotting in the needle.
10 Slip a sterile gauze square (3 × 3-in) under the needle (double if necessary) to anchor it in the proper position.	10 To prevent needle orifice from pressing against vein wall and the needle from piercing vein wall.
11 Anchor needle in position using adhesive strips; fasten a loop of tubing to prevent pull on needle.	11 Effective taping allows some mobility for the patient and retains safe inflow of solution.
12 Regulate flow rate of solution.	12 Proper monitoring of solution will prevent overloading of the circulatory system.

Follow-up Phase

1 Gently loosen adhesive tape and fixation near injection site.
2 Place a sterile gauze square over needle or cannula where it enters vein; withdraw needle (or cannula) and *exert pressure at site*. If bleeding persists, apply a gauze square or Band-Aid and elevate part.
3 Remove adhesive marks with solvent.
4 Record:
   a. Nature of therapy and time given.   d. Any problems.
   b. Type of solution and rate of flow.   e. Patient's reaction.
   c. Total amount of solution.

GUIDELINES: Intravenous Infusion with Insertion of Plastic Catheter (Mounted on Metal Needle)

NOTE: See Nursing Alert, p. 91.

Equipment

Infusion set containing (sterile):
  Rubber tourniquet
  Gauze squares

Foil wrapped alcohol sponges or iodine-base antiseptic
Hollow intravenous needle with catheter (Teflon, Silastic or polyvinylchloride) attached to rigid hub

NOTE: Thorough hand washing followed by donning of sterile gloves is recommended.

Procedure

As described on p. 98, than as follows:

Doctor's/Nursing Action	Reason
1 When needle has punctured vein wall, gently push needle 1.2 cm (0.5 in) farther.	1 To ensure entry of catheter into vein lumen.
2 Hold needle in place; slowly advance catheter hub until it is in desired place.	2 Caution: After catheter is advanced, do not reinsert metal needle since it could cut catheter.
3 Slowly remove needle while holding catheter hub in place.	3 If catheter is not held in place, it is possible to pull catheter out of vein.
4 Apply pressure on vein beyond catheter with the small or ring finger (Fig. 4.5).	4 This will reduce blood leakage while removing needle and connecting tubing to infusion set.
5 Connect infusion tubing to hub of catheter.	
6 Apply iodine-base ointment.	6 To prevent infection.
7 Tape catheter after covering injection site with a sterile dressing.	7 To prevent catheter movement which could irritate vein and lead to phlebitis.
8 Loop tubing and fasten to arm.	8 To prevent any tension on tubing from affecting or moving catheter in the vein.

Follow-up

1 Frequent inspection of venepuncture site.	1 To ensure proper functioning of infusion.
2 Record date of insertion, size and type of catheter.	2 This is done on the patient's chart as well as on adhesive tape near infusion puncture site.
3 Change dressing and apply antiseptic ointment every 24 hours.	3 To minimize possibility of infection.
4 Change catheter every 24 hours.	4 Preferably the entire set is changed every 24 hours; the longer an intravenous set is in use, the greater the possibility of contamination by either airborne micro-organisms or those introduced via manipulation of equipment.

GUIDELINES: Intravenous Infusion by Insertion of Catheter
Through Needle (IntraCath.)
NOTE: See Nursing Alert, p. 91.

Equipment

Infusion set containing (sterile):
   Rubber tourniquet
   Gauze squares
   Foil wrapped alcohol sponges or iodine-base antiseptic
   Intravenous needle with plastic catheter through needle

NOTE: Thorough hand washing followed by donning of sterile gloves is recommended.

Procedure

As described on p. 98 than as follows:

Doctor's/Nursing Action	Reason
1 When needle has punctured vein wall, gently thread catheter through needle until desired length of catheter in vein has been achieved.	1 To ensure entry of catheter into vein.
2 Place index finger over vein (with catheter in place) and withdraw needle.	2 To hold catheter in proper position.
3 Apply pressure at puncture site for several seconds.	3 To control bleeding.
4 Slide needle shield to cover bevel of needle.	4 This will prevent cutting of the catheter by the needle.
5 An effective splint for the needle (and its junction with catheter) is made by taping a wooden tongue blade to needle and catheter.	5 This will prevent kinking of catheter and possibility of its breaking at bevel of needle.

Nursing Alert: If insertion of catheter through the needle is unsuccessful, remove both catheter and needle *at the same time.* **Otherwise, if catheter is pulled through needle,** *it may break and slip into the circulatory system.*

Follow-up

1 Frequent inspection of venepuncture site will ensure proper functioning of infusion.	
2 Record date of insertion, size and type of catheter.	2 This is done on the patient's chart as well as on adhesive tape near puncture site.
3 Change dressing and apply antiseptic ointment every 24 hours.	3 To minimize infection possibility.

Doctor's/Nursing Alert	Reason
4 Change catheter every 24 hours.	4 Preferably the entire set is changed every 24 hours; the longer an intravenous set is in use the greater the possibility of contamination either by airborne micro-organisms or via manipulation of equipment.

GUIDELINES: Use of Winged Infusion Set (Venepuncture) 'Butterfly'

Winged Infusion is the puncturing of a vein with a needle which has a pair of plastic wings attached to a flattened hub (Fig. 4.10).

NOTE: See Nursing Alert, p. 91.

Advantages

1 Wings can be folded upwards for easy manipulation and control of needle during insertion into vein.
2 The absence of a hub allows needle to be manoeuvred close to skin surface.
3 Usually this type of commercially prepared set has a shorter needle with a short bevel that lessens possibility of puncturing the opposite vein wall.
4 Following insertion of the needle, the wings are released; they spread flat against patient's skin and provide two anchor surfaces for taping. Absence of hub reduces possibility of pressure irritation.

Procedure

As described on p. 98, then as follows:

Doctor's/Nursing Action	Reason
1 Position wing set so that bevel of needle is up.	1 This permits proper introduction of needle through skin into vein.

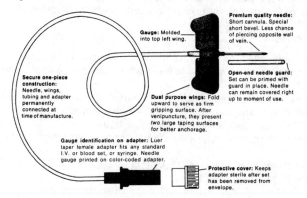

Figure 4.10. 'Butterfly' winged infusion set.

Doctor's/Nursing Action	Reason

2   Note gauge of needle on left wing.

    2   Most sets are marked for easy recognition of needle gauge.

3   Pinch wings firmly together between thumb and index finger.
    Needle is held firmly and comfortably for insertion.

4   Follow usual procedure, described on p. 98, for inserting needle.

5   Advance needle cautiously into vein; simultaneously, lift wings up slightly —to avoid piercing opposite vein wall.

6   Release tourniquet and release wings; hold flat against patient's skin and permit fluid to flow temporarily.
    This will anchor needle in vein and permit checking of flow of fluid.

7   Apply tape parallel to needle on each side. Make a protective loop and fasten to arm with tape—to anchor needle position.

GUIDELINES: Administration of Intravenous Drugs Into an Established Intravenous Infusion

This may be achieved by a Y-type infusion set giving two types of fluid—one containing the drug to be given over a longer period of time, the other containing the normal intravenous fluid. Or the drug may be given as a 'bolus' injection using a two-way tap connection or via a Butterfly needle with an extension for giving drops.

Features and Advantages

1   Drugs may be given on an intermittent basis through a 'keep-open' infusion.
2   The secondary bottle contains the medication; this may be single dose or multiple dose.
3   When desired, the primary infusion is clamped off and the prescribed amount of medication from the secondary bottle is administered.
4   A check-valve performs the following functions:
    a. Permits the primary infusion to flow after the medication has been administered.
    b. Prevents air from entering the system.
    c. Prevents secondary fluid from 'running dry'.
    d. Permits less mixing of primary fluid with secondary solution.
5   Higher flow rates can be achieved by elevating either of the receptacles.

Equipment

Infusion set with Y-type connection
Gauze squares and iodine-based antiseptic or alcoholic squares
Tourniquet
Tape

Procedure

Follow procedure as for administering intravenous fluids according to using the cubital fossa, plastic catheter or intracath. Observe both drip chambers and adjust rates according to doctor's instructions.

Intravenous Bolus

Intravenous Bolus refers to the administration of a medication from a syringe and needle directly into an ongoing intravenous infusion, or an intravenous needle (e.g. Butterfly) specifically inserted for this purpose, i.e., directly into a vein. All drugs given using this method must be given *slowly* and the patient is carefully observed throughout the procedure.

NOTE: Intravenous medication is often restricted to intensive care and special units and is administered by specially prepared personnel.

Advantages

1   Avoids incompatibility problems that may occur when several medications are mixed in one bottle.
2   Reduces patient discomfort because there are fewer intramuscular and intravenous injections.
3   Provides for immediate absorption of drugs; the effects are rapid and observable.
4   Permits rapid concentration of a medication in the patient's bloodstream.

Precautions and Recommendations

1   Determine patient's condition and his ability to accept the drug.
    Perhaps a more dilute medication is indicated.
    For example: Does patient have heart disease, limited cardiac output, diminished urinary output, pulmonary congestion?
2   Most medications require dilution because of their irritating effect on veins.
    A good policy is to use a syringe that can accommodate about 3 ml more than the prescribed amount of medication.
    Example: If 2 ml of medication are to be given, use a 5 ml syringe. When connected to the intravenous line, withdraw the additional 3 ml of intravenous fluid making a total of 5 ml (2 ml of medication plus 3 ml of intravenous fluid).
3   Administer medication *slowly*. The shortest time to spend in emptying a syringe should be 1 min; the longest could be 6 or 7 min. Slow administration provides an opportunity to observe the patient; if untoward effects occur, stop the injection.
4   Check the list of incompatible medications; often the local hospital pharmacy prepares this list in collaboration with the medical staff based on medications used by the local hospital. Frequent updating is needed because of new drugs and research.

5   Watch for major patient reactions such as anaphylaxis, respiratory distress, tachycardia, bradycardia, seizures. Also note 'minor' side effects such as nausea, flushing, vomiting, skin rash, confusion, gastrointestinal distress.

If a major reaction occurs or if a minor one is increasing in severity, stop the medication and notify the doctor.

6   Be familiar with antidotes for side effects and be prepared to administer them if prescribed:

Example: Skin reactions—Benadryl   Vomiting—Metochlorpropromide
               Anaphylaxis—Epinephrine   Diarrhoea—Lomotil

Emergency medications should be available in 'crash boxes'.

7   Cardiopulmonary resuscitative procedures should be familiar to nurses giving intravenous bolus medications.

Procedure Methods

1   Directly into the vein (see Guidelines: Venepuncture, p. 98, doctor's role).

2   Into intravenous tubing using two-way tap. Two-way taps vary in direction of flow and a careful check must be made of the make in use. The principle lies in shutting off the intravenous infusion whilst the drug is being given.

a. As with venepuncture, aseptic technique is rigidly observed.

b. The tubing is carefully swabbed with alcohol before it is punctured.

c. Ensure the intravenous infusion is running adequately.

d. Check precautions and recommendations as on p. 107.

e. Turn tap to obstruct intravenous flow of fluid.

f. Insert drug slowly, observing patient.

3   Into Butterfly type needle (see Fig. 4.10).

a. A winged needle is positioned in a vein; to the winged hub is attached a 9–10 cm (3.5 in) length of plastic tubing.

b. At the end of this short tubing is a permanently attached latex reseal injection site.

c. This is used to inject medications or withdraw periodic blood samples.

For indwelling needle sets or catheters for intermittent procedures, provision should be made to *heparinize* the venepuncture set (Heprinse). If this is not done, there is risk of occlusion of the lumen due to accumulation of fibrinous material. Sufficient heparin is injected to fill the needle and tubing. After each drug administration, replace the heparinized saline.

Complications of Intravenous Therapy

Infection

A local reaction due to contamination; this may spread systemically.

1. Causes (Fig. 4.11):

a. Fluid contamination; this may be due to faulty preparation, crack in flask, puncture in plastic container, fluid additives.

b. The longer the intravenous catheter is left in the patient, the greater is the risk of infection.

c. Failure to cleanse skin rigorously—to removed dead skin, dirt, mucus, etc., before applying antiseptic agent to infusion site.

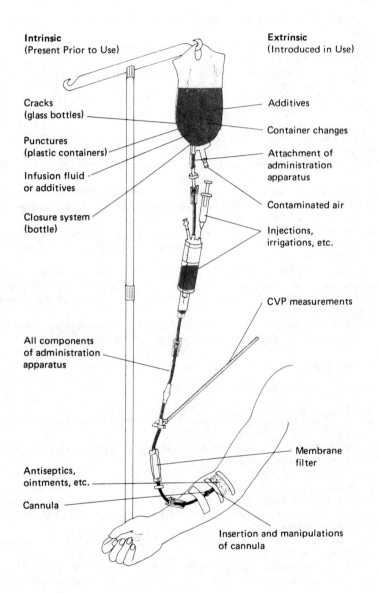

Intrinsic
(Present Prior to Use)

Extrinsic
(Introduced in Use)

Cracks
(glass bottles)

Additives

Container changes

Punctures
(plastic containers)

Attachment of
administration
apparatus

Infusion fluid
or additives

Contaminated air

Closure system
(bottle)

Injections,
irrigations, etc.

CVP measurements

All components
of administration
apparatus

Membrane
filter

Antiseptics,
ointments, etc.

Cannula

Insertion and manipulations
of cannula

Figure 4.11.   Potential mechanisms for contamintion of intravenous infusion systems. (Maki, D G (1976.) Preventing infection in intravenous therapy, Hospital Practice, April.

d. Failure to wash hands thoroughly before and after every patient contact by hospital personnel.

e. Use of contaminated hand lotion following hand washing by personnel coming in contact with patient.

f. May be transmitted within the patient from another infected part of his body to the catheter site.

g. The practice of irrigating or otherwise manipulating an occluded, leaking or infiltrated catheter may provide the opportunity for introducing contaminants.

2   Preventive nursing measures:

a. Practise rigid aseptic technique in starting an infusion; use sterile disposable gloves and consider the procedure a minor operation.

b. Thoroughly cleanse the infusion site; follow this with an iodine-base antiseptic.

c. Take care to anchor the catheter/cannula firmly in order to prevent excessive movement that might traumatize the cannulated vein and possibly facilitate entry of organisms at infusion site.

d. Record date of catheter or cannula insertion on patient's chart and also near dressing. This will serve to indicate how long the set has been in place and when it should be replaced.

e. Check (daily) the cannulated vein by gentle palpation to detect evidence of tenderness or pain; note any unexplained fever. If these are present, remove dressings and examine for signs of inflammation. Discontinue infusion if they are present.

f. The use of winged (scalp-vein) needles with smaller bores appears to be associated with less infection than use of plastic catheters.

Mechanical Failures

Solution flow slowing down or stopping, etc.

1   Causes:

a. Needle may be lying against the side of the vein, cutting off fluid flow. (Patient may have moved his arm.)

b. Level of intravenous receptacle may change rate of flow (gravity):

(1) Higher—more rapid.

(2) Lower—less rapid.

c. Needle may be clogged due to clotting.

d. Regulator of flow rate may be faulty; the clamp with a tapered v-shaped groove seems to provide greater dependability than the regular clamp.

2   Nursing assessment and approach:

a. Note whether there is swelling at needle site; if oedema is present, it suggests infiltration (see below).

b. Remove tape and check for kinking of tubing.

c. Rotate needle slightly—the bevel of the needle may be lying against wall of vein.

d. Move the patient's arm to a new position.

e. Elevate or lower needle to prevent occlusion of bevel of needle; if necessary to maintain a slightly different position use a gauze pad or cotton ball as a prop and maintain position by placing a few adhesive straps.

f. Try pulling the needle or catheter back a short distance since it may be occluded at a bifurcation.

g. Check patency of needle by lowering the receptacle below level of needle; a flashback of blood from the patient into the intravenous tubing indicates patency.

h. Never flush out a cannula or needle by injecting sterile saline with a syringe and needle directly into tubing since it may force a blood clot into circulation.

i. If none of the preceding steps produces the desired flow, the needle should be removed and the infusion restarted.

Nursing Alert: Sterile distilled water is never added to an intravenous set-up because it is hypotonic.

Pyrogenic Reaction

A generalized reaction due to contaminated equipment or solutions (less apparent with disposable equipment).

1 Symptoms (occur about 30 min to 1 hour after start of infusion):
   a. Abrupt temperature elevation, chills.
   b. Face flushing, sudden pulse rate change.
   c. Complaints of backache, headache.
   d. Nausea and vomiting.
   e. Hypotension—vascular collapse.
   f. Cyanosis—vascular collapse.
2 Preventive nursing measures:
   a. Use indwelling catheters only when absolutely necessary; infection increases significantly with the length of duration of venous catheterization.
   b. For long-term infusions, infusion site is changed every 48 hours; mark catheter to indicate when it is to be changed.
   c. For long-term catheterization, a larger needle (i.e., a No. 14 needle with No. 16 catheter 20 cm or 8 in long) in external jugular or subclavian vein directed to superior vena cava seems to minimize complications.
      (1) Less disparity in diameters of tube and vessel.
      (2) Rapid dilution of irritating fluids.
3 Nursing treatment measures:
   a. Discontinue infusion.
   b. Check vital signs; reassure patient.
   c. Notify doctor.
   d. Save equipment for further laboratory study.
   e. Record name, lot number and information, i.e., manufacturer of solution and any medications that have been added.

Infiltration

Dislodging of needle will cause fluid to infiltrate tissues.

1 Symptoms at site:
   a. Oedema, blanching of skin—also check undersurface of arm for puffiness.
   b. Discomfort, depending on nature of solution.
   c. Fluid flows more slowly or stops.

   d. Note temperature of skin; since solution is much cooler than patient, infiltration site will feel cool to touch.
   e. With a vasoconstrictor, such as noradrenalin (Levophed), infiltration can cause serious injury leading to necrosis and sloughing of tissues.
2 Nursing preventive measures:
   a. Fasten needle securely.
   b. Limit arm movement by splinting properly.
   c. Check tubing for kinking.
   d. Avoid looping of tubing below bed level.
3 Nursing treatment measures:
   a. Stop infusion
   b. Notify doctor.
   c. Place a sterile 3-in × 3-in gauze pad over needle and vein; withdraw needle and apply firm pressure over venepuncture site for several minutes.
   d. Apply warm compresses to increase fluid absorption.
   e. Restart infusion elsewhere.
   f. Use plastic cannula to reduce trauma when site is moved.
   g. If noradrenalin (Levophed) was used:
   (1) Notify doctor of infiltration.
   (2) Prepare antidote—phentolamine (Rogitine). When this is injected liberally into site, tissue necrosis and sloughing may be prevented.

Circulatory Overload

Patient receives an excessive amount of solution (happens more frequently in elderly patients or in infants).

1 Symptoms:
   a. Headache, flushed skin, rapid pulse.
   b. Venous distension.
   c. Increased blood pressure.
   d. Increased venous pressure.
   e. Coughing, shortness of breath, increased respirations.
   f. Syncope, shock.
   g. Pulmonary oedema leading to dyspnoea and cyanosis.
2 Nursing preventive measures:
   a. Know whether patient has existing heart condition—more prone to develop acute pulmonary oedema.
   b. Monitor solution flow.
   c. Place patient in semisitting position during infusion.
   d. Be especially attentive to the elderly or the infant.
3 Nursing treatment measures:
   a. Stop the infusion; notify doctor.
   b. Raise patient to sitting position—will ease the breathing problem.

Drug Overload

Patient receives an excessive amount of fluid containing drugs.

1 Toxic concentrations of drug are concentrated in the brain and heart.

2   Symptoms:
  a. Dizziness, fainting leading to shock.
  b. Specific symptoms related to the offending drug.
3   Nursing preventive measures—monitor flow rate carefully.
4   Nursing treatment—related to the nature of the medication.

Thrombophlebitis

1   Causes:
  a. Overuse of a vein, which may cause vasospasm; this may lead to inflammatory process and infection.
  b. Irritating infusion solution (strong acids or alkalies, hypertonic glucose solutions and certain drugs such as cytotoxic agents, methacillin, barbiturates).
  c. Clot formation in an inflamed vein.
  d. Anatomic location—veins of the lower extremity (relatively sluggish blood flow) are more vulnerable than those of the upper extremity.
  e. Length of time the cannula is in place—the longer the cannulation, the greater the possibility of infection.
  f. Polyvinylchloride catheters appear to be associated with infection more often than steel needles.
  g. Catheter diameter; large-bore catheters are more often associated with phlebitis than small-bore.
2.   Symptoms:
  a. Tenderness at first, then pain along course of the vein.
  b. Oedema and redness at injection site.
  c. Arm feels warmer than other arm.
3   Nursing treatment measures:
  a. Apply cold compresses immediately to relieve pain and inflammation.
  b. Later follow with moist warm compresses to stimulate circulation and promote absorption.

Air Embolism

Air may enter the circulatory system.

Nursing Alert: Recognize the high possibility of air embolism when doctors pump in blood (e.g., 500 ml in 10 min) since this builds high pressure in blood receptacle.

1   Symptoms:
  a. Hypotension, cyanosis, tachycardia.
  b. Increased venous pressure, loss of consciousness.
2   Nursing preventive measures:
  a. Replace initial bottle before it is completely empty with a fresh, full bottle; check attachment to be certain it is tight.
  b. In 'Y'-type sets, tightly clamp the nearly empty bottle to prevent air from being sucked into the tubing.
  c. Allow fluid to flow through tubing and needle or catheter to force air out—before starting infusion.

3   Nursing treatment measures:
   Unless prompt action is taken, patient may die within minutes.
   a. *Immediately* turn patient on left side with head down—air will rise into right ventricle and allow blood to pass into the lungs. The trapped air will be slowly dissipated through pulmonary system.
   b. Administer oxygen.

Nerve Damage

May result from tying the arm too tightly to the splint.

1   Symptoms:
   Numbness of fingers or hands.
2   Nursing preventive measures:
   Place padding around arm where bandage is to be applied.
3   Nursing treatment measures:
   a. Massage arm and move shoulder through its range of motion.
   b. Instruct patient to open and close hand several times each hour.
   c. Physiotherapy may be required.

CARE OF THE WOUND

A *wound* is a break in the continuity of tissue.

Classification

According to the manner in which it is made:

Incised—made by a clean cut with a sharp instrument, e.g., a surgeon's incision with a scalpel.
Contused—made by blunt force, which does not break through the skin but causes considerable soft tissue damage, e.g., a rock when thrown bruises a person.
Lacerated—made by an object which tears tissues, producing jagged irregular edges, e.g., blunt knife, jagged wire, glass.
Stab puncture—made by a pointed instrument, such as an ice pick, bullet, knife stab, nail.

Surgical Classification

Clean—an aseptically made wound, as in surgery, in which all bleeding vessels have been ligated (tied).
Contaminated—exposed to excessive amounts of bacteria, e.g., unprepared colon surgery, dirty laceration. These wounds are not grossly infected but have been exposed to bacteria (contaminated) and have higher risk of infection.
Infected—a wound which may not be closed may contain devitalized or infected material.
Debridement—the process whereby devitalized or necrotic tissue is cut out and flushed clean with saline solution.

Physiology of Wound Healing

First Intention Healing (Primary Union)

Healing which takes place aseptically with a minimum of tissue damage and tissue reaction; this is the ideal sought by the surgical staff; surgically closed (sutures or surgical tapes).

Second Intention Healing (Granulation)

Wounds which are left open to heal spontaneously; not surgically closed. They need not be infected.

1   If infected, pus forms; drainage is accomplished by incision and perhaps insertion of drains.
2   Necrotic material disintegrates and sloughs off.
3   Cavity fills with a red, soft, sensitive tissue which bleeds easily.
4   Buds, called granulation tissue, enlarge to fill area formerly destroyed and thus form a scar.

Third Intention Healing (Secondary Suture)

1   Occurs when a wound breaks down and is resutured or when a wound has been kept open and fills with granulation tissue and then is closed with sutures (two faces of granulation tissue are brought together in apposition).
2   Scar tissue formation is deeper, wider and more pronounced.

Factors Affecting Wound Healing

Local Factors (important)

1   Tension on wound edges.
2   Local vascularity, i.e., adequacy of blood supply to wounded tissue.
3   Presence or absence of contamination.
4   Oedema.
5   Dead space—allows collection of blood and serum, preventing apposition and favouring infection.

Systemic Factors (less important)

1   Adequate nutrition through proper diet.
    Protein and vitamin C are particularly effective in promoting healing.
2   Administration of whole blood—to maintain adequate levels of red blood cells.
3   Age.
    Tissues of younger individuals heal more rapidly than those of older persons.
4   Other—steroid treatment, diabetes mellitus.
5   Neoplasms.

The Purposes of Dressings

1   To protect the wound from mechanical injury.
2   To splint or immobilize the wound (Fig. 4.12).
3   To absorb drainage and fluid wastes.

4 To promote homoeostasis and minimize accumulation of fluid, as in a pressure dressing.
5 To prevent contamination from bodily discharges.
6 To provide physical and psychological comfort for the patient as well as a physiological environment conducive to wound healing.
7 To debride a wound.
8 To inhibit or kill organisms by using dressings that contain antiseptic medications.
9 To support a fractured or reconstructed area.

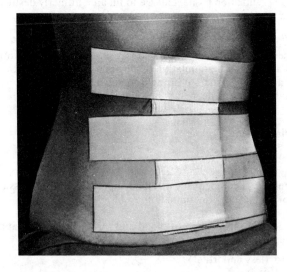

Figure 4.12. Laparotomy dressings are of many types, depending on the nature of the operation; the most frequent use of adhesive tape on the abdomen is in the application of postoperative dressings. For the ordinary laparotomy, 5 or 8 cm (2 or 3 in) wide strips of adhesive tape are usually applied transversely in close arrangement over the dressing; the ends of such strips should extend to at least the midaxillary line in order to provide good support and fixation. The illustration shows an effective method of securing a standard abdominal dressing. Some surgeons cover the dressing solidly with adhesive tape, but others question this practice on the grounds that it interferes with transpiration of water vapour from the area around the wound and thus may produce maceration and aid in the development of infection. (© Johnson & Johnson. Used by special permission of Johnson & Johnson, the copyright owners, and not to be reproduced for any purpose without Johnson & Johnson's permission.)

10   To provide information about the nature of the progress of the underlying wound.

Wound Healing Without Dressings

Preferred by some surgeons; may be desirable for a simple, clean wound.

Advantages

1   Permits better observation and early detection of problems.
2   Promotes cleanliness and facilitates bathing.
3   Eliminates conditions necessary for growth of organisms.
    a. Warmth.
    b. Moisture.
    c. Darkness.
4   Avoids adhesive tape reaction.
5   Facilitates patient activity.
6   Is economical.

Disadvantages

1   Psychologically, a patient may object to an exposed wound.
2   Wound is more vulnerable to injury.
3   Bedding and clothing may catch on stitches.

GUIDELINES: Changing a Surgical Dressing

Surgical Dressing Technique

The procedure of changing dressings, examining and cleansing the wound, utilizing principles of asepsis.

1   This may be performed by one nurse alone, the doctor or two nurses.
2   The condition of the wound is noted in order to understand the nature of the patient's surgical recovery.
3   The healing process is facilitated by keeping the wound clean.
4   The date for removal of stitches (Fig. 4.13) or clips depends on the wound and the surgeon's instructions.

Equipment

Sterile

Pack containing scissors, forceps, galli-pots, gauze and cotton wool swabs. (Some of these items may be packed individually)
Antiseptic solution
Gloves—Disposable may be used
For a wound with drainage tube—add sterile safety pin if shortening is required.
Equipment for irrigating the wound may be required

Unsterile

Bag for discarded dressing
Adhesive tape of the appropriate size.

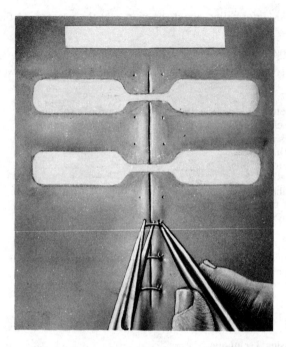

Figure 4.13.   Suture removal. It is always well to use butterfly strips or paper tapes (e.g. Steristrips) after stitches are removed to prevent separation of the edges and the possible formation of a wide scar due to lateral traction of the tissues. The strips should be left on for at least 1 week covered by a protective gauze dressing kept in place only by long narrow strips of tape. The strips shown in this figure are butterfly closures, which are sterile, waterproof and ready for use. NOTE: When a stich is removed the scissors are slipped under and to the left or right as far as possible. Stitch is grasped at knot with forceps and pulled out. (© Johnson & Johnson. Used by special permission of Johnson & Johnson, the copyright owners and not to be reproduced for any purpose without Johnson & Johnson's permission.)

Procedure

Preparatory Phase

1   Inform the patient that his dressing is to be changed. Explain procedure to him. Have him lying in the bed.
2   Avoid changing dressings at mealtime.
3   Ensure his privacy by drawing the curtains or closing the door; expose the dressing site.
4   If the dressings have foul odour, perhaps they can be changed in a separate treatment area that is adequately ventilated.
5   Prevent undue exposure of the patient; respect his modesty and prevent him from becoming chilled.
6   Wash your hands thoroughly; this should be done before and after each patient.

Nursing Action	**Reason**

Removing Adhesive Tape

1 Remove tape along longitudinal axis, slowly and gently.	1 Removing tape in same plane is less injurious and less painful.
2 Peel back edges by holding skin taut and pushing away from tape.	2 It is less traumatic to push skin away from tape than to pull tape from skin.
3 Remove tape near a wound by pulling towards the wound.	3 Pulling away from a wound may tear some of the delicate newly formed tissues.
4 Use a suitable solvent, e.g., 'Zoff' if the tape does not pull away easily.	4 This will prevent soreness and painful removal.

Removing Old Dressing

Method A (using disposable gloves)

1 Don sterile disposable gloves; remove top dressings carefully and discard into plastic bag.	1 Dressings are not to be handled by ungloved hands because of the possibility of transmitting pathogenic organisms.
2 Gradually loosen last dressing and observe skin and wound site.	2 If dressings adhere, moisten them with sterile saline and slowly withdraw dressing.
3 Remove and discard disposable gloves into plastic bag.	3 This will go to the incinerator later.

Method B (using a sterile plastic bag)

1 After washing hands, open package containing sterile plastic bag.	1 Bag should extend several centimetres (inches) above wrist.
2 Put right hand into sterile bag being careful not to touch outside of bag (this bag acts as a sterile glove).	2 Bag acts as a glove to protect hand from the dressings.
3 Pick up all soiled dressings as above and hold them in right hand; use left hand to grasp top edge of bag and pull it down over the hand and dressings.	3 This encloses soiled dressings in a plastic container; this bag can be used to receive cotton balls or dressings used to clean wound.

Cleansing the Simple Wound

1 Use aseptic technique.	1 To prevent contamination of a clean wound or to prevent further contamination of a 'dirty' wound. Also to prevent transmission of pathogenic organisms to clean area.
2 Open sterile pack containing scissors, forceps, swabs, etc.	

Nursing Action	Reason
3 Open any accessory packs required including pack of sterile fluid.	
4 Using forceps (or gloved hands) cleanse wound using a fresh swab each time and in one direction. Dry with fresh dry swab.	4 Applying a one-way direction prevents recontamination of the wound. Leaving the wound moist aids suitable media for pathogenic organisms.
5 Apply gauze and dressing suitable for the wound.	
6 Secure dressing with tape.	

Follow-up Care

1 Make patient comfortable.	
2 Dispose of soiled dressings in proper receptacle. Discard disposable items and clean equipment which is to be reused.	2 To prevent transmission of pathogenic organisms.
3 Record nature of procedure and condition of wound as well as patient reaction.	

GUIDELINES: Dressing a Draining Wound

Reinforcement of Dressings

Draining wounds may require frequent changes of dressings. Outer layers may be removed and fresh dressings applied without disturbing wound site. (a) Saturated dressings cause discomfort to the patient. (b) Dressing edges may become dry, hard and scratchy. (c) Odour may be unpleasant.

Auxiliary Aids to Facilitate Dressing Changes

Montgomery Straps (rarely used)

Strips of adhesive tape, the edges of which have been folded back for a short distance with a small hole cut in the folded portion and threaded with gauze strips or cotton tape. Two opposing strips are brought together and the tapes tied.

Many-tailed Binder

A many tailed binder which when applied snugly (starting at the lower end) produces a comfortable and conforming support for the patient (Fig. 4.14).

The binder should be placed low enough on abdomen to provide abdominal support without impeding respiration.

Removal of Adherent Dressings

1 To prevent the discomfort of removing dry, sticking dressings, moisten the dressing with cleansing solution.
2 Provide a disposable towel to catch any excess fluid.

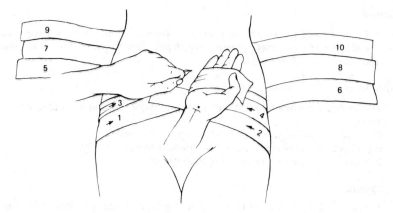

Figure 4.14.   Procedure for applying a many-tailed binder. (From Fuerst, E V, and Wolff, L, Fundamentals of Nursing, 5th edition, J B Lippincott.)

Anchoring and Gradual Withdrawal of Drainage Tubes

1   With each dressing change, the drainage tube is often pulled out of the wound a few centimetres and the excess tube is cut.
2   Hollow hard rubber or polyethylene tubes are used occasionally to drain a cavity. The tube is usually anchored with a suture.
3   Penrose or corrugated drainage tube with a safety pin.
    For the drain, such as a penrose, which is drawn out of the wound a few centimetres each day, a safety pin is positioned to prevent the drainage tube from slipping back into the wound (abdomen).
    The pin should be placed in its new position *prior* to cutting the drain.

Skin Care

1   Drainage is often irritating to surrounding skin tissues, particularly if it contains gastrointestinal secretions.
2   Apply protective ointment if prescribed (caution—ointments may cause maceration and may prevent drainage).
    a. Paraffin gauze.
    b. Zinc oxide ointment.
3   Recognize value of portable wound suction in maintaining cleanliness of surrounding tissues (p. 122).
4   Attach drainage tubing to suction bottle.
    Check tubing frequently for kinking or looping which would restrict flow of drainage.

GUIDELINES: Using Portable Wound Suction (Redivac, HemoVac, Porto-Vac)

Portable wound suction is a suction system which gently removes exudate and debris from a wound by means of a perforated catheter connected to a portable suction apparatus.

Purpose

To speed healing of the wound by removing fluids that could retard tissue granulation and by exerting negative pressure which permits two layers of tissue to adhere and thus eliminates dead space.

Advantages

1 Tubing rarely becomes occluded because it is siliconized and has multiple perforations.
2 Pressure exerted is gentle and even; suction is quiet.
3 Equipment is lightweight, permitting patient to move easily.
4 It is easy to measure amount of wound drainage.

Equipment

1 A long (0.25–0.5 cm) (0.125–0.25 in) malleable stainless steel introducing needle with a cutting edge on one end and a fine screw thread at the other.
2 A long 0.25 cm (0.125 in) calibre, siliconized, noncollapsible, polyethylene catheter with many small perforations in the centre.
3 A noncollapsible, siliconized, polyethylene connecting tube. The wound catheter fits snugly into the lumen of this tube.
4 A vacuum source (evacuator) consisting of an unbreakable plastic container with rigid ends and collapsible sides (may be a size to collect 200, 400 or 800 ml of fluid).
   Box has one cuffed hole into which the connecting tube fits snugly and an airhole supplied with a plug. This box may be of accordion-like collapsible plastic or it may have steel coil springs on the inside to hold the ends of the box apart.
5 A plastic Y-connector which fits between wound catheters and connecting tube and allows two wound tubes to be connected to one evacuator if desired.

Method of Inserting Drainage Tube(s)

1 In the operating room, the surgeon places the perforated drainage tubing in the desired wound area.
2 A stab wound is made with the needle end and excess tubing is drawn through the wound (stab wound is preferred because a more tightly sealed porthole is created; if the wound opening is used, drainage may seep through the incision line).
3 Needle is cut off and tubing is attached via adaptor to evacuator tubing (Fig. 4.15).

Method of Initiating Suction

Nursing Action	Reason
1 Connect tubes to evacuator.	
2 Squeeze ends of box together.	2 This will expel air.
3 Plug air hole.	3 To create a negative pressure.
4 As spring expands, a negative pressure of approximately 45 mmHg is produced.	4 Any fluid and blood in tissues is sucked into evacuator. Negative pressure is not great enough to suck

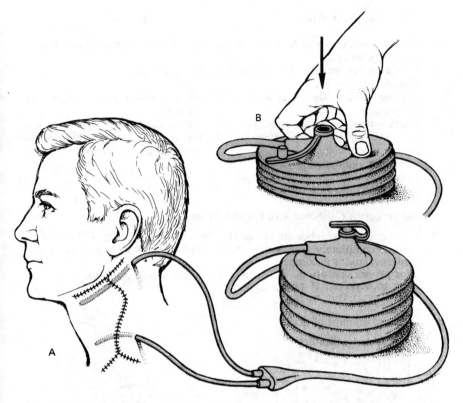

Figure 4.15.   a. Two perforated catheters are draining the incisional area following a radical neck dissection. By means of a Y-tube, drainage is drawn into a portable wound suction receptacle. When full, open top plug of receptacle and empty. b. To re-establish negative pressure, compress receptacle as indicated and replace plug; suction drainage will resume.

Nursing Action	**Reason**
	the soft tissues into the holes of the catheters.
5 When evacuator is full (200, 400 or 800 ml—depending on size of evacuator), it is time to empty.	5 Negative pressure has been fully dissipated.

Emptying Evacuator

1 Carefully remove plug, maintaining its sterility.	
2 Empty contents of evacuator into calibrated container.	2 Measure drainage.
3 Place evacuator on flat surface.	3 To permit adequate compression.

Nursing Action	**Reason**
4 Cleanse opening as well as plug with an alcohol sponge.	4 To maintain cleanliness of outlet.
5 Compress evacuator completely (Fig. 4.15).	5 To remove air.
6 Replace plug while evacuator is compressed.	6 To re-establish negative pressure (suction).
7 Check system for proper operation.	7 Look for fluid entering receptacle.
8 Secure evacuator to bedding; if patient is ambulatory, fasten evacuator to his clothing.	8 This permits patient to move without disturbing closed suction.
9 Record character and amount of drainage.	

Wound Irrigation Combined with Portable Wound Suction

1 Perforated wound tubes are placed side by side in wound (Fig. 4.16a). One is connected to irrigating fluid (or antibiotic solution), the other to portable wound suction.
2 At least 30% of the perforated section of one tube should be positioned parallel to the perforated area of the other.

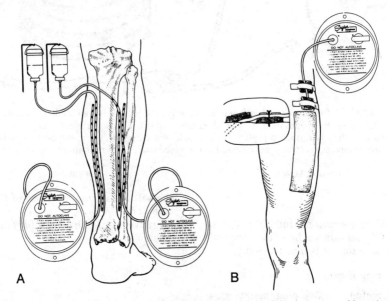

A   B

Figure 4.16.   a. An example of an efficient antibiotic drip and suction system. Note that the perforated wound tubes lie parallel to each other (intake and output). b. When drainage of long duration is anticipated, the wound drainage tubing can be fixed (so that it will not slip out of the wound) by a stainless steel wire suture (size 40 or 50) as the magnified drawing indicates. The drainage tubing is cushioned on a pad of gauze. (Courtesy of Zimmer, Warsaw, Ind, USA.)

3   If tubes are to remain for some time, a suture (usually stainless steel wire) is used (note arrow in Fig. 4.16b).
4   Having the drainage tube exit through a stab wound (away from main incision line) makes it convenient to manipulate, inspect and remove the drainage tube without disturbing the wound dressing.
5   After drip fluid has been stopped, all remaining tubes should have suction applied for at least 48 hours.

Tube Removal

1   At conclusion of use, discard tubing and evacuator by placing in a paper bag and depositing in container for incineration.
2   See Guideline: Changing a Surgical Dressing (p. 117).

Wound Infection

Infection in a wound occurs when there is growth of bacteria; infection may be limited to a single area or may affect a patient systemically.

Factors Affecting the Extent of an Infection

1   The kind, virulence and quantity of contaminating micro-organisms.
2   Presence of foreign bodies or devitalized tissue.
3   Location and nature of the wound.
4   Amount of dead space or presence of haematoma.
5   Immunity response of the patient.
6   Presence of ischaemia leading to wound compression.
7   Conditions of the patient, such as whether he is elderly, alcoholic, diabetic, malnourished.

Clinical Manifestations

1   Local:
       Induration (hardening of area), erythema, pain.
2   Systemic:
       Elevated temperature.

Nursing Alert: A useful rule of thumb guide is that an elevated temperature occurring within 24 hours suggests pulmonary infection; within 48 hours suggests urinary tract infection; after 72 hours suggests wound infection.

Preventive Medical and Nursing Measures

Preoperative

1   Encourage patient to achieve an optimum nutritional level.
       If hypoproteinaemic with weight loss, provide oral or parenteral alimentation.
2   Reduce preoperative hospitalization to barest minimum to avoid acquiring 'hospital infection'.
3   Treat current infections.

4   Avoid skin injury during preoperative surgical preparation.
    The interval of time between shaving and the operation should be reduced to a minimum.
5   Cleanse operative site with detergent-antiseptic.
6   When possible avoid shaving, to prevent nicks and scratches; utilize depilatory creams.
7   Administer systemic antibiotics if prescribed.

Postoperative

1   Maintain meticulous aseptic technique in caring for dressings, catheters, drains.
2   Encourage turning, coughing, early ambulation as soon as feasible.
3   Remove urinary bladder catheter as soon as patient can manage without it.
4   Administer antibiotics locally or systemically when they do the most to prevent infections; avoid prolonged administration which can encourage the growth of resistant strains of bacteria.

SUTURING

GUIDELINES: Suturing for Simple Wound Closure

This is usually carried out by a doctor, but a nurse may be instructed and required to carry out suturing in an accident and emergency or obstetric department.

Purpose

To close a small wound using nonabsorbable sutures such as black silk or dermal suture.

Equipment

Sterile gloves
Sterile suture set containing:
    Drape with aperture
    Needle holder for curved needles
    Needles: cutting edge—straight and/or curved
    Toothed forceps
    Scissors to cut sutures
    Suture material
    Dressings
Saline solution to cleanse suture line
Antiseptic solution or soap and water to cleanse area surrounding wound

Procedure (Fig. 4.17)

Nursing Action	Reason
1 Thoroughly cleanse small wound using detergent-germicidal soap.	1 To remove foreign bodies, debris, crusted blood; to minimize the possibility of contamination.

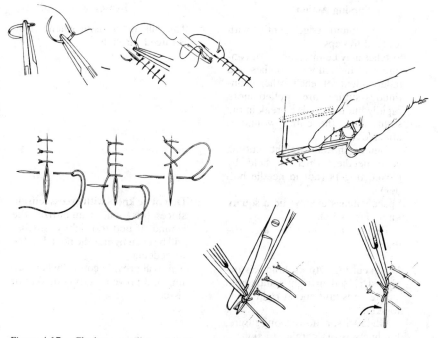

Figure 4.17. Closing a small wound using nonabsorbable sutures.

Nursing Action	**Reason**
2 Apply an antiseptic which will be nonirritating to exposed subcutaneous tissues.	2 To reduce microbial contamination.
3 Don sterile gloves and apply drape with opening centred over wound.	3 This will present a sterile field.
4 Usually a straight cutting edge-needle is preferable for suturing skin.	4 Less motion is required with a straight needle; if wound is deeper, a curved needle is more effective.

5 Thread needle with desired suture material.
  37·5 cm (15 in) is a convenient suture length; when threaded, allow 30 cm (12 in) on one side of needle and 7·5 cm (3 in) on the other.
  A curved needle is threaded from inner curve outward.
  This method helps prevent suture from falling out of needle.	

Nursing Action	Reason
6 Grasp wound edge gently with toothed forceps.	6 This will anchor tissue when needle is forced through.
7 Stitches may be interrupted or continuous. Interrupted stitches are independent of each other; continuous sutures are applied more rapidly but if there is a break in the suture line, the entire wound is affected. Figure shows straight cutting edge needle, which is held by gloved fingers (not in needle holder).	
8 Space stitches evenly; tie a square knot (Fig. 4.18). *Tissues need only be approximated.*	8 Do not tie knots with excess tension since this will traumatize the wound. If tied too tightly, stitches will be even tighter the next day due to oedema.
9 When cutting sutures, hold scissors almost closed in right hand; hold suture ends taut and at right angle to skin. Glide scissors down along suture, holding scissors parallel to skin.	9 This will provide control when cutting and prevent cutting of skin or tissue.
10 Cut stitch, leaving 0.65 cm (0.25 in) tails extending from knot.	10 To prevent knot from becoming undone; such a cut stitch will be easy to grasp when it is time for stitch removal.
11 Continue with stitches to close wound.	
12 Cleanse suture line with saline dampened gauze; apply dressing and tape.	12 Remove dried blood to lessen irritation to skin.

GUIDELINES: Suture Removal

The timing of stitch removal (of nonabsorbable stitches) depends on the location of the stitch on the body: head and neck, 3–5 days; chest and abdomen, 5–7 days; lower extremities, 7–10 days.

Equipment

Stitch removal tray or dressing pack containing:
  Swabs
  Forceps
  Scissors or stitch cutter
  Dressings

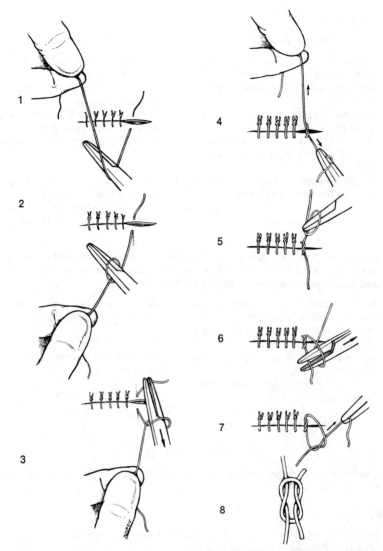

Figure 4.18. Tying a square knot. 1. After the suture is drawn through both sides of the wound, allow a short end of suture to remain. 2. Remove curved needle from holder and with the long end of the suture make a loop around the needle holder, starting with the holder in front of the suture. 3. Grasp the short end of the suture with the needle holder, which is through the loop. 4. Pull the suture through the loop and carefully tie the first part of the knot using the needle holder to pull one end. Traction is exerted parallel to the skin, with short end towards you. 5. To complete the square knot, reverse the suture ends so that the short end is away from you. 6. Tie second part of knot. 7. Again tighten by pulling ends parallel to skin. 8. Square knot is completed.

Procedure

Nursing Action	Reason
1 Cleanse the stitch area carefully and thoroughly using swabs wrung out in antiseptic solution. Repeat using a fresh, dry swab.	1 Stitches provide pathways for micro-organisms to invade tissues; therefore, skin surface must be rendered as clean as possible.
2 Use hydrogen peroxide if there are dried blood encrustations.	2 In the process of liberating oxygen, peroxide will loosen dried serum.
3 Grasp the knot of the suture with a pair of smooth forceps and gently pull upwards.	3 This will pull stitch away from skin.
4 Cut the shortened end of the stitch as close to the skin as possible.	4 This will allow the stitch to be pulled free of wound so that only that part of the stitch which is under the skin touches subcutaneous tissues.

Nursing Alert: Note that no segment of the stitch which is on the surface of the skin should be drawn below the skin surface. To permit this would introduce skin surface contaminants subcutaneously with risk of infection.

5 For continuous suture removal, cut the suture at each skin orifice on one side and remove the suture through the opposite side.	5 The objective here again is to avoid subcutaneous contamination.
6 If there is any oozing, apply a small dressing.	6 Any orifice is a potential site for infection.
7 Avoid injury to the tender and newly healed wound.	

BANDAGES AND SLINGS

Use of bandages and slings may be occasionally required in the first aid or accident and emergency situation.

Purpose

A *bandage* is applied to keep a dressing in place over a wound.
A *sling* is applied to immobilize an arm.

General Procedure:

1 Face the individual who is to have a bandage applied.
2 (If right-handed) The person applying the bandage holds the roll in the right hand and the starting end in the left hand.
3 Cover a dressing with a bandage that extends 5 cm (2 in) above and below dressing; do not begin or end a bandage over the wound.

Types of Bandages (Figs 4.19–4.23)

Butterfly Strip

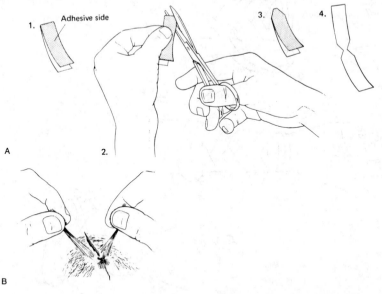

Figure 4.19.   a. To make a butterfly strip, fold a strip of 1.5 cm (0.5 in) wide adhesive tape back on itself (1 and 2); cut off the corners evenly at the folded end to form broad nicks (3) when the strip is unfolded (4). b. Tying hair to close a cut. (Blosser, J (1975) Wilderness medicine, Emergency Medicine, 7: 38. Artist: Shirly Baty).

Finger Bandage

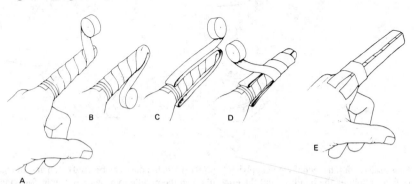

Figure 4.20.   Bandaging a finger is effectively done using a spiral and recurrent loop technique. Note that the final dressing is completed using narrow strips of adhesive.

Spiral Reverse Bandage for Arm and Leg

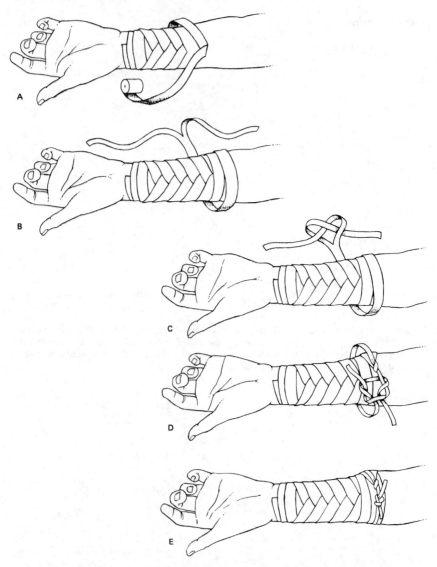

Figure 4.21.   a. The technique of applying a spiral reverse bandage can be used on an arm or leg. b. After applying the bandage, cut the end tail down the middle to provide two ends for tying around the arm. c. A simple tie prevents the bandage from splitting further. d. The two ends are used to encircle the arm and are tied in a square knot. e. The final knot is placed so that the weight of the extremity is not resting on it, thereby causing pressure.

Pressure Bandage of Ear

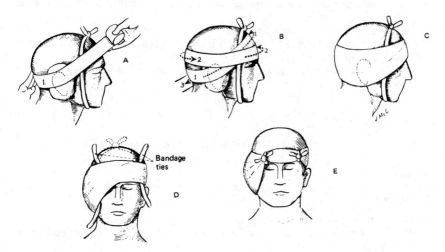

Figure 4.22. Application of pressure bandage of ear. (Ferguson, L K, Surgery of the Ambulatory Patient, J B Lippincott.)

Triangular Sling

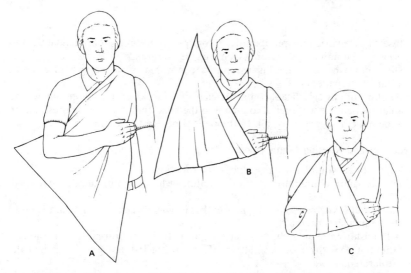

Figure 4.23. A triangular sling makes a comfortable sling. Note that the elbow is covered snugly and that the entire arm is supported, including the hand.

4   Apply bandage from the distal to the proximal; from medial to lateral.
5   Apply bandage turns evenly and securely; overlap each turn by two thirds the width of the bandage.
6   Separate skin surfaces such as fingers.
7   Assess the area bandaged for signs of constriction of circulation; if constriction is evident, reapply bandage.
8   Select width and quality of bandage to suit the area being bandaged.

POSTOPERATIVE DISCOMFORTS

Vomiting

Incidence

1   Occurs in many postoperative patients.
2   Results from an accumulation of fluid or food in the stomach before peristalsis returns.
3   May occur as a result of abdominal distension which follows manipulation of abdominal organs.
4   Induced during anaesthesia from inadequate ventilation.
5   Likely to occur if the patient believes preoperatively that he will vomit (psychological induction).
6   May be a side effect of narcotics.

Preventive Measures

1   Insert nasogastric tube preoperatively for operations on gastrointestinal tract to prevent abdominal distension which triggers vomiting.
2   Determine whether patient is susceptible to morphine since it may induce vomiting in some patients.
3   Be alert for any significant comment such as "I just know I will vomit under the anaesthetic". Report such a comment to the anaesthetist who may prescribe an antiemetic drug and also talk to the patient before the operation.

Treatment and Nursing Management

1   Support the wound during retching and vomiting.
2   Discard vomitus and refresh patient—mouthwash for mouth, clean linen for bed, etc.
3   Suspect idiosyncrasy to a drug if vomiting is worse when a medication is given (but diminishes thereafter).
4   Administer antiemetic medication such as metochlorpropromide (Maxolon).
5   Offer hot tea with lemon or small sips of a carbonated beverage such as ginger ale, if tolerated.
6   Report excessive or prolonged vomiting so that the cause may be investigated.
7   Detect presence of abdominal distension, hiccups, suggesting gastric retention.

Restlessness and Sleeplessness

Promoting Factors	Relief Measures
1 Discomfort such as back pain, headache and thirst.	1 Massage the back gently using an emollient lotion. Administer acetylsalicylic acid as prescribed.
2 Tight dressings or drainage-soaked dressings.	2 Change dressings and check for tightness.
3 Urinary retention.	3 Utilize nursing measures to initiate micturition (see p. 145).
4 Abdominal distension.	4 Insert rectal tube to relieve flatus—stimulates peristalsis and propels gas to rectum (Fig. 4.24).
5 Noise and environmental stimuli.	5 Keep noise level at a minimum. Limit visitors. For rest periods provide privacy, darkness and quiet.
6 Worry and anxiety.	6 Attempt to find cause of concern. Provide time to talk with the patient and permit him to vent his feelings. Seek advice of spiritual counsellor or psychologist if necessary. Offer sedatives or hypnotics as required.

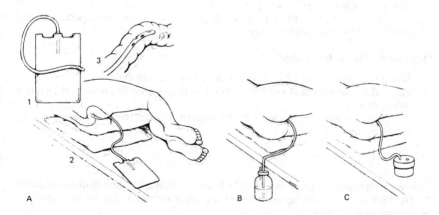

Figure 4.24.   Rectal intubation. a. (1) Rectal tube is attached to plastic bag; (2) tube in place, patient lying on left side; (3) enlargement of lower colon showing gas bubbles which will be tapped by rectal tube. b. Tubing connected to a water bottle with vent. c. Tubing connected to a plastic receptacle.

Thirst

Causes

1 Inhibition of secretions by preoperative medication with atropine.
2 Fluid lost via perspiration, blood loss.
3 Increased salt intake (intravenous or orally).

Nursing Management

1 Administer fluids by vein or by mouth if tolerated.
2 Offer sips of hot tea with lemon juice to dissolve mucus.
3 Apply a moistened gauze square over lips occasionally to humidify inspired air.
4 Allow patient to rinse mouth with mouthwash; lemon juice and glycerin swabbing of the mouth is also refreshing.
5 Obtain boiled sweets or chewing gum to help in stimulating saliva flow and in keeping the mouth moist.

Constipation

Causes

1 Trauma and irritation to the bowel during surgery.
2 Local inflammation, peritonitis or abscess.
3 Long-standing bowel problem: this may lead to faecal impaction.

Preventive Measures

1 Early ambulation to aid in promoting peristalsis.
2 Adequate fluid intake to keep stool soft.
3 A high fibre diet, e.g., bran, fruit, whole grain foods, to promote peristalsis and maintain adequate fluid balance.

Treatment (Faecal Impaction)

1 Insert a gloved finger and break up the impaction manually.
2 Administer an oil enema of 180–200 ml to help soften the mass and facilitate evacuation.
3 Inject 30–60 ml of peroxide of hydrogen into rectum; the foaming action may break up the faecal masses.

Pain

Pain is a subjective symptom in which the patient exhibits a feeling of distress caused by stimulation of certain nerve endings; usually it indicates that tissue damage is beginning to take place.

Clinical Manifestations

1 Autonomic. Outpouring of adrenalin:
   a. Elevation of blood pressure.

    b. Increase in heart and pulse rate.
    c. Rapid and irregular respiration.
    d. Increase in perspiration.
2 Skeletal muscle.
    Increase in muscle tension or activity.
3 Psychological:

    a. Increase in irritability. ⎫ Patient's reaction depends upon:
    b. Increase in apprehension. ⎪ 1 Previous experience.
    c. Increase in anxiety. ⎬ 2 Anxiety or tension.
    d. Attention focused on pain. ⎪ 3 State of health.
    e. Complaints of pain. ⎭ 4 His ability to concentrate away from the problem or be distracted.

Physiological and Psychological Observations

1 Pain is one of the earliest symptoms which the patient expresses upon return to consciousness.
2 Maximal postoperative pain occurs between 12 and 36 hours after surgery and usually disappears by 48 hours.
3 Anaesthetic agents which are soluble are slow to leave the body and therefore control pain for a longer time than agents which are insoluble; the latter produce rapid recovery, but the patient is more restless and complains more of pain.
4 Older persons seem to have a higher tolerance for pain than younger or middle-aged persons.
5 There is no documented proof that one sex tolerates pain better than the other.
6 Psychological conditioning of the patient affects pain tolerance.
7 The quality of nurse–patient interaction may have a greater influence on relief from pain than does the medication.
8 The nurse may reduce the patient's need for pain relief by making him more comfortable physically; frequent change of position, back rubs, talking to him and letting him express his concern can help lower his anxiety level.
9 Patients who have had abdominal or chest surgery are more likely to need narcotics. The exchange of respiratory gases can be reduced by pain that causes reflex chest-muscle contraction.
10 Potent drugs such as morphine may produce depression of the patient's respiratory centre thereby reducing rate and depth of breathing; also, such drugs tend to constrict bronchiolar smooth muscles and increase tracheal bronchial secretions—leading to atelectasis and pneumonia.

Nursing Management

1 Assess the nature, location and duration of pain and record these evaluations.
    a. Ask the patient to point to the pain centre.
    b. Find out what the patient *means* by pain.
    c. Determine whether the pain is associated with an activity, such as turning or taking a deep breath.
    d. Encourage the patient to describe the pain in his own words, e.g., stabbing, consistent, dull.

   e. Investigate possible causes of pain such as bandage or adhesive which is too tight or cast which is too snug.
2 Evaluate the patient's response to his pain.
   a. Observe the patient's facial expression and bodily movements as he experiences the pain.
   b. Is he pain-free when distracted by visitors or television?
   c. Does he appear to complain in anticipation of the next dose of medication?
   d. Help patient to express his angry feelings about pain and discomfort.
3 Employ comfort measures in caring for the patient.
   a. Provide therapeutic environment—proper temperature and humidity, ventilation, visitors.
   b. Increase patient's bodily comfort by adding blanket if he is cold, and vice versa.
   c. Massage his back in soothing strokes—move him easily and gently.
   d. Offer diversional activities, soft radio music, or favourite quiet television programme.
   e. Provide for fluid needs by giving a cool drink, offering a bedpan.
4 Initiate measures to reduce the likelihood of pain.
   a. Encourage the patient to turn frequently.
   b. Massage pressure areas; support vulnerable areas—strategic placement of pillow, anchoring a footboard, placing a pillow between legs in the Sims's lateral position.
   c. Determine patient's need to micturate and need for relief from intestinal distension.
   d. Loosen constricting dressings.
   e. Keep bedding clean, dry and free from crumbs.
   f. Maintain the patient in correct physiological position.
   g. Encourage patient to verbalize—to ease pain reaction, raise threshold.
   h. Give analgesic drugs as prophylaxis to prevent pain.
5 Relieve localized pain.
   a. Carefully support the painful area and elevate painful extremities.
   b. Apply medications or counterirritants gently; use hot or cold applications as prescribed.
   c. Encourage and assist the patient to follow prescribed exercise programme.
6 Recognize the power of suggestion; mention that relief of pain will take place when a 'reasonable' method is selected and used.
   a. Combine chosen method of pain relief with verbal assurance that it will help.
   b. Explain why the method chosen will help in relieving pain—positive assurance has been recognized as enhancing the effect of the 'reasonable' action.
   c. Indicate to the patient that you understand that he has pain, that you have time to listen and to help him, and that you care.
7 Administer pain-relieving agents as prescribed.
   a. Administer tranquillizers to relieve anxiety.
   b. Use narcotic analgesics when postoperative pain justifies such medication.
   c. Provide soporifics for sleep induction.
   d. Administer muscle-relaxant and antispasmodic medications for uncontrolled muscle tension

e. Utilize specific medications for specific conditions such as relief of nausea, relief of undesirable coughing, relief of headache.

8 Recognize desired effects and untoward reactions of all medications given.

   a. Observe patient for desired effect of medication.

   b. Be alert to toxic manifestations and hypersensitivity reactions.

   c. Be knowledgeable regarding drug interactions.

   d. Note signs of respiratory embarrassment, adverse vital signs, rashes.

POSTOPERATIVE COMPLICATIONS

Shock

Shock is a response of the body to peripheral circulatory failure.

Classification

1 *Oligaemic* (haematogenic)—shock resulting from loss of plasma or whole blood; this may be external or internal. When 10% of the blood volume is lost, *hypovolaemic* shock occurs.

2 *Bacteraemic* (septic or toxic shock)—characterized by a change in the capillary endothelium, permitting loss of blood and plasma through capillary walls into surrounding tissues; no actual fluid volume is lost from the body.

3 *Cardiogenic*—observed when there is interference with heart pumping action, as might occur in myocardial infarction, cardiac tamponade, which results in inadequate vascular circulation.

4 *Neurogenic* (vasogenic)—marked vasodilation and reflex inhibition which results in sluggish circulating system, depriving vital centres of proper blood supply.

5 *Psychic*—results from extreme pain or deep fear.

Altered Physiology and Clinical Manifestations

1 Loss of effective circulating blood volume—initiates metabolic and physiologic reactions resulting in poor tissue perfusion.

2 Pituitary hormones are released:
ACTH (adrenocorticotropic)—stimulates the adrenal cortex to secrete glucocorticoids.
ADH (antidiuretic)—stimulates kidney tubules to absorb more fluid.

3 Adrenalin and noradrenalin promote capillary vasoconstriction—increases flow through vital centres but diminishes flow through peripheral tissues. Later, peripheral vasoconstriction produces *pale, cold, clammy skin*.

4 Acidosis due to tissue hypoxia causes lung to compensate—increased rate and volume.

5 Heart rate accelerates; diastole lessens.
   Coronary perfusion occurs during diastole; with lessened perfusion, cardiac output falls, resulting in *reduced systolic pressure, lowered pulse pressure*, and generalized vasoconstriction.

6 Weak, thready pulse and subnormal temperature.

7 Lip cyanosis and surrounding pallor.

8 At first patient appears *nervous* and *apprehensive*; later, *apathy develops* and *sensations are dulled*.

Effects of Shock

1   Anoxia (hypoxia)—lack of oxygen in the body.
2   Anoxaemia (hypoxaemia)—decreased amount of oxygen in the blood.
3   Oliguria—decreased kidney secretion and urinary output.
4   Anuria—absence of urinary secretion.
5   Thrombosis with subsequent emboli due to blood stasis.

Treatment and Nursing Management

Chief Objective

To restore circulating blood volume.

Prevention

1   Prepare adequately the mental as well as the physical condition of the patient.
2   Anticipate any complications that may arise during and after surgery.
3   Have blood available if there is any indication that it may be needed.
4   Measure accurately any blood loss.
5   Keep operative trauma to a minimum; minimize postoperative disturbance of the patient.
6   Anticipate progression of symptoms upon earliest manifestation.
7   Monitor vital signs frequently until they are stable.
8   Assess vital sign deviations; evaluate blood pressure in relation to other parameters.
9   Institute therapy immediately following an injury, etc., which is likely to lead to shock.
10 Recognize that blood pressure limits vary with individuals; in some patients 90/60 may be normal whereas in others it may indicate severe shock.

Definitive Management

1   Keep the airway patent!
    a. Use an airway or place an endotracheal tube.
    b. Remove oral and tracheal secretions.
    c. Institute resuscitative measures if necessary.
2   Arrest haemorrhage.
    Ascertain where haemorrhage is occurring; if external, utilize pressure control.
3   Place patient in most physiologically desirable position for shock (Fig. 4.25).
    a. Elevate the head on a pillow.
    b. Keep trunk horizontal.
    c. Elevate lower extremities about 20–30°, keeping knees straight.

Nursing Alert: Do not use Trendelenburg head-low position because (1) after initial increase of blood to the head, a reflex compensatory action takes place causing vasoconstriction and thereby decreasing blood supply to the brain; and (2) viscera tend to fall against the diaphragm causing increased resistance to breathing and inadequate ventilation.

4 Call medical officer who will ensure an adequate venous return by:

 a. Inserting intravenous catheter for infusion in upper extremities; two may be required.

 b. Placing a central venous pressure (CVP) catheter in or near right atrium (see Fig. 1.3 of Volume 2, Chapter 1 and Guidelines, p. 13).

 (1) Notice direction and degree of change from initial reading.

 (2) Utilize route established by CVP catheter for emergency fluid volume and electrolyte replacement.

 c. Starting plasma expanders if needed until whole blood is available.

 d. Beginning blood transfusion when blood is available.

5 The medical officer may obtain blood for determinations of pH, P_{O_2}, P_{CO_2} and haematocrit.

 a. pH—may indicate acidosis resulting from anaerobic metabolism.

 b. P_{CO_2}—assesses function of pulmonary alveolar membrane.

 c. P_{O_2}—determines level of oxygen tension.

 d. Haematocrit—reveals losses due to obstruction or peritonitis.

6 The medical officer may request a urinary catheter to be inserted to monitor hourly urinary output.

 Objective is to maintain a 1 ml/kg/h urinary volume output to ensure adequate kidney perfusion.

7 Antibiotics may be prescribed in order to offset infection which can occur due to stagnant hypoxia in wounds and in peripheral tissues.

 Large doses of penicillin, streptomycin or broad-spectrum chemotherapeutic agents may be used.

8 Support the defence mechanisms of the patient.

 a. Comfort and reassure patient if he is conscious.

 b. Resort to sedation and analgesia with discriminating judgement.

 c. Keep the patient warm, but do not apply too much external covering since it will produce unnecessary vasodilation resulting in more fluid loss.

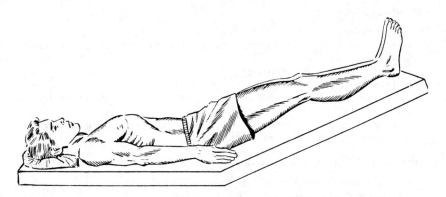

Figure 4.25. Proper positioning of patient who shows signs of shock, if not contraindicated by previous condition. Elevate the lower extremities about 20° keeping the knees straight, trunk horizontal and head slightly elevated.

9   Recognize signs of impending cardiac failure—increasing CVP, distended neck veins, pulmonary râles, etc. The medical officer will initiate prophylactic digitalization.
        Rapid-acting medications in the very young and very old (digoxin) may be used.
10   Throughout entire panorama of impending shock, continue flow sheet, recording of vital signs, observations and interventions.

Haemorrhage

Haemorrhage is the escape of blood from a blood vessel.

Classification

General

1   *Primary*—occurs at the time of operation.
2   *Reactionary*—occurs within the first few hours after surgery.
        Blood pressure returns to normal and causes loosening of poorly tied vessels and flushing out of weak clots from untied vessels.
3   *Secondary*—occurs some time after surgery.
        Due to infection which exudes the clot in the end of a major vessel.

According to Blood Vessels

1   *Capillary*—slow general oozing from capillaries.
2   *Venous*—bleeding which is dark in colour and bubbles out.
3   *Arterial*—bleeding which spurts and is bright red in colour.

According to Location

1   *Evident or External*—visible bleeding on the surface.
2   *Concealed or Internal*—bleeding which cannot be seen.

Clinical Manifestations

1   Apprehension, restlessness, thirst; cold, moist, pale skin.
2   Pulse increases, respirations become rapid and deep ('air hunger'), temperature drops.
3   With progression of haemorrhage.
    a. Decrease in cardiac output.
    b. Rapidly decreasing arterial and venous blood pressure as well as haemoglobin.
    c. Pallor around the mouth, spots appear before the eyes, ringing in the ears.
    d. Patient grows weaker until death occurs.

Treatment and Nursing Management

1   Treat the patient as described for shock (p. 139).
2   Inspect the wound as a possible site of bleeding.
        If an extremity is bleeding, apply a gauze-pad pressure dressing.
3   Call for the medical officer who will administer blood cross-matched or blood substitute until blood is available.

Nursing Alert: In giving fluids by vein recognize that, in the case of haemorrhage, giving too large a quantity or administering fluids too rapidly may elevate the blood pressure sufficiently for haemorrhage to begin again.

Femoral Phlebitis or Thrombophlebitis

Phlebitis often occurs after operations on the lower abdomen or during the course of septic conditions such as ruptured ulcer or peritonitis. (See Volume 2, Chapter 1, Conditions of the Cardiovascular System).

Causes

1   Injury.
    a. Damage to vein resulting from tight straps or leg holders during surgery.
    b. Compression of a blanket roll under the knees.
2   Fluid loss or dehydration leading to a rise in haematocrit.
3   Lowered metabolism and circulatory depression after surgery leading to slowing of blood flow.
4   Combinations of the above.

Clinical Manifestations

1   Left leg appears to be affected more frequently than right.
2   Pain or cramp in the calf, progressing to painful swelling of entire leg.
3   Slight fever, chills, perspiration.
4   Marked tenderness over anteromedial surface of thigh.
5   Intravascular clotting without marked inflammation may develop leading to phlebothrombosis.

Nursing Alert: A complaint of slight soreness of the calf is never ignored. The danger inherent in femoral thrombosis is that a clot may be dislodged and produce an embolus.

Treatment and Nursing Management

Prophylaxis

1   Hydrate the patient adequately postoperatively to prevent blood concentration.
2   Encourage leg exercises and ambulate the patient as soon as permitted by the surgeon. (Exercises are taught preoperatively—see p. 77.)
3   Avoid any restricting devices such as tight straps that can constrict and impair circulation.
4   Prevent the use of bed rolls, knee garters, even 'dangling' over the side of the bed, because there is danger of constricting the vessels under the knee.

Active Therapy

1   The medical officer will initiate anticoagulant therapy either intravenously, intramuscularly or by mouth (see p. 77).
2   Prevent swelling and stagnation of venous blood by wrapping the legs from the toes to the groin with elastic bandage or elastic stockings.

Pulmonary Complications

Preventive Measures

1   Report any evidence of upper respiratory infection to the surgeon.
2   Aspirate secretions that might cause respiratory embarrassment.
3   Recognize the predisposing causes of pulmonary complications:
   a. Infections—mouth, nose, throat.
   b. Aspiration of vomitus.
   c. History of heavy smoking, chronic respiratory disease.
   d. Obesity.
   e. Irritating effect of ether on mucous membranes.

Complications

1   *Atelectasis*—collapse of pulmonary alveoli caused by a mucous plug closing a bronchus.
2   *Bronchitis*—inflammation of bronchi causing a cough with considerable mucous secretion.
3   *Bronchopneumonia*—a chest complication with elevated temperature, pulse and respiratory rate plus a productive cough.
4   *Lobar pneumonia*—onset of a chill followed by a high temperature, pulse and respiration elevation, flushed cheeks, respiratory embarrassment.
5   *Hypostatic pulmonary congestion*—more common in the debilitated or elderly patient whose weakened heart and vascular system permit stagnation of secretions at base of lungs.
6   *Pleurisy*—knife-like pain in the chest on the affected side, particularly on intake of a deep breath, and elevated temperature, pulse and respirations.
   (For greater detail see Volume 2, Chapter 3, Conditions of the Respiratory System.)

Treatment and Nursing Management

1   Appraise the patient's progress very carefully on a daily basis for the first postoperative week to detect early signs and symptoms of respiratory difficulties.
   a. Slight temperature, pulse and respiration elevations.
   b. Apprehension and restlessness.
   c. Complaints of chest pain, signs of dyspnoea or cough.
2   Promote full aeration of the lungs.
   a. Turn the patient frequently.
   b. Encourage the patient to take 10 deep breaths hourly.
   c. Assist the patient in coughing in an effort to bring up mucous secretions.
   d. Encourage the patient to ambulate as early as the doctor will allow.
3   Initiate specific measures for particular pulmonary problems.
   a. Provide cool mist or steam (electric vaporizer) for the patient who exhibits signs of bronchitis.
   b. Encourage the patient to take fluids and expectorants if he appears to be developing pneumonia.
   c. Administer antibiotics to patients with pulmonary infections.

d. Prevent abdominal distension—causes pulmonary and circulatory embarrassment.

e. Provide analgesics for discomfort.

f. Note that the patient who has pleurisy with effusion may need chest aspiration; have equipment ready and be prepared to assist.

g. Be prepared to administer oxygen to assist in aeration of the lungs for oxygenation of blood.

Pulmonary Embolism

An *embolus* is a foreign body in the bloodstream—usually a blood clot that has become dislodged from the original site. When such a clot is carried to the heart from the systemic circulation it is forced into the pulmonary artery or one of its branches.

Clinical Manifestations

1 Sharp, stabbing pains in the chest.
2 Anxiousness and cyanosis.
3 Pupillary dilatation, profuse perspiration.
4 Rapid and irregular pulse becoming imperceptible—leads rapidly to death.
5 Dyspnoea.

Immediate Treatment

1 Administer oxygen and inhalations with the patient in an upright sitting position.
2 Reassure and quiet the patient.
3 Administer morphine to control panic, if not contraindicated in patients with respiration difficulties.

Urinary Difficulties

Retention of Urine

1 *Incidence*—occurs most frequently after operations on the rectum, anus, vagina or lower abdomen; often precipitated by pethidine given for postoperative pain.
2 *Nursing measures:*
   a. Assist patient to sit or even stand up (if permissible) since many patients are unable to micturate while lying in bed.
   b. Provide the patient with privacy.
   c. Utilize the psychological aid of running the tap water—frequently the sound or sight of running water relaxes the spasm of the bladder sphincter.
   d. Catheterize only when all other measures are unsuccessful.
      (1) May lead to possible bladder infection.
      (2) Subsequent catheterizations are often required.

Nursing Alert: Recognize that when a patient micturates very small amounts (30–60 ml every 15–30 min) this may be a sign of overdistended bladder ('overflow of retention').

Urinary Incontinence

1 *Cause*—loss of tone of the bladder sphincter.
2 *Incidence*—occurs as a complication in the aged after surgery.
3 *Recovery*—disappears as patient gains strength and muscle tone.
4 *Management:*
  a. Offer a bedpan hourly.
  b. Provide extra padding under patient; use special disposable pants.
  c. Initiate a consistent plan for special care of the skin to avoid skin breakdown.

Intestinal Obstruction

Causes

1 May occur following surgery on lower abdomen and pelvis, especially when there is drainage.
2 A loop of intestine may kink because of inflammatory adhesions.
3 A loop of intestine may become involved in the drainage tract.
4 Paralytic ileus—due to handling intestine during operation.

Clinical Manifestations

1 Most commonly occurs between the third and fifth postoperative day.
2 Sharp, colicky abdominal pains with pain-free intervals.
3 Pain is localized and should be noted since it may become more generalized later; location may pinpoint source of difficulty.
4 Peristaltic activity can be assessed by listening to the abdomen with a stethoscope.
5 Pain-free intervals grow shorter as time advances.
6 With completion of obstruction, intestinal contents back up into stomach and cause vomiting (faecaloid).
7 Abdominal distension and perhaps hiccups occur, but no bowel movements, if obstruction is complete; if obstruction is partial or incomplete, diarrhoea may occur.
8 Following simple enema, returns are clear, indicating very small amount of intestinal contents has reached large intestines.
9 If obstruction is not relieved, vomiting continues, distension becomes more pronounced, pulse increases, shock develops and death occurs.

Treatment

1 Relieve abdominal distension by passing a nasogastric tube and aspirating contents.
2 Administer electrolytes per intravenous infusion as prescribed.
3 Consider surgical intervention if obstruction continues unresolved.

Hiccup (Singultus)

Hiccups are intermittent spasms of the diaphragm causing a sound ('hic') that results from the vibration of closed vocal cords as air rushes suddenly into the lungs.

Cause

Irritation of phrenic nerve between spinal cord and terminal ramifications on under-surface of diaphragm.

1 *Direct*—distended stomach, peritonitis, abdominal distension, chest pleurisy or tumours pressing on nerves.
2 *Indirect*—toxaemia, uraemia.
3 *Reflex*—exposure to cold, drinking very hot or very cold liquids, intestinal obstruction.

Treatment

1 Remove the cause if possible.
   a. Gastric lavage for gastric distension.
   b. Adhesive strapping in pleurisy.
   c. Removal of drainage tubes causing irritation.
2 When removal of cause is not possible, favourite simple remedies may be tried.
   a. Holding breath while taking large swallow of water.
   b. Applying finger pressure on the eyeballs through closed lids for several minutes.
   c. Inhaling carbon dioxide (breathing in and out of a paper bag).
3 Medications may be prescribed (chlorpromazine, Benzedrine, quinidine or barbiturates). The degree of success with these drugs varies widely.
4 Introduce a catheter (No. 16F) into the patient's pharynx about 7–10 cm (3–4 in); rotate gently and jiggle back and forth; this action interrupts impulses from vagus nerve and hiccups stop (Fig. 4.26).
5 For intractable hiccups, an extreme procedure is surgical crush of the phrenic nerve.

Wound Complications

Haemorrhage and Haematoma

Manifestations

1 Inspect dressings frequently during first 24 hours postoperatively.
   a. Note evidence of bright red blood on dressings.
   b. Look for bulging which may indicate bleeding and clot formation (haematoma) under the skin.
   c. Examine bedding directly underneath incision site for evidence of trickling ooze.
   d. Check drainage bottle for undue amount of red drainage.
2 Check vital signs for evidence of bleeding—elevated pulse, apprehension, air hunger (see p. 142).

Treatment

1 Notify doctor.
2 If bleeding continues, it may be necessary for the patient to return to surgery to have bleeding vessel ligated, to remove large haematoma, to resuture wound.

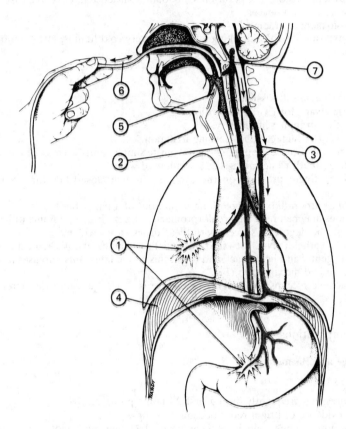

Figure 4.26.   Controlling hiccups. Irritations in chest or abdomen (1) are transmitted by the vagus nerve (2). The reflex arc is completed by the transmission of the impulses to the diaphragm by the phrenic nerve (3). This causes contraction of the diaphragm (4) resulting in sudden intake of breath, which in turn is suddenly interrupted by rapid closure of the glottis (5). This is the hiccup. Introduction of a No. 16F catheter into the nasopharynx about 7.5–10 cm (3–4 in) (6) stimulates the pharyngeal branches of the vagus nerve (7) and interrupts the reflex arc, stopping the hiccups.

Infection

Causative Organisms

1   *Staphylococcus aureus.*
2   *Escherichia coli.*
3   *Proteus vulgaris.*
4   *Pseudomonas aeruginosa.*
5   Anaerobic bacteria, e.g., *Bacteroides fragilis.* Anaerobes have become more prominent in wound infections, particularly following bowel surgery; a characteristic odour can be detected. Often this infection is detected only if anaerobic cultures are performed.

Prophylaxis

1   Strict asepsis when wound is made and later during wound management.
2   Housekeeping cleanliness and pertinent patient instruction concerning dressings.

Clincial Manifestations

1   Wound tenderness and swelling—apparent in 36–48 hours.
2   Elevated pulse and temperature.

Treatment

1   Surgeon removes one or more stitches, separates wound edges and examines for infection using a probe.
2   A culture is taken and sent to the bacteriology laboratory.
3   Wound irrigation may be done; have asepto syringe and saline available.
4   A drain (rubber or gauze) may be inserted.
5   Antibiotics are prescribed.
6   Hot wet dressings may be suggested.

Rupture (Dehiscence, Disruption, Evisceration, Abdominal Catastrophe)

Causes

1   The wounds of elderly patients do not heal as readily as those of younger patients.
2   Pulmonary and cardiovascular diseases contribute to wound breakdown since they impede delivery of nutritional essentials to the wound (circulatory and pulmonary difficulties).
3   Abdominal distension, infection, poor nutritional status and systemic diseases, e.g., diabetes.

Prophylaxis

1   Apply a binder (Fig. 4.14) for heavy or elderly patients or those with weak or pendulous abdominal walls.
2   Encourage proper nutrition with emphasis on adequate amounts of protein and vitamin C.

Clinical Manifestations

1   Patient complains that something suddenly gave way in his wound.
2   In an intestinal wound, the edges of the wound may part and the intestines may

gradually push out—observe for drainage of peritoneal fluid on dressings (clear or serosanguineous fluid).

Treatment

1 Notify surgeon immediately.
2 If intestines are exposed, cover with sterile moist dressings.
3 Keep patient on absolute bed rest.
4 Instruct patient to bend his knees—relieves tension on abdomen.
5 Assure the patient that his wound will be properly cared for; keep him quiet and relaxed.
6 Prepare patient for surgery and repair of the wound.

Postoperative Psychological Disturbances

Delirium is a mental aberration which occurs only occasionally in some postoperative patients.

Classification

Toxic

1 *Incidence*—occurs in combination with symptoms of general toxaemia, e.g., peritonitis, sepsis.
2 *Symptoms*—acutely ill, restless patient with elevated temperature and pulse, flushed face, bright and roving eyes—indicates mental confusion.
3 *Treatment:*
   a. Administer fluids to aid in elimination of toxins.

NOTE: Not all delirious patients can tolerate fluids. It is also inappropriate to administer fluids if it may lead to cerebral fluid retention and delirium; treatment in this instance is fluid restriction.

   b. Control infection by giving the proper antibiotics.

Traumatic

1 *Incidence*—develops following sudden trauma, particularly in the highly nervous person.
2 *Symptoms*—manifests itself by wild excitement, hallucinations, delusions or melancholic depression.
3 *Treatment:*
   a. Administer tranquillizing medications; chloral hydrate, paraldehyde.
   b. This state of delirium begins and ends abruptly.

Delirium Tremens

1 *Incidence*—patients who have used alcohol excessively are poor surgical risks and take anaesthetic agents poorly.
2 *Symptoms*—postoperatively, after continued abstinence from alcohol, patient shows signs of delirium tremens.
   a. Restless, nervous, easily irritated.

b. Sleeps poorly, disturbed by unreal dreams, momentarily appears to be in a strange place and does not know nursing or medical staff.

c. Later, loses control of mental functions; his mind is filled with haunting hallucinations that torment him constantly.

d. Additional symptoms include sleeplessness, excessive perspiration and marked tremor of the limbs. Patient eventually becomes stuporous.

3   *Medical and nursing management:*

a. Administer sedatives to keep the patient quiet and comfortable; stimulation may be required by older alcoholics in the form of whisky or strychnine.

b. Give glucose intravenously and concentrated vitamins by mouth to control nutritional deficiencies.

c. Recommend that the patient remains in bed; it may be necessary to restrain him so that injuries are minimized. (Bear in mind that restraining should be a last resort since this often makes such a patient quite rebellious.)

d. Encourage ambulation as soon as the surgical condition permits.

e. See also Alcoholism.

FURTHER READING

Books

Bordicks, K G (1980) Patterns of Shock—implications for nursing care, 2nd edition, Macmillan

Ellis, H and Wastell C (1980) General Surgery for Nurses, 2nd edition, Blackwell Scientific

Fish, E J (1979) Surgical Nursing, 10th edition, Balleère Tindall

Fream, W C (1978) Notes on Surgical Nursing, 2nd edition, Churchill Livingstone

Henderson, M A (1980) Essential Surgery for Nurses, Churchill Livingstone

Macfarlane, D A and Thomas L P (1980) Textbook of Surgery, 4th edition, Churchill Livingstone

McFarland, J (ed) (1980) Basic Clinical Surgery for Nurses and Medical Students, 2nd edition, Butterworth

Moroney, J (1978) Surgery for Nurses, 14th edition, Churchill Livingstone

Nash, D F E (1980) The Principles and Practice of Surgery for Nurses and the Allied Professions, 7th edition, Arnold

Roaf, R. and Hodkinson, L J (1978) Basic Surgical Care, 2nd edition, Pitman

Smith, D W and German C P H (1978) Care of the Adult Patient, 4th edition, J B Lippincott

Taylor, S (1977) Principles of Surgery and Surgical Nursing, 3rd edition, Hodder & Stoughton

Articles

Daws, J V (1981) Learn before you practice. Two training programmes for nurses to administer intravenous additives, Nursing Times, 77: 83–84

Davies, B D (1981) Communications in nursing. Pre-operative information given in relation to patient outcome, Nursing Times, 77: 599–601

Ferguson, V (1981) Informed consent: given the facts, Nursing Mirror, 153; 35–36
Marks, M (1981) Intravenous therapy—the extended role of the nurse, Nursing
    Focus, 2 (11): 377–387
Westaby, S (1981–1982) Wound care, Nursing Times, 77: series nos 1–6

Chapter 5

EMERGENCY NURSING

EMERGENCY MANAGEMENT*

Emergency management refers to the care given to patients with urgent and critical needs.

Principles of Assessment and Emergency Management

Underlying Consideration

Injuries or conditions interfering with vital physiologic function take precedence. Treat the potentially life threatening problems first.

Objectives:

To preserve life.
To prevent deterioration before definitive treatment can be given.
To restore patient to useful living.

1   Maintain a patent airway, employing resuscitation measures if necessary.
      Assess for chest injuries with subsequent airway obstruction.
2   Control haemorrhage and its consequences.
3   Assess and restore cardiac output.
4   Prevent and treat shock; maintain or restore effective circulation.
5   Carry out a rapid assessment of the patient's physical condition; the clinical course of the injured or seriously ill patient is not static.
6   Protect wounds with sterile dressings.
7   Splint suspected fractures (including fractures of cervical spine in patients with head injuries).
8   Check to see if patient has a Medic Alert or similar identification designating allergies, etc.
9   Start taking and recording patient's vital signs, blood pressure, etc.

Obtaining Data (History)

If possible, a brief history of the accident/illness is taken from the patient or the person accompanying him—relative, ambulance man, neighbour.

---

* This section will deal mainly with emergency management of trauma and other conditions not found elsewhere in this book. Management of acute heart conditions is found in Chap. 1, Vol. 2, and management of acute respiratory problems in Chap. 3, Vol. 2.

1 What were the circumstances, forces, location and time of injury?
2 What was the health status of the patient before the accident or illness?
3 Is there a past history of illness?
4 Is patient currently taking any medications—especially hormones, insulin, digitalis, anticoagulants?
5 Does he have any allergies?
6 Does he have any bleeding tendencies?
7 Is he under a general practitioner.
8 When did he eat his last meal? (Important if an anaesthetic is to be given.)

Psychological Management of Patients and Families in Emergencies

Underlying Consideration

Body trauma is an insult to physiological and psychological homoeostasis; it requires both physiologic and psychologic healing.

Objective

To prevent psychological incapacity following trauma.

1 Understand and accept the basic anxieties of the acutely traumatized patient. Be aware of the patient's fear of death, mutilation and isolation.
2 Understand and support the patient's feelings concerning his loss of control (emotional, physical and intellectual).
3 Be prepared to handle all aspects of acute trauma; know what to expect and what to do—alleviates nurse's anxieties and increases patient's confidence.
4 Maintain and convey optimism and concern for the welfare of the patient.
5 Caution the family not to be shocked or horrified by the patient's condition; encourage them to reassure the patient that they value him.
6 Accept the rights of the patient and family to have their own feelings.
7 Maintain a calm and reassuring manner—helps emotionally distressed patient or family to mobilize their psychological resources.
8 Assist the family to cope with sudden and unexpected death. Some helpful measures include the following:
   a. Take the family to a private place.
   b. Talk to all of the family together.
   c. Assure family that everything possible was done.
   d. Allow family to talk about the deceased and what he meant to them—permits ventilation of feelings of loss.
   e. Avoid volunteering unnecessary information (patient was drinking, etc.).
   f. Avoid giving sedation to family members—may mask or delay the grieving process which is necessary to achieve emotional equilibrium and prevent prolonged depression.
   g. Allow family members to view the body if they wish to do so (if body is not mutilated).

Airway Management and Artificial Ventilation

Artificial ventilation is accomplished by means of mouth-to-mouth and mouth-to-nose resuscitation (described in Guidelines which follow), a bag-mask unit or tracheal intubation. Artificial ventilation is instituted on a person who is not breathing; if he is unresponsive and without a palpable carotid or femoral pulse, external cardiac massage should be started. (Airway management and artifical ventilation are discussed in detail under Respiratory Insufficiency and Failure, Chap. 3, Vol. 2.)

GUIDELINES: Giving Mouth-to-Mouth and Mouth-to-Nose Resuscitation*

Action	Reason

Performance Phase

OPEN THE AIRWAY

1 Place the patient on his back.

2 Tilt the patient's head backwards as far as possible by placing one hand beneath the patient's neck and the other hand on his forehead.

3 Lift the neck with one hand and tilt the head backwards by pressure with the other hand on the patient's forehead.

4 If the head cannot be tilted back successfully, place your fingers behind the angles of the patient's jaw and forcefully displace the mandible forward while tilting the head backwards and using your thumbs to retract the lower lip—to allow patient to breathe through his mouth as well as his nose (jaw thrust technique).

VENTILATE THE PATIENT

Mouth-to-Mouth Ventilation

1 Keep one hand behind the patient's neck.

2 Pinch the patient's nostrils together with the thumb and index finger of the other hand while also continuing to exert pressure on the forehead to maintain the backward tilt.

Reason column:

2 In an unconscious, supine patient, the base of the tongue falls against the posterior wall of the pharynx, obstructing airflow into the trachea.

3 This extends the neck and lifts the tongue away from the posterior pharynx; the mouth opens, and the obstruction of the airway is relieved, since the tongue no longer occludes the back of the throat.

4 This provides additional forward displacement of the lower jaw.
If the patient does not breathe spontaneously after this manoeuvre, search for presence of vomit or of a foreign body in the mouth. Start artificial ventilation.

Absence of ventilation is determined by minimal or absent respiratory effort, failure of chest or upper abdomen to move, and inability to detect air movement through mouth or nose.

1 This maintains the head in a position of maximum backward tilt.

2 If the jaw thrust technique is used, keep the patient's mouth open with your thumbs and seal his nose by placing your cheek against it.

* From (1974) Standards for Cardiopulmonary Resuscitation (CPR) and Emergency Cardiac Care (ECC), JAMA, 227: 837–851.

Action	Reason
3 Open your mouth wide. Take a deep breath. Make a tight seal with your mouth around the patient's mouth and blow into his mouth.	
4 For the *initial* ventilatory manoeuvre, give the patient four quick full breaths without allowing time for full lung deflation between breaths.	
5 Remove your mouth from the patient's and allow him to exhale passively.	5 Watch the patient's chest fall.
6 Repeat this cycle once every 5 s as long as respiratory inadequacy persists (12 ventilations per minute).	6 Adequacy of ventilation is ensured by: **a.** Seeing the patient's chest rise and fall. **b.** Feeling in your own airway the resistance and compliance of the patient's lungs as they expand. **c.** Hearing and feeling the air escape during exhalation.

Mouth-to-Nose Ventilation

This is performed when it is impossible to open the patient's mouth, when it is impossible to ventilate through his mouth, when his mouth is seriously injured, or when it is difficult to achieve a tight seal around the mouth.

Performance Phase

1 Tilt the patient's head with one hand on the forehead while using the other hand to lift the lower jaw.	1 This manoeuvre seals the lips.
2 Take a deep breath. Seal your lips around the patient's nose and blow in until you feel his lungs expand.	
3 Remove your mouth from the patient's nose and allow him to exhale passively.	3 Watch his chest fall when he exhales. It may be necessary to open the patient's lips to allow air to escape during exhalation since the soft palate may cause nasopharyngeal obstruction.
4 Repeat the cycle every 5 s (12 ventilations per minute).	

HAEMORRHAGE

Emergency Management

Objective

To maintain an adequate circulating blood volume.

1 Cut the patient's clothing away quickly and carry out a rapid physical examination.

2   Apply firm pressure over the wound or the artery involved (Fig. 5.1); almost all bleeding can be stopped by direct pressure. Unchecked arterial bleeding produces death.

3   Apply a firm pressure dressing. Elevate the injured part to stop venous and capillary bleeding. Immobilize an injured extremity to control blood loss.

4   An intravenous cannula is inserted to provide means of blood replacement.
    a. Blood samples are withdrawn for analysis, grouping and cross-matching.
    b. Fluid replacement including isotonic electrolyte solutions, plasma and blood (depending on clinical estimates of type and volume of fluids lost).
    c. Rate of infusion depends on severity of blood loss and clinical evidence of hypovolaemia.

5   The following steps are taken for internal bleeding:
    a. Whole blood plasma expanders are given at the rate of blood loss.
    b. Prepare patient immediately for the operating theatre.

6   Apply a torniquet only as a last resort when the haemorrhage cannot be controlled by any other method.
    a. Apply the tourniquet; tie it tightly enough to control arterial blood flow.
    b. Tag the patient (with a skin marking pencil or on adhesive tape to his forehead) with a 'T' and a message stating location of the tourniquet and the time applied.
    c. Loosen the tourniquet every 20 min for 1–2 min to prevent irreparable vascular or neurologic damage. If there is no arterial bleeding, remove the tourniquet and again try pressure dressing.
    d. In the event of a traumatic amputation, leave the tourniquet in place until the patient is in the operating theatre.

7   Watch for cardiac arrest; patients who haemorrhage are candidates for cardiac arrest caused by hypovolaemia with secondary anoxia.

SHOCK

Shock is the condition in which there is loss of effective circulating blood volume; inadequate organ and tissue perfusion result, leading to derangements of cellular function.

Clinical Manifestations

1   Decreasing arterial pressure (systolic pressure usually falls more rapidly than diastolic pressure).
2   Increasing pulse rate.
3   Cold, clammy skin; prostration.
4   Pallor; circumoral pallor.
5   Alterations of mental status.
6   Suppression of kidney function.

Emergency Management

Objectives

To restore and maintain tissue perfusion.
To correct physiological abnormalities.

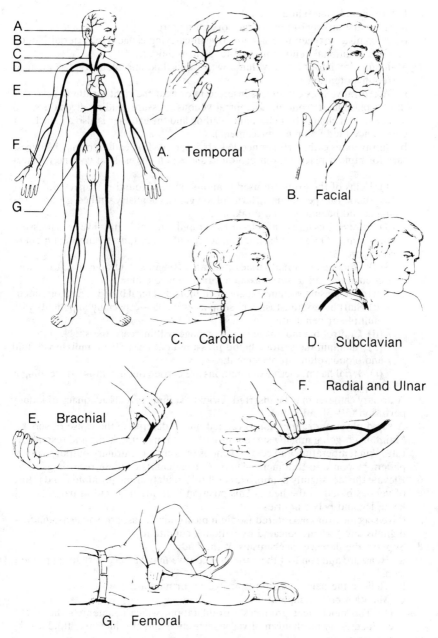

A.   Temporal

B.   Facial

C.   Carotid

D.   Subclavian

F.   Radial and Ulnar

E.   Brachial

G.   Femoral

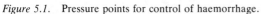

Figure 5.1.   Pressure points for control of haemorrhage.

1   Establish and maintain airway.
    a. Clear the airway of mucus and foreign material.
    b. Administer oxygen to augment oxygen-carrying capacity of arterial blood.
    c. Give additional ventilatory assistance as required.
2   Maintain circulatory blood volume with rapid fluid and blood replacement to correct hypotension.
    a. A central venous catheter is inserted in or near the right atrium to serve for fluid replacement (continuous central venous pressure reading gives direction and degree of change from baseline reading and the catheter is also a vehicle for emergency fluid volume replacement).
    b. Intravenous catheter(s) or needles are inserted. Two catheters may be necessary for rapid replacement in profound shock; emphasis is on volume replacement.
       (1) Veins of the arms are used if an abdominal wound is suspected.
       (2) Blood for specimens (arterial blood gases, chemistry studies, group, cross match and haematocrit) are taken.
       (3) Intravenous infusion is started at a rapid rate until central venous pressure rises 5 cm H_2O above baseline measurement or until there is improvement of condition.
          (a) Glucose in normal saline or lactated Ringer's solution is used to restore circulation and to serve as an adjunct to whole blood.
          (b) Use plasma volume expanders if indicated until blood can be obtained.
          (c) Start blood transfusion as soon as available—especially in patients with multiple or penetrating injuries.
          (d) Control haemorrhage; haemorrhage will increase the shock state.
          (e) Maintain the systolic blood pressure at at least 80–90 mmHg via fluid and blood volume replacement.
          (f) Serial haematocrit examinations are carried out if continued bleeding is suspected.
3   A urinary catheter may be inserted. Urinary volume reveals adequacy of kidney perfusion (30–50 ml/hour).
4   A rapid physical examination is carried out to determine the cause of shock.
5   Maintain on-going nursing surveillance of blood pressure, heart and respiratory rate, skin temperature and central venous pressure, and urinary output to assess patient response to treatment—keep accurate charts of these recordings.
6   Elevate the feet slightly to improve cerebral circulation and promote rapid return of venous blood to the heart. This position is contraindicated in patients with head, leg and pelvic injuries.
7   Give specific drugs as ordered (sodium bicarbonate, vasopressors, vasodilators, digitalis, etc.) when indicated by patient's condition.
8   Support the defence mechanisms of the body.
    a. Reassure and comfort the patient—sedative may be necessary for apprehension.
    b. Relieve the pain by cautious analgesics or narcotics.
    c. Maintain body temperature:
       (1) Too much heat produces vasodilatation, which counteracts the body's compensatory mechanism of vasoconstriction and also increases fluid loss by perspiration.

(2) A patient who is in septic shock should be kept cool since high fever will increase cellular metabolic effects of shock.

WOUNDS

Wounds (injury to tissues) vary from minor lacerations to severe crushing injuries.

Underlying considerations

Life threatening problems such as airway obstruction, haemorrhage and shock must be dealt with before the wound is treated.

Emergency Management

Objectives

To control haemorrhage.
To avoid complications.
To promote rapid healing.
To minimize scarring and prevent deformity.

1   Inspect the wound using sterile techniques—to determine the extent of damage to underlying structures.
   a. Shave around wound (with exception of eyebrows).
   b. Cleanse around wound—Savlon or other agent.
   c. The doctor may infiltrate with local anaesthesia intradermally through the wound margins or by regional block.
2   Cleanse and debride the wound.
   a. Irrigate gently and copiously with isotonic saline—to remove surface dirt.
   b. Remove devitalized tissue and foreign matter.
   c. Small bleeding vessels are clamped and tied.
3   The wound is sutured if primary closure is indicated (depends on nature of wound, length of time since injury was sustained, degree of contamination, vascularity of tissues).
   a. Subcutaneous fat is approximated loosely with a few sutures to close off dead space.
   b. Epidermis is closed; sutures placed close to wound edge with skin edges carefully levelled to prevent uneven scar surfaces.
4   Apply dressing—to protect wound; may serve as a splint and as a reminder to patient that he has sustained an injury.
5   Alternatively wound may be packed loosely and allowed to heal secondarily with gross contamination.
6   Give tetanus and antibiotics prophylactically if indicated.

Tetanus Prophylaxis in Wound Management

All wounds need adequate examination and toilet which should include the removal of all dead and potentially dead tissue and all foreign bodies.

Specific Tetanus Prophylaxis

All wounds can be divided into 'clean' and 'dirty'. A 'dirty' wound is any wound sustained out of doors that draws blood, was inflicted more than 6 hours previously or was inflicted while dealing with raw meat, skins or animals. A 'clean' wound is one which is inflicted indoors less than 6 hours previously. Patients can be divided into four groups according to their immune state.

A—Patients who are immune because their tetanus prophylaxis is up-to-date and their last injection was not more than 5 years previously.

B—Patients who have been immunized and have had a booster dose within the last 10 years.

C—Patients who have been immunized but have not had a booster dose for 10 years or more.

D—Patients who have never had a complete course of tetanus toxoid.

Tetanus Prophylaxis Procedure

Clean Wound	Immune State	Dirty Wound
Nil	A	Nil
Tetanus toxoid booster	B	Tetanus toxoid booster
Tetanus toxoid booster	C	Tetanus toxoid booster and antibiotic
Course of tetanus toxoid	D	Course of tetanus toxoid and antibiotic

1   Course of tetanus toxoid—for complete active immunization a full course of three injections of absorbed tetanus vaccine is given. The initial dose of 0.5 ml; a booster dose of 0.5 ml is given 6–12 weeks later and a final booster dose of 0.5 ml 6–12 months later. Immunity will not have reached a satisfactory level until after the second injection. After a course of three injections, immunity will be satisfactory for 5 years but depends on the severity of the injury.

Antibiotic Prophylaxis

Antibiotic prophylaxis will be either penicillin or erythromycin. A course giving adequate serum levels for 3–5 days is suggested. Triplopen 1.25 megaunits is often used for patients who are not allergic to penicillin.

Immediate Passive Protection (Humotet)

When immediate passive protection is required human tetanus immunoglobulin can be given (250 i.u. in 1 ml is an average dose). If given with tetanus vaccine, it must be injected into a different site with a different syringe and needle. Indications for the use of 'Humotet' are all highly tetanus-prone wounds, e.g., penetrating wounds, wounds with dead tissue, wounds which occur in association with farm or garden dirt or animal faeces.

Anaphylactic Shock

Adrenaline injection (BP) should be available during prophylactic procedures for treatment of anaphylactic shock. In adults 0.5–1 ml intramuscularly is given. In children the dosage varies according to age.

INTRA-ABDOMINAL INJURIES

Intra-abdominal injuries may be either penetrating or blunt.

Penetrating Abdominal Injuries

Penetrating abdominal injuries (gunshot wounds, stab wounds, etc.) are frequently serious and usually require surgery.

Emergency Management

Objectives

To control the bleeding.
To maintain the blood volume until surgery can be performed.

1 Keep the patient on the stretcher since movement may fragment a clot in a large vessel and produce massive haemorrhage.
   a. Cut the clothing away from the wound.
   b. Assess respiratory and cardiac status.
   c. Tabulate the number of wounds.
   d. Look for entrance and exit wounds.
2 Assess for signs and symptoms of haemorrhage. Haemorrhage frequently accompanies abdominal injury, especially if the liver and spleen have been traumatized.
3 Control the bleeding and maintain the blood volume until surgery can be performed.
   a. Apply compression to external bleeding wounds.
   b. Intravenous catheter(s) are inserted for rapid fluid replacement to restore circulatory dynamics.
   c. Upper extremity veins are used to avoid pumping fluids out through a wound in the inferior vena cava.
   d. Watch for occurrence of shock after an initial positive response to transfusion therapy; this is often the first sign of internal haemorrhage.
4 Aspirate the stomach contents with nasogastric tube—also helps detect gastric wounds and prevents lung complications from aspiration.
5 Cover protruding abdominal viscera with sterile saline dressings to protect viscera from drying.
   a. Flex patient's knees since this position will prevent further protrusion.
   b. Withhold oral fluids to prevent increased peristalsis and vomiting.
6 Insert indwelling urethral catheter to ascertain the presence of haematuria and to monitor the urinary output.
7 Keep records of the patient's vital signs, urinary output, central venous pressure readings (when indicated) and neurological status.

8   Prepare for X-ray to determine if there is peritoneal penetration:
   a. Purse string suture placed around wound.
   b. Small rubber catheter or Intracath is introduced through wound.
   c. Contrast medium introduced through catheter; x-rays are made and will reveal if peritoneal penetration has taken place.
9   Carry out tetanus prophylaxis as directed (p. 162).
10   Give broad spectrum antibiotic as directed to prevent infection since bacterial contamination is a frequent complication (depending on history and nature of wound).
11   Prepare for surgery if patient shows evidence of shock, bleeding, wound haemorrhage, free air, burst abdomen, haematuria, etc.

Blunt Abdominal Trauma

Underlying Considerations

1   Trauma to the abdomen is frequently associated with extra-abdominal injuries—chest, head and extremities.
2   The incidence of delayed trauma-related complications is greater than that associated with penetrating injuries; this is especially true of blunt injuries involving the liver, kidneys, spleen and pancreas.

Clinical Manifestations

1   Pain; pain on movemement.
2   Rebound tenderness; maximal point of tenderness.
3   Guarding.
4   Diminishing or absent bowel sounds.

Emergency Management

1   Take a detailed history (frequently unobtainable, inaccurate and misleading); obtain all possible data about the following:
   a. Method of injury.
   b. Time of onset of symptoms.
   c. Passenger location (driver frequently sustains spleen/liver rupture).
   d. Recent food intake.
   e. Bleeding tendencies.
   f. Concurrent disease. Medications.
   g. Past medical problems.
   h. Immunization history, with attention to tetanus.
   i. Allergies.
2   The medical officer will carry out examination (inspection, palpation, auscultation and percussion of the abdomen).
   a. Look for chest injuries, especially fracture of lower ribs.
   b. Avoid moving the patient until initial assessment is done—movement may fragment a clot in a large vessel and produce massive haemorrhage.
   c. Inspect front, flanks and back for bluish discoloration, asymmetry, abrasions, contusions.

d. Assess for signs and symptoms of haemorrhage; haemorrhage frequently accompanies abdominal injury, especially if the liver has been traumatized.

e. Note tenderness, guarding, rigidity, spasm.

f. Look for increasing abdominal distension.

Measure abdominal girth at umbilical level upon admission—serves as a baseline from which changes can be determined.

g. Auscultate for bowel sounds.

h. Note loss of dullness over solid organs (liver; spleen)—indicates presence of free air; dullness over regions normally containing gas indicates presence of blood.

i. Rectal examination/vaginal examination—for diagnosis of injury to pelvis, bladder and intestinal wall.

j. Avoid giving *narcotics* during observation period—may mask clinical picture.

3 Monitor vital signs frequently and carefully—may be the only clue to intra-abdominal bleeding.

4 Obtain baseline laboratory studies.

a. Urinalysis—as a guide to possible urinary tract injury; to monitor urine output.

b. Serial haemoglobin and haematocrit levels—their trend reflects presence or absence of bleeding.

c. White blood cell count elevated with rupture of spleen.

d. Serum amylase—rising level may indicate pancreatic injury.

e. Electrolytes.

5 Obtain abdominal and chest x-rays.

6 Assist with insertion of nasogastric tube—to prevent vomiting and subsequent aspiration; helpful in decompressing (removing air) gastrointestinal tract.

7 Patient may be admitted for observation or exploratory laparotomy.

CRUSH INJURIES

Crush injuries occur when a person is crushed beneath debris, run over or compressed by machinery.

Clinical Manifestations

1 Oligaemic shock—due to extravasation of blood and plasma into injured tissues after compression has been released.

2 Paralysis of part, erythema and blistering of skin—damaged part (usually an extremity) becomes swollen, tense, hard.

3 Renal dysfunction—prolonged hypotension causes kidney damage and acute renal insufficiency.

Emergency Management

1 Control shock.

2 Observe carefully for acute renal insufficiency—injury to back may cause severe kidney damage.

3 Splint major soft tissue injuries to control bleeding and pain.

4 Elevate the extremity.

5 Administer medication for pain and anxiety, as prescribed.

CHEST INJURIES

Injuries to the chest can be dire emergencies and are potentially life-threatening because of disturbances to cardiorespiratory physiology. See Chap. 3, Vol. 2 for a more complete discussion of chest injuries.

Emergency Management (Fig. 5.2)

Objective

To restore normal cardiorespiratory function as rapidly as possible.

Airway Assessment

1   Undress patient completely in order to evaluate respiratory pattern and to look for other injuries; multiple injuries frequently occur with chest injuries.
2   Is the chest wall intact?
3   Are there active respiratory movements and lung expansion?
4   What is the respiratory rate?
5   Is there shortness of breath, inspiratory or expiratory stridor, cyanosis or pain?
6   Determine if the patient is ventilating properly. Auscultate both sides of the chest.
7   Are the neck veins distended?—May indicate cardiac temponade.
8   Is there swelling of neck and face?—Swelling due to torn bronchus or laceration of lung may cause subcutaneous emphysema.
9   Palpate the abdomen in all thoracic injuries; look for rigidity and tenderness over liver, spleen, kidneys.
10 Look for fracture of the pelvis and long bones since these fractures may cause haemorrhage and shock.
11 *Priorities:*
    a. Ensure the airway.
    b. Perform a rapid physical examination to detect associated injuries.
    c. Assist with insertion of a tube into the chest cavity if indicated.
    d. Elevate the head and chest unless the patient is in shock.
    e. Prepare for blood transfusion; patients with severe thoracic injuries need blood to replace that which has been lost in the pleural cavity.

Sucking Wounds

Air passes through hole in the chest wall (from stab or bullet wound, etc.), causing the lungs to collapse and the mediastinum to shift. There is an audible passage of air from the wound during inspiration and expiration.

1   Instruct the patient to exhale.
2   Cover the wound with tulle gras and a pressure bandage applied by circumferential strapping—prevents further shifting of mediastinum and allows for airtight closure of wound; tulle gras dressing helps seal the leak.
3   The medical officer will insert chest tube connected to a water-seal and controlled suction drainage system—pneumothorax almost invariably accompanies these wounds.
    a. The skin is cleansed and infiltrated with a local anaesthetic by the doctor.

EMERGENCY MANAGEMENT OF PATIENT WITH CHEST INJURIES

Objective: Restore Normal Cardiopulmonary Function
as Rapidly as Possible

Assess Patient to Determine Physiological Status

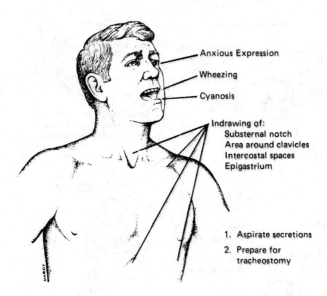

— Anxious Expression

— Wheezing

— Cyanosis

Indrawing of:
Substernal notch
Area around clavicles
Intercostal spaces
Epigastrium

1. Aspirate secretions
2. Prepare for
   tracheostomy

Clinical Assessment   Emergency Management

Flail Chest

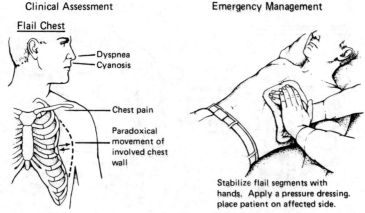

— Dyspnea
— Cyanosis

Chest pain

Paradoxical
movement of
involved chest
wall

Stabilize flail segments with
hands. Apply a pressure dressing,
place patient on affected side.

Figure 5.2.   Emergency management of patient with chest injuries. Objective: to restore cardiopulmonary function as rapidly as possible.

Clinical Assessment   Emergency Management

Hemothorax

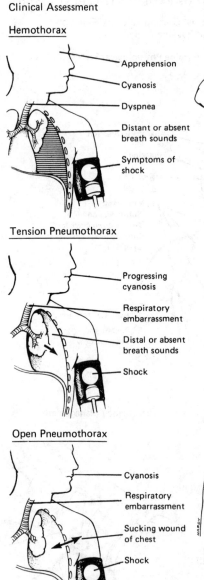

- Apprehension
- Cyanosis
- Dyspnea
- Distant or absent breath sounds
- Symptoms of shock

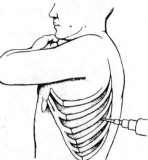

Drain hemothorax with needle and syringe. Prepare for emergency thoracotomy.

Tension Pneumothorax

- Progressing cyanosis
- Respiratory embarrassment
- Distal or absent breath sounds
- Shock

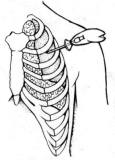

Insert large bore needle into pleural cavity, with finger cot to act as flutter valve.

Open Pneumothorax

- Cyanosis
- Respiratory embarrassment
- Sucking wound of chest
- Shock

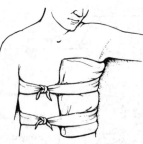

Instruct patient to exhale forcefully. Place occlusive dressing firmly in place. Make wound airtight.

Figure 5.2. (cont.)

b. A small incision is made between the fifth and sixth intercostal space in the midaxillary line.

c. The chest tube is inserted and sutured in place.

d. Chest tube is attached to a closed water-seal drainage system to evacuate blood and air and to measure blood loss.

4 Continue to assess respiratory status. Treat the patient symptomatically until surgical closure of the chest wall wound can be carried out.

Flail Chest

Usually results from multiple rib fractures, which cause instability of the chest wall and subsequent respiratory impairment.

1 Immobilize the flail portion of the chest by stabilizing it with the hands and then applying a pressure dressing with adhesive strapping (Fig. 5.2).

2 Prepare for tracheotomy or endotracheal intubation plus mechanical ventilation with volume-controlled ventilator to expand the lungs and give adequate oxygenation and to promote stability of the chest wall.

3 Place patient on his injured side; ensure that injury is compressed—by padding or a sandbag.

4 Assist with insertion of tube into the chest cavity.

5 A central venous catheter is inserted.

a. Blood is taken for haemoglobin, haematocrit determinations, typing and cross matching.

b. Monitor central venous pressure.

c. Administer intravenous fluids as indicated.

6 Arterial blood for blood gas analysis is taken to determine the physiological effects of the flail chest.

Tension Pneumothorax

Occurs when air enters the pleural cavity and produces displacement of the heart and mediastinum to the uninvolved side (with resultant severe cardiorespiratory embarrassment).

1 Assess the patient.

a. Assess for dyspnoea, chest pain, tachycardia and diminished or absent breath sounds on the involved side.

b. Test for fremitus (vibration) by placing a hand on the thorax and asking the patient to speak. Lack of fremitus when the patient speaks indicates a large accumulation of air.

c. Listen for tympany (drumlike resonant sound) when the patient's chest is tapped.

d. Secure portable chest x-ray as directed.

2 Assist with insertion of a chest drain to which a Heimlich flutter valve is attached to prevent back flow of fluid and air into the pleural space.

Haemothorax

An accumulation of fluid and blood in the pleural cavity which can cause collapse of the lung and hypovolaemia or shock.

1 Assess the patient.

   a. Note any increase in pulse rate, decrease in blood pressure, signs of bleeding and shock.
   b. An absence of breath sounds on the affected sides at the base and in the midlung fields may indicate haemothorax.
2 Assist with the insertion of a chest tube at the fifth and sixth intercostal space in the midaxillary line. Attach the tube to a water-seal drainage system.
3 Blood volume is restored by giving blood and fluids.
4 Prepare for emergency thoracotomy for operative control of bleeding, particularly if large haemothorax is present.

Ruptured Bronchus

1 Assess for respiratory distress, haemoptysis and subcutaneous and mediastinal emphysema.
2 Assist with closed chest drainage.
3 Prepare for surgical intervention to repair bronchus.

Cardiac Tamponade

Compression of the heart resulting from excessive fluid within the pericardial sac. It is the result of intrapericardial injury secondary to blunt or penetrating trauma.

1 Assess for distant heart sounds, *distended neck veins,* falling blood pressure, pulsus paradoxus and reluctance on the part of the patient to lie down.
2 Assist with pericardiocentesis.
3 Monitor the electrocardiogram (ECG) and central venous pressure.
4 Prepare for thoracotomy if there is continuing evidence of bleeding into the pericardium.
5 Blood is taken for cross match for possible blood transfusion.
6 Hypovolaemia is corrected with intravenous fluids.

HEAD INJURIES

Head injuries are classified as open or closed injuries. About 15–20% of all patients who come to emergency departments for treatment have some form of head trauma. (See Chap. 1, Vol. 3 for a more complete discussion of treatment of head injuries.)

Emergency Management

Nursing Alert: Exercise care when moving the patient's head and neck. Fracture of the cervical spine frequently accompanies a head injury.

1 Maintain the airway and exchange of air—hypoxia and hypercapnia can increase brain swelling and cell damage.
   a. Keep the patient semiprone with head to one side after making certain there is no cervical spine injury. Prone position facilitates drainage from the tracheobronchial tree and minimizes aspiration of nasopharyngeal and gastric secretions.
   b. Clear the respiratory passages via suctioning.
   c. Ensure adequate oxygenation and humidification. (Hypoxia of the brain,

which leads to increased intracranial pressure, is the most frequent cause of death following head injury.)

d. Obtain a portable x-ray of lateral cervical spine prior to intubation to rule out cervical spine fracture. A laryngostomy may be considered if patient is in acute respiratory distress.

e. Assist with endotracheal intubation if patient is comatose (after determining that a cervical neck injury is not present).

f. Utilize assisted ventilation if necessary. (The brain is very sensitive to lack of oxygen.)

2 Control haemorrhage and shock.

a. Shock is rarely the result of head injury—it usually has some other cause.

b. Marked intracranial bleeding in an adult usually produces hypertension.

3 Determine the baseline condition of the patient—serves as a basis for comparison as patient's condition changes.

a. Assess level of responsiveness. Record exactly what patient does and can do on command.

b. Determine the presence of headache, double vision, nausea, vomiting, papilloedema, retinal haemorrhage.

c. Assess pupil size and reaction to light.

d. Measure blood pressure, pulse, respirations.

e. Assess for signs of rising intracranial pressure—deterioration in level of responsiveness, slowing of pulse, rising systolic pressure, increasing pulse pressure, changes in pattern of respiration, dilating, nonreacting pupils.

f. Assess motion and strength of extremities.

g. Assess for injuries to other organ systems.

4 Look for changes in patient's condition. (*Change in level of responsiveness is the most sensitive sign of improvement or deterioration.*)

5 Utilize intracranial monitoring (if available)—for recognition of increased intracranial hypertension and to help guide the use of hyperosmotic agents (mannitol, glycerol) to lower elevated intracranial pressure.

6 Prepare for computed tomography or angiography—gives information useful for achieving a precise diagnosis.

7 Prepare for surgical intervention—for depressed fracture, bleeding, etc.

SPINAL CORD INJURY

Spinal cord injury may vary from a mild cord concussion with transient numbness to an immediate and permanent quadriplegia. The most common sites are the cervical areas C-5, C-6 and C-7 and the junction of the thoracic and lumbar vertebrae (T-12, L-1).

Any person with a head, neck or back injury should be suspected of having a potential spinal cord injury until the suspicion is proved groundless.

Clinical Manifestations

1 Total sensory loss and motor paralysis below level of injury.

2 Loss of bowel and bladder control; usually urinary retention and bladder distension.

3   Loss of sweating and vasomotor tone below level of cord lesion.
4   Marked reduction of blood pressure—from loss of peripheral and vascular resistance.
5   Neck pain.
6   Priapism—persistent erection of penis.

Emergency Management

1   Immobilize the patient. Keep him on the transfer board or on a hard, flat stretcher (Fig. 5.3).

Nursing Alert: A spinal cord injury can be made worse during the acute phase of injury. Proper handling is an immediate priority.

    a. Do not move the spine; keep the back straight—flexion or extension can aggravate the cord injury.
    b. Keep the head and neck in a neutral position.
    c. Move the patient on a stretcher or transfer board.
        (1) Carry out x-ray procedures while patient is on the board. A lateral cervical spine film is usually done to count all seven vertebral bodies.
        (2) Transfer patient to Stryker frame after initial evaluation.
2   Assess and examine patient for level of spinal cord injury and assiciated injuries; the presence of spinal shock may make assessment difficult.
    a. Test for strength and motion of extremities.
        (1) Request patient to flex and extend elbows and to squeeze fingers of examiner.
        (2) Request patient to move hips, knees, ankles, toes.
        (3) Observe pattern of respirations—intercostal muscle paralysis causes paradoxical movement of chest and abdomen.
        (4) Observe for priapism (persistent erection of penis)—a sign of spinal cord injury.
    b. Test for sensory impairment—prick the skin with a pin.
    c. Test the biceps, triceps, quadriceps and Achilles reflexes.
    d. Record vital signs.
    e. Look for the presence of associated injuries.
3   Assess the patient's respiratory exchange. Prepare for tracheotomy if there is a high cervical lesion.

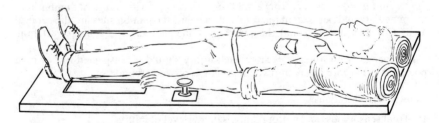

Figure 5.3.   When transporting a patient with a cervical injury of spine, assign someone to stabilize the patient's head. (From (1967) *Am J Orthoped*, 9(2): 36–37.)

4 Introduce nasogastric tube—to prevent and treat paralytic ileus, gastric and intestinal distension.
5 Catheterize the patient—patient with spinal cord injury cannot empty his bladder.
6 Start intravenous infusion.
7 Prepare patient for skeletal traction (Crutchfield tongs) if he has a cervical spinal cord injury—to obtain anatomic alignment and reposition dislocated facets.
8 Prepare for surgical intervention (controversial)—for mechanical decompression of cord, interruption of haemorrhagic cord necrosis, etc.

MULTIPLE INJURIES

Underlying Considerations

1 *Evidence* of gross trauma may be slight or may be completely absent. The injury regarded as the least significant may be the most lethal.
2 Any injury interfering with a vital physiologic function is an immediate threat to life and has highest priority for immediate treatment (obstructed airway, haemorrhage).
3 The patient should be completely undressed and a rapid physical examination should be carried out as quickly as possible after the airway has been established.
4 Mortality in patients with multiple injuries is related to the severity of the injuries and the number of systems and organs involved.

Emergency Management (Fig. 5.4)

Objectives

To determine the extent of injuries.
To establish priorities of treatment.

Carry out a *rapid* physical examination to determine if patient is breathing, bleeding or in shock; determine the status of his responsiveness and if he has severe wounds or fracture deformities.

1 Establish an open airway.*
   a. Ask conscious patient if he is having difficulty in breathing. Ask if he has chest pain.
   b. Apply suction to clear the trachea and bronchial tree.
   c. Insert oropharyngeal airway—to prevent occlusion by tongue.
   d. Ventilate the patient (bag-mask system).
   e. Prepare for endotracheal intubation if adequate airway cannot be maintained.
   f. Suspect serious intrathoracic injuries if respiratory distress continues after adequate airway has been established. See p. 166–170 for management of chest injuries.
   g. Administer oxygen if required.

* Imperative lifesaving procedures are performed simultaneously by the emergency team.

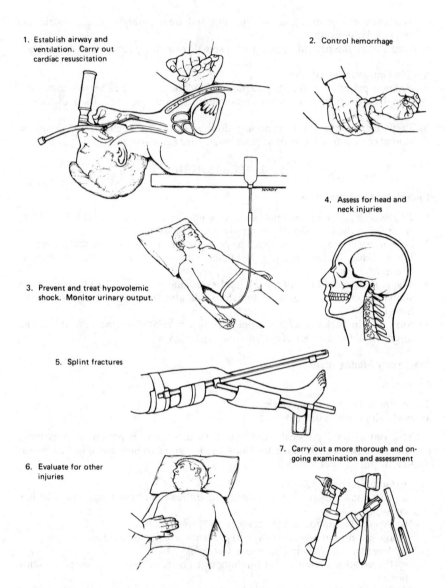

1. Establish airway and ventilation. Carry out cardiac resuscitation

2. Control hemorrhage

3. Prevent and treat hypovolemic shock. Monitor urinary output.

4. Assess for head and neck injuries

5. Splint fractures

6. Evaluate for other injuries

7. Carry out a more thorough and ongoing examination and assessment

Figure 5.4. The patient with multiple injuries. Any injury that interferes with vital physiological functions and poses an immediate threat to life takes priority for immediate treatment. Imperative lifesaving procedures are performed simultaneously by the emergency team.

2   Assess cardiac function and treat cardiac arrest—hypoxia, metabolic acidosis and chest trauma may precipitate cardiac arrest.*
   a. For cardiac arrest, start closed chest compression and ventilation.
   b. If chest wall is unstable (flail chest), emergency thoracotomy and manual compression may be necessary.
   c. Sodium bicarbonate is given (intravenously) to compensate for acidosis if indicated—severely traumatized patients with respiratory and circulatory embarrassment will have some degree of metabolic acidosis.
3   Control haemorrhage.*
   a. Apply pressure over bleeding points if haemorrhage is overt.
   b. Expect significant blood loss in patient with fracture of shaft of femur, with multiple fractures or with major pelvic trauma.
   c. Use tourniquet(s) for massive arterial bleeding from extremities which cannot be halted with pressure.
   d. Prepare for immediate surgical intervention if patient is bleeding internally.
4   Prevent and treat hypovolaemic shock.
   a. At least two intravenous catheters (or needles) are inserted; blood for laboratory studies is taken as directed (typing and cross matching, baseline complete blood count, electrolytes, blood urea nitrogen, glucose, prothrombin time).
   b. A central venous catheter is introduced to monitor patient's response to fluid infusion and to prevent fluid overload.
   c. Monitor urinary output (via catheter)—gives indication of adequacy of fluid replacement.
   d. Intravenous infusions are started in both upper extremities (if necessary); assist with venous cut-down as directed.
   e. Balanced saline solution (lactated Ringer's solution) is given in sufficient quantity to maintain blood pressure until blood is available.
   f. Balanced saline solution is given rapidly enough to keep central venous pressure readings at 5–15 cm H_2O; monitor rate and direction of change (important parameters).
   g. Monitor ECG.
   h. Carry out on-going clinical evaluation to observe for improvement or deterioration; improvement in level of responsiveness, skin warmth, speed of capillary filling, etc., shows reversal of shock state.
   i. Prepare for immediate surgical intervention if patient does not respond to fluids or blood. Inability to restore blood pressure and circulatory volume in patient usually indicates major internal bleeding.
5   Assess for head and neck injuries (p. 170).
   Make definite statements concerning baseline neurologic status of patient (level of responsiveness, size and reactivity of pupils, motor power, reflexes).
6   Splint fractures to prevent further trauma to soft tissues and blood vessels and to relieve pain; note presence or absence of pulses in fractured extremities.
7   Assess patient for gastrointestinal injuries.
   a. Examine patient repeatedly for abdominal pain, muscular rigidity, tenderness, rebound tenderness, diminished bowel sounds, hypotension and shock.

* Imperative lifesaving procedures are performed simultaneously by the emergency team.

   b. Assist with insertion of nasogastric tube if upper gastrointestinal bleeding is suspected or if gaseous distension of stomach develops—will decrease incidence of vomiting and aspiration.

   c. Prepare for laparotomy if patient shows continuing signs of haemorrhage and deterioration.

8   Continue to monitor urinary output hourly—reflects cardiac output and state of perfusion of visceral organs.

   a. Assess for haematuria and oliguria.

   b. Record measurements on a chart.

9   Evaluate patient for other injuries and institute appropriate treatment including tetanus immunization. (See wound treatment, p. 161.)

10   Carry out a more thorough physical examination after resuscitation and management of above priorities.

FRACTURES

A fracture is a break in the continuity of the bone. Fractures are classified as either open or closed. In open fractures, the broken ends are in direct contact with the exterior and can therefore become infected.

Immediate Treatment of Fractures in the Casualty Department

1   Give immediate attention to the patient's general condition, especially if the patient is admitted with multiple injuries.

   a. Assess respiratory function.

   (1) Look for respiratory difficulties, e.g., oedema due to facial and neck injuries, accumulation of secretions in the respiratory tract, etc.

   (2) Examine chest for sucking chest wounds, flail chest, etc.

   (3) Have tracheal intubation or emergency tracheotomy equipment ready.

   b. Control haemorrhage.

   (1) Control bleeding by covering with a dressing and applying direct pressure.

   (2) Suspect internal haemorrhage (pleural, pericardial or abdominal) in the event of continuing shock and in the presence of injuries to chest and abdomen.

   c. Treat for shock. This is usually the result of blood loss in patients with fractures.

   (1) Watch for fall in blood pressure, cold clammy skin and rapid thready pulse.

   (2) Heavy blood loss may accompany fractures of the femur and pelvis.

   (3) Prepare to assist with the setting up of an intravenous infusion. Plasma or plasma expanders may be used. Intravenous fluid will help to maintain the blood pressure.

   (4) Blood is taken for grouping and cross matching and a blood transfusion is commenced as soon as blood is available.

   (5) Administer oxygen as required.

   (6) Give analgesics as prescribed to control pain (splinting the limb and controlling pain are essential in treating shock accompanying fractures).

   d. Look for evidence of head, chest and other injuries.

2   Inspect the fractured part(s).
   a. Cut away clothing as necessary.
   b. Observe the entire body using a methodical head-to-toe system—inspect for lacerations, bruising, swelling and deformities.
   c. Look for angulation (bending), shortening and rotation.
   d. Check the state of the limb:
      (1) That the circulation to the limb is intact.
      (2) That the sensations of the limb are normal.
      (3) Which movements of the limb are affected.
      (4) The amount of swelling and bruising.
      (5) The amount of skin damage if an open fracture.
   e. Handle the fractured limb gently and as little as possible.
3   Apply a sterile dressing if the fracture is an open one.
4   For detailed account of treatment of individual fractures, see Volume 3, Chapter 4, Musculoskeletal Conditions.

BURNS

First Aid Management

Stop burning process to prevent further tissue destruction.

1   Remove patient from source of burn or smoke.
2   Remove clothing when saturated with boiling water. Clothing charred by flames is best removed in the casualty department with scissors.
3   Cover with clean sheets—for patient with extensive thermal injuries.
4   Immerse small areas of burns in cold water for 10 min—inhibits capillary permeability and thereby suppresses or prevents oedema, blister formation and tissue destruction.
   a. Reimmerse part for additional 10 min if pain resumes.
   b. Immersions may be repeated for a period of 40 min.
5   Keep patient warm.

Chemical Burns

1   Irrigate copiously with large quantities of running water (except for burns caused by phosphorus).
2   Cover with loosely applied clean cloth.

Electrical Burns

Electrical energy affects all tissues that it traverses—may cause sepsis and gangrene of extremity due to thrombosis of the blood vessels.

1   Remove electrical source with a nonconductor such as dry wood.
2   Treat for coma, circulatory and respiratory collapse.

Treatment of Burns in the Casualty Department

Objectives

To maintain ventilation and circulation.
To prevent or treat shock and acute renal failure.

To relieve pain and prevent infection.
To prevent the depth of injury from increasing.

General

1   Assist with assessment of thermal injuries to determine the extent of burns and their probable depth.
2   Determine the history.
   a. Circumstances of accident.
   b. Approximate duration of exposure to heat.
   c. Age and previous health condition (e.g., diabetes, renal disease, etc.).
   d. Time, place and mechanism of injury.
   e. Mental status.
   f. Care given patient before coming to casualty department.
3   Carry out rapid physical examination.
   a. Assess for hoarseness of voice and respiratory stridor (in patients with head and neck burns).
   b. Look for other injuries especially in patients burned from automobile accidents or explosions.
4   Use rigid asepsis (cap, mask, gown, sterile gloves) when indicated.
5   Replace fluids.
   a. Blood is taken for grouping, cross matching and blood gas samples.
   b. Intravenous fluids are commenced and a cutdown is sometimes necessary through unburned skin.
   (1) Patient loses significant intravascular protein, salt and water during the first few hours after burn, plasma volume is greatly reduced.
   (2) See Fluid Therapy Protocol Following a Burn (p.363).
   (3) Record fluids given on the appropriate chart.
6   Combat shock—due to local blood vessel damage with increased capillary permeability and loss of fluid into injured tissues.
   a. Insert indwelling urinary catheter to assess urine volume, pH, specific gravity, sugar, acetone. Measure volume hourly. Observe for haemoglobinuria.
   b. Assess patient for fractures, bleeding, head, chest and abdominal injuries, haemothorax, cardiac tamponade.
   c. Give definite treatment for shock.
7   Assist in care of the burn wound.
   a. Avoid further damage and contamination. Take swabs for bacteriological examination.
   b. Assist in performance of escharotomy (incision through eschar) since circumferential eschar on chest or extremities act as a tourniquet and will cause compression of the blood vessels.
8   Give analgesic as indicated (intravenous, in small doses).
   a. Patients with extensive superficial burns will complain of pain because of irritated hypersensitive nerve endings.
   b. Occasionally patients with deep burns may require no medication during shock period because of destruction of nerve endings in burned tissue.
9   Start a record of vital signs.
10   Systemic antibiotics may be given—for burn wound sepsis.
11   Administer tetanus immune globulin (Humotet) for immediate protection or toxoid if previously immunized.

12   Insert nasogastric tube to allow evacuation of air from stomach and prevent gastric dilatation; patient with extensive burns is likely to have decreased gastrointestinal motility.
13   Children with burns covering more than 10% of the body surface and adults with more than 15% will require hospital admission and intravenous fluids.
14   Patients with critical burns should be treated at a burn centre or in a burn unit.

Electrical Burns

1   Determine points of entrance and exit of current—to ascertain the organs that may be damaged.
2   Debride entrance and exit wounds.
   a. Remove charred and devitalized skin.
   b. Assist with fasciotomy, if oedematous, to relieve pressure on blood vessels.
3   Monitor for cardiac irregularities—death may ensue from ventricular fibrillation.
4   Watch for complications of myoglobinuria—large amounts of myoglobin pigment result from electrical muscle destruction.

Inhalation Burns

1   Establish adequate airway, maintain adequate oxygenation, especially for patients with major burns and for the elderly.
2   Prepare for endotracheal intubation or early tracheotomy in the following circumstances:
   a. Patients with deep burns of face, neck and respiratory tract; injuries from inhalation of gases.
   b. Stridor and inadequate respiratory exchange.
   c. Patient unable to handle tracheobronchial secretions.
3   Give oxygen as required since carbon monoxide poisoning may accompany inhalation burns.

EYE INJURIES

Basic Assumptions

1   All ocular injuries are potentially serious.
2   Suspect a penetrating ocular injury with every eye wound until suspicion is proved incorrect.
3   Record visual acuity as soon as possible on every eye patient; this is a reflection of the basic integrity of the eye.

Emergency Management

Corneal Abrasion

Injury to the cornea which goes no deeper than the epithelium.

1   Instil Amethocaine 0.25% solution as requested—to relieve pain and facilitate eye examination.
2   Stain the cornea with fluorescein—to detect existence of an abrasion and its extent.

    a. Gently touch conjuctiva of lower lid with edge of fluorescein paper strip.
    b. The exposed (damaged) layers of epithelium will take the stain and turn green; undamaged areas remain unstained.
3 Apply pressure bandage firmly but gently over eye—to put eye at rest and to prevent movement of the eyelid, with resultant irritation of abraded corneal area.
4 Give oral analgesic as necessary—abrasions of the cornea are painful.
5 Advise patient to rest his eyes for 24 hours for greater comfort; the corneal epithelium usually heals in 24–48 hours.
6 Instruct the patient to return to ophthalmologist the following day for dressing change and inspection of eye for evidence of infection or ulcer formation.

Contusion

Black eye; haemorrhage into the orbit from trauma; hyphema (haemorrhage into anterior chamber of eye).

1 Contusions usually clear slowly and without treatment.
    a. Apply cold compresses intermittently for first 24 hours to control pain and swelling.
    b. Apply warm compresses (after 24 hours) intermittently.
2 Place patient on bed rest with both eyes bandaged for hyphema.

Foreign Bodies Lodged in Cornea

Treatment by ophthalmologist or emergency department doctor.

1 Instil sterile anaesthetic into the conjunctival sac—to facilitate examination.
2 Ophthalmologist will remove superficial particles with a moist cotton-tipped applicator; foreign body removed with a spud or similar instrument using a slit lamp for magnification.
3 Apply eye patch and reinforce instruction to return to ophthalmologist the following day to determine if healing is underway.

Penetrating Injuries to the Eye

1 Cover eye with sterile dressing and call ophthalmologist.
    a. Intraocular foreign bodies should be removed as soon as possible; they cause damage by disintegration or become encapsulated by fibrous tissue.
    b. Apply eye patch lightly—pressure of pad may cause further penetration.
2 Give sedative–analgesic combination as directed; have patient lie quietly until ophthalmologist arrives.
3 Give tetanus prophylaxis for any penetrating eye injury.
4 Give oral antibiotics in high doses as directed—blood aqueous barrier resists penetration.

Burns of the Eye

Cause drying of the cornea with resulting chronic conjunctivitis and corneal ulceration.

1 *Thermal burns* (associated with face or body burns).
    a. Call ophthalmologist.

b. Thermal burns are treated in the same way as burns of skin structures.
2 *Chemical burns*—may be either acid or alkali in nature. Both cause intense pain and inflammation.
   a. *Irrigate eye with copious amounts of water*—holding the patient's eye directly under running water with lids retracted by gauze flats is the best way to irrigate the eye when immediate irrigation is required.
   b. Irrigate for 20–30 min.
   c. Repeat irrigation every 15–20 min (using regular eye irrigation equipment) until patient is seen by ophthalmologist.
   d. Control severe pain thereafter with systemic analgesics as prescribed.
   e. Patient may be hospitalized for treatment to enhance healing.

HEAT STROKE

Heat stroke is a medical emergency caused by failure of the heat-regulating mechanisms of the body when the temperature–humidity index is high. Persons who are not acclimatized to heat exposure, the elderly and those with cardiovascular problems are particularly vulnerable.

Clinical Manifestations

Headache and visual disturbances
Dizziness and nausea
Hot, flushed, dry skin
Weak, rapid and irregular pulse

Sudden loss of consciousness
High fever
Cessation of sweating
Muscle cramping

Emergency Management

Objective

To reduce high temperature as rapidly as possible.
1 Reduce the body temperature (rectal) to 39°C (102.2°F) as rapidly as possible, using one or more of the following methods.
   a. Place the patient on a hypothermia blanket if one is available.
   b. Place the patient in a cool environment.
   c. Remove all clothing. Sponge patient liberally with water at room temperature—or
   d. Place patient in a tub of cool water.
   e. Give chilled saline enemas if temperature does not come down.
   f. Place electric fan so that it blows on patient since air movement increases evaporation.
2 Administer oxygen by face mask if cyanosis is present. Intubate patient with cuffed endotracheal tube and attach to ventilator if necessary to support failing cardiorespiratory systems.
3 Start intravenous infusion as directed; give slowly because of danger of pulmonary oedema.

4   Give antipyretic and chlorpromazine (intravenously) as directed.
5   Give supportive care for convulsions.
6   Measure urinary output—acute tubular necrosis s a complication of heat stroke.
7   Correct metabolic acidosis.
8   Advise patient to avoid immediate re-exposure to high temperatures (after his condition has stabilized). Patient may remain hypersensitive to high temperatures for considerable length of time.

COLD INJURIES AND HYPOTHERMIA

Underlying Considerations

1   The extent of injury from exposure to cold is not always known when the patient is seen initially. A frozen extremity appears white, yellow-white or mottled blue-white and is hard, cold and insensitive to touch.
2   Colour changes (purple: cyanosis) after rewarming may be transient *or* they may indicate pressure within the fascial compartment.

Emergency Management

Objective

To restore normal body temperature.

1   Do not allow the patient to walk if lower extremities are involved.
2   Remove all constrictive clothing.
3   Rewarm extremity rapidly in warm-water bath of 32–41°C (90–106°F)—early thawing appears to give better chance for maximum tissue preservation.
   a. Handle part gently to avoid further mechanical injury.
   b. Protect thawed part; do not rupture blebs.
   c. Administer analgesic for pain if necessary—thawing process may be quite painful.
4   Carry out physical examination—to look for concomitant injury (soft tissue injury, fracture, dehydration, alcoholic coma, fat embolism).
5   Restore electrolyte balance; check for acidosis.
6   Give tetanus prophylaxis if indicated by associated trauma.

Hypothermia in the Elderly

Hypothermia in the elderly is a common occurrence in the winter months. The patient, often a woman living alone, sustains a fall or has an acute illness, which immobilizes her in a cold flat or house, unable to get help. It may be a varying length of time before help arrives. By this time, the patient is often dehydrated, undernourished and confused, and may have numerous social problems.

Objective

To restore normal body temperature by gradual warming.

1   Place the trolley in a warm part of the department and remove the patient's clothing. Show care and consideration as the patient is often upset by the state in which she finds herself, but has been unable to prevent.

2 Wash and clean the patient as necessary.
3 Cover with a polythene 'space blanket' which will retain most of the body heat.
4 Place an ordinary blanket on top.
5 Clean mouth if required, check swallowing reflex and administer warm drinks.

In severe cases:

1 Oxygen with artificial respiration may be required.
2 Ventricular fibrillation may be treated by a defibrillator and cardiac massage.
3 If the patient is dehydrated, intravenous fluids will be administered, e.g., 5% dextrose.
4 If necessary a central venous pressure line is established.
5 Hydrocortisone sodium succinate 100–200 mg stat may be given intravenously followed by 100 mg 4 hourly.
6 Antibiotics are given if respiratory infection is present.
7 Catheterization may be necessary to check kidney function.

ANAPHYLACTIC REACTION

Anaphylactic reaction is a sudden, generalized systemic (and frequently fatal) reaction occurring within seconds to minutes after exposure to causative agent, namely, foreign sera, drugs or insect venoms.

Altered Physiology

1 An anaphylactic reaction is the result of an antigen–antibody interaction in a sensitized individual who, as a consequence of previous exposure, has developed a special type of antibody (immunoglobin) that is specific for this particular allergen.
2 The antibody immunoglobulin IgE is responsible for the great majority of immediate type human allergic responses—the individual becomes sensitive to a particular antigen after production of IgE to this antigen.

Causes

Penicillin, sera, other drugs, bee and wasp stings, or almost any repeatedly administered parenteral or oral therapeutic agent.

Clinical Manifestations

1 Diffuse erythema and feeling of warmth (with or without itching).
2 Respiratory difficulty—choking sensation, difficulty in swallowing, tightness or pain in chest, wheezing and shortness of breath, hoarseness, respiratory stridor.
3 Hives on face and upper chest—appear within first few seconds after injection. (With massive facial angio-oedema, expect that upper respiratory oedema may occur.)

4   Severe abdominal cramps, nausea, vomiting, urinary and bowel incontinence.
5   Vascular collapse; cyanosis, pallor, imperceptible pulse—circulatory failure leading to coma and death.

Emergency Management

1   Establish an airway.
   a. Turn face to one side; support angles of mandible.
   b. Insert oropharyngeal or endotracheal tube; apply oropharyngeal suction for excessive secretions.
   c. Employ resuscitative measures (especially for patients with stridor and progressive pulmonary oedema).
   d. If glottic oedema is present, an incision through the cricothyroid ligament will provide an airway.
   e. Use positive pressure oxygen therapy by mask and compression bag.
   f. Use closed chest cardiac massage if necessary.
2   Give epinephrine as directed—to provide rapid relief of hypersensitivity reaction. This should be done while another person is establishing the airway.
   a. Give subcutaneously if not in shock; intravenously if in vascular collapse.
   b. The dosage may be repeated as directed.
   c. Apply tourniquet above injection site if anaphylactic reaction followed injection or insect sting—to delay absorption of the antigen.
   d. Infiltrate injection site with epinephrine as directed.
   e. Remove tourniquet for up to 5 min temporarily every 15–20 min.
3   Give antihistamine drugs, e.g. chlorpheniramine maleate (Piriton) intramuscularly or intravenously if the patient requires adjunctive treatment—useful when asthma is present.
4   Administer hydrocortisone intravenously if the patient is having a prolonged reaction—helpful in preventing later relapses.
5   Give vasopressor agent intravenously under close observation for extreme hypotension. Titrate according to blood pressure.
6   Give aminophylline intravenously *slowly* over a 10-min period; useful for patients with severe bronchospasm and asthmatic symptoms.
7   If patient is convulsing, give intravenous injection of short-acting barbiturate or diazepam (Valium) over several minutes.

Preventive Measures and Health Teaching

1   Be aware of the danger of anaphylactic reactions.
2   Ask about patient's previous allergies to medications; if positive, do not give the medication or injection.
3   Question patient before giving a foreign serum or other type of antigenic agent to determine if he has had it at some earlier time.
4   Question patient concerning previous allergic reactions to food or pollen.
5   Avoid giving drugs to patients with hay fever, asthma and other allergic disorders unless absolutely necessary.
6   Avoid giving parenteral medications unless absolutely necessary; anaphylactic reactions are more likely to occur when therapeutic agent is given parenterally.

7 Do skin testing before administering foreign serum.
   a. Skin testing can precipitate anaphylaxis in highly susceptible individuals.
   b. A negative skin test does not always indicate safety.
   c. Have epinephrine on hand to control acute untoward reactions.
8 If patient is being treated as an outpatient, keep him in office, hospital or clinic at least 30 min after injection of any agent.
9 Caution patients who are sensitive to insect bites to carry first aid kits or kits equipped to treat insect stings. Instruct patient to report any untoward reaction that develops after he leaves the clinic, etc.
10 Encourage allergic individual to wear identification tag.

POISONING

Poison is any substance which when ingested, inhaled, absorbed, applied to the skin or developed within the body, in relatively small amounts, produces injury to the body by its chemical action.

Swallowed Poisons

Objectives of Emergency Treatment

1 To remove or inactivate the poison before it is absorbed.
2 To give supportive care to maintain vital organ systems.
3 To use the specific antidote to neutralize the poison.
4 To give treatment to hasten the elimination of the absorbed poison.

General Aspects of Management

1 Try to discover the nature of the poison. Call the National Poisons Information Service if an unknown toxic agent has been taken or if it is necessary to identify an antidote for a known toxic agent.
2 Maintain the airway.
   a. Administer oxygen for respiratory depression, unconsciousness, cyanosis, shock.
   b. Administer artificial respiration if respiration is depressed; positive expiratory pressure applied to airway may help keep alveoli inflated.
   c. Assess for central nervous system depression.
3 Consider gastric lavage or induce vomiting as the situation dictates. This can be of doubtful value if attempted more than 4 hours after ingestion except for the recovery of salicylates which can be achieved up to 24 hours and tricyclics up to 8 hours.
4 Treat shock appropriately (see p. 160).
5 Support the patient having convulsions; many poisons excite the central nervous system; the patient may convulse because of oxygen deprivation.
6 Give analgesics for pain with caution; severe pain causes vasomotor collapse and reflex inhibition of normal physiologic function.
7 Monitor central venous pressure as indicated.

8   Monitor fluid and electrolyte balance.
9   Reduce elevated temperature.
10 Give specific therapy. Administer special chemical antidote (if indicated) or specific pharmacologic antagonists as early as possible.
11 Provide constant nursing surveillance and attention to the patient in a coma; coma from poisoning results from interference with brain cell function or metabolism.
12 Assist with forced diuresis, haemodialysis or peritoneal dialysis to shorten period of unconsciousness in the event of barbiturate and other hypnotic or tranquillizer poisoning.
13 Assist in securing specimens of blood, urine, stomach contents or vomitus.

Corrosive Poisons

Types of Corrosive Poisons

1   Acid and acid-like corrosives; sodium acid sulphate (toilet bowl cleaners), acetic acid (glacial), sulphuric acid, nitric acid, oxalic acid, hydrofluoric acid (rust removers), iodine, silver nitrate.
2   Alkali corrosives—most common are sodium hydroxide (lysol; drain cleaners), dishwasher detergents, sodium carbonate (washing soda), ammonia water, sodium hypochlorite (household bleach).

Clinical Manifestations

1   Severe pain; burning sensation in mouth and throat.
2   Painful swallowing or inability to swallow.
3   Vomiting.
4   Destruction of oral mucosa.

Nursing Alert: Do not induce vomiting if victim has consumed a strong acid, alkali or other corrosive or hydrocarbon solvent. Do not induce vomiting if patient is in a coma, is unconscious or is having convulsions.

Emergency Management

If the patient can swallow after ingestion of a *corrosive poison*, he may be offered milk as an emollient agent.

Noncorrosive poisons

1   Remove poison from patient's stomach immediately by inducing vomiting. Either:
    a. Induce vomiting by giving ipecacuanha or inserting the index finger or the blunt end of a spoon or spatula on the back of the patient's throat; or
    b. Carry out gastric lavage if less than 4 hours since ingestion, but not if a corrosive substance is involved.
2   A patient who has ingested hydrocarbons should have a chest x-ray done to assess for damage, e.g., chemical pneumonia.
3   Instruct family to bring unused poison to hospital for identification.

Other Common Poisons

Iron

Iron is very dangerous in small children. Desferrioxamine mesylate solution (2 g to 1 l) is used for gastric lavage. A solution of desferrioxamine mesylate 10 g to 50 ml water should be left in the stomach and 2 g given intramuscularly. Desferrioxamine mesylate is a chelating agent rendering the iron harmless.

Paracetamol

Paracetamol can cause liver damage, often fatal, occurring several days after taking as little as 20–30 tablets (10–15 g). It can occur without jaundice. Plasma paracetamol concentrations dictate the amount of antidote to be given, e.g., methionine, acetylcysteine or cysteamine, which all afford protection against liver damage if given within 10–12 hours of ingestion.

Paraquat

Paraquat is a weedkiller and is extremely toxic if taken in the concentrated form. That available for domestic use is usually much weaker. The systemic effects of swallowed concentrated paraquat are painful ulceration of the tongue, lips and fauces within a few hours accompanied by nausea and vomiting. Later convulsions, dyspnoea with pulmonary oedema and acute renal failure may also occur. Obtain a specimen of urine, which should confirm the diagnosis, but a more accurate level of concentration will be shown in the plasma paraquat levels. Gastric lavage is carried out and a solution of Fullers earth and magnesium sulphate is left in the stomach. Oral administration of Fullers earth over a period of 24 hours is continued. In severe cases a forced diuresis combined with charcoal haemoperfusion may also be used.

GUIDELINES: Assisting with Gastric Lavage

Gastric lavage is the aspiration of the stomach contents and washing out of the stomach by means of a gastric tube.

Purposes

1   To remove unabsorbed poison after poison ingestion.
2   To diagnose gastric haemorrhage and for the arrest of haemorrhage.
3   To cleanse the stomach before endoscopic procedures.
4   To remove liquid or small particles of material from the stomach.

Nursing Alert: Gastric lavage is always dangerous, especially after acid or alkali ingestion, in the presence of convulsions or after ingestion of hydrocarbons or petroleum distillates. It is dangerous after ingestion of strong corrosive agents.

Equipment

Stomach tubes (large lumen)
Large irrigating syringe with adapter
Large plastic funnel with adapter to fit stomach tube

Water soluble lubricant
Tap water or appropriate antidote (milk, saline solution, sodium bicarbonate solution, fruit juice, activated charcoal*)
Bucket for aspirate
Mouth gag; nasotracheal or endotracheal tubes with inflatable cuffs
Containers for specimens

Procedure

Action	Reason
1 Remove dental appliances and inspect oral cavity for loose teeth.	
2 Measure the distance between the bridge of the nose and the xiphoid process. Mark with indelible pencil or tape.	
3 Lubricate the tube with water soluble lubricant.	
4 If the patient is comatose he is intubated with a cuffed nasotracheal or endotracheal tube. Have doctor present.	4 A cuffed endotracheal tube prevents aspiration of gastric contents.
5 Place the patient in a left lateral position with the head, neck and trunk forming a straight line. After the lavage tube is passed, the head of the table is lowered. Have standby suction available.	5 This position prevents fluid from running into the trachea and keeps reflux vomitus from being aspirated.
6 Pass the tube via the oral (or nasal) route while keeping the head in a neutral position. Pass the tube to the adhesive marking or about 50 cm (20 in).	6 The depth of insertion of the tube will vary with the height of the patient. If the tube enters the larynx instead of the oesophagus the patient will experience coughing and dyspnoea.
7 Submerge free end of tube below water level at the moment of patient's exhalation.	7 If tube is inadvertently in the lungs, the water will bubble with each exhalation.
8 Aspirate the stomach contents with syringe attached to the tube before instilling water or antidote. Save the specimen for analysis.	8 Aspiration is carried out to remove the stomach contents.
9 Remove syringe. Attach funnel to the stomach tube or use 50-ml	9 Overfilling of the stomach may cause regurgitation and aspiration

---

* Activated charcoal will absorb significant quantities of many drugs and chemicals and thus retards absorption from the gastrointestinal tract.

Action	Reason
syringe to put lavage solution in gastric tube. Volume of fluid placed in the stomach should be small.	or force the stomach contents through the pylorus.
10 Elevate funnel above the patient's head and pour approximately 120–300 ml of solution into funnel.	10 If the syringe method is used, the turbulence from the pressure of the syringe will cause the fluid to mix with the stomach contents and assist in washing all of the mucosal surface. It is possible for poison/drugs to be trapped in the rugae of stomach.
11 Lower the funnel and siphon the gastric contents into the bucket.	
12 Save samples of first two washings.	12 Keep first washings isolated from other washings for possible analysis.
13 Repeat lavage procedure until the returns are relatively clear.	
14 At the completion of lavage: **a.** Stomach may be left empty. **b.** Antidote may be instilled in tube and allowed to remain in stomach. **c.** Aperient may be put down tube.	
15 Pinch off tube during removal or maintain suction while tube is being withdrawn.	15 Pinching off the tube prevents aspiration and the initiation of the vomiting reflex. Keeping the patient's head lower than the body also gives this protection.
16 Give the patient an aperient if ordered.	16 An aperient may be given if the poison has no corrosive action on the bowel. The aperient will help remove unabsorbed material from the intestine.

Inhaled Poisons

Carbon Monoxide Poisoning

May occur as an industrial or household accident or as an attempted suicide.

Underlying Principles

1 The effect of carbon monoxide is to render the haemoglobin useless as an oxygen-carrying chemical, because it unites so firmly with the pigment in place of oxygen. As a result, tissue anoxia occurs.

2   Carbon monoxide causes damage by hypoxia:
   a. Patient may appear intoxicated (result of cerebral hypoxia).
   b. Skin may be cherry red or cyanotic and pale—skin colour is *not* a reliable sign.
3   History of exposure to carbon monoxide should justify immediate treatment.

Emergency Management

Objectives

To reverse cerebral and myocardial hypoxia.
To hasten carbon monoxide elimination.

1   Give 100% oxygen at atmospheric or hyperbaric pressures to reverse hypoxia and accelerate elimination of carbon monoxide.
2   Observe the patient constantly—psychoses, spastic paralysis, visual disturbances and deterioration of personality may persist following resuscitation and may be symptoms of permanent central nervous system damage.

Skin Contamination Poisons

Emergency Management

1   Drench skin with water (shower, hose).
2   Apply stream of water on skin while removing clothing.
3   Cleanse skin thoroughly with water; rapidity in washing is most important in reducing extent of injury.

Injected Poisons

Stinging Insects

Bee, hornet, wasp.

Nursing Alert: A patient may have an extreme sensitivity to *Hymenoptera* stings (bees, hornets, wasps). This constitutes an acute emergency. Stings of the head and neck are especially serious although stings in any area of the body can result in anaphylaxis.

Clinical Manifestations

Anaphylactic shock (p. 183).

1   Severe fall in blood pressure.
2   Difficult breathing.
3   Oedema of face, lips.
4   Urticaria.
5   Itching.
6   Bronchial constriction.
7   Diarrhoea, abdominal cramps.

Emergency Management and Health Teaching

1 Give epinephrine as requested.
2 See p. 183 for treatment of anaphylactic shock.
3 Patients known to be sensitive to *Hymenoptera* venom should carry an emergency kit with tourniquet, epinephrine, syringe and needles, an aerosol inhalator containing epinephrine and oral antihistamine tablets.
   a. Instruct the patient to take epinephrine immediately if he is stung.
   b. Flick stinger off with the fingernail, if possible.
   c. Do not squeeze venom sac—may cause additional venom to be injected.
4 Instruct the patient to avoid the following:
   a. Localities with stinging insects (camp and picnic sites).
   b. Going barefoot outdoors—some insects may nest on ground.
   c. Perfumes and bright colours—attract bees.

Snake Bite

Snake bites are fairly uncommon in the UK. The adder is the only poisonous snake native to the British Isles. Snake venoms are complex poisons. The toxic effects of snake venoms include agitation, restlessness, abdominal colic, diarrhoea and vomiting. In the UK each region has a special hospital designated to store snake antivenom. Advice should be sought from these hospitals regarding treatment and care.

The most common snake to be found is the grass snake, the bite of which is harmless, except for the local effects which include a mild inflammatory reaction with pain swelling.

1 The patient should be laid on a trolley. Reassure—victims of snake bites are extremely frightened individuals.
2 Ask the patient to describe the snake in detail if possible.
3 Examine the site of the bite—usually the ankle or hand and it usually consists of two puncture marks.
4 Record temperature, pulse, respiration and blood pressure.
5 Clean the site of the bite.
6 Give antitetanus toxoid.
7 If the snake is known to be a grass snake, the patient can be discharged. If the snake was unidentified, the patient is usually admitted overnight for observation.

Food Poisoning

Food poisoning is a sudden, explosive illness which may occur after ingestion of contaminated food or drink.*

Emergency Management

1 Determine the source and type of food poisoning.
   a. Have family bring suspected food to medical facility.

* Botulism, a serious form of food poisoning, is discussed on p. 241 since the treatment differs and the patient requires continuing surveillance.

b. Take the history:
  (1) How soon after eating did the symptoms occur? Immediate onset suggests chemical, plant or animal poisoning.
  (2) What was eaten in the previous meal? Did the food have any unusual odour or taste?—Most foods causing bacterial poisoning do not have unusual odour or taste.
  (3) Did vomiting occur? What was the appearance of the vomit?
  (4) Did diarrhoea occur?—Usually absent with botulism, shellfish or other fish poisoning.
  (5) Are any neurologic symptoms present?—Occur in botulism, chemical, plant and animal poisoning.
  (6) Does the patient have fever?—Seen in salmonella, favism (ingestion of fava beans) and some fish poisoning.
  (7) What is the patient's appearance?
2 Monitor vital signs on a continuing basis.
   a. Assess respiration, blood pressure, central venous pressure (if indicated), and muscular activity.
   b. Weigh the patient for future comparisons.
3 Support the respiratory system. Death from respiratory paralysis can occur with botulism, fish poisoning, etc.
4 Maintain fluid and electrolyte balance—electrolytes and water are lost as a result of vomiting and diarrhoea.
   a. Watch for oligaemic shock—from severe fluid and electrolyte losses.
   b. Assess for apathy, rapid pulse, fever, oliguria, anuria, hypotension, delirium.
   c. Carry out blood electrolyte studies—sodium, potassium, chloride, arterial blood gas determinations, pH, carbon dioxide.
   d. Get stool specimen for culture and sensitivity and for ova and parasite tests if indicated.
5 Correct and control hypoglycaemia.
6 Control the nausea.
   a. Give sips of weak tea, carbonated drinks, tap water for mild nausea.
   b. Give clear liquids 12–24 hours after nausea and vomiting subside.
   c. Graduate to a low residue bland diet.
7 Control the diarrhoea—diarrhoea may be desirable to rid body of ingested toxins.
   a. Give atropine, meperidine (Pethidine) or codeine as ordered.
   b. Apply warm compresses and moist, mild heat to abdomen—for comfort.
   c. Give antidiarrhoeal agents as ordered—to absorb and bind toxins.

DRUG ABUSE

Drug abuse is the use of drugs for other than legitimate medical purposes. The clinical manifestations may vary with the drug used but the underlying principles of management are essentially the same. Adopt a supportive, empathetic and realistic relationship with the patient.

Acute Drug Reaction

Priorities

1 Maintain adequate airway.
2 Support respiration.
3 Correct hypotension.

Emergency Management

1 Maintain the patient's respirations.
   a. Use a cuffed endotracheal tube and provide assisted ventilation in a severely depressed patient with absent vomit or cough reflexes.
   b. Measure arterial blood gases—for hypoxia due to hypoventilation, acid-base derangements, etc.
   c. Give narcotic antagonist if indicated.
2 Remove the drug from the stomach as soon as possible (if drug has been ingested).
   a. Induce vomiting if patient is seen *early* after ingestion.
   b. Use gastric lavage if the patient is unconscious or if there is no way to determine when the drug was ingested.
      (1) In patients with absent vomit or cough reflexes, carry out this procedure only after intubation with cuffed endotracheal tube to prevent aspiration of stomach contents.
      (2) Activated charcoal may be useful adjunct to therapy and is used after vomiting or lavage.
3 Consider haemodialysis or peritoneal dialysis for potentially lethal poisoning.
4 Try to maintain a free flow of urine since the drug or metabolites are excreted by the kidneys.
5 Do a thorough physical examination to rule out insulin shock, meningitis, sub-dural haematoma, stroke, trauma.
   a. Look for needle marks, constricted pupils.
   b. There is a high incidence of infectious hepatitis among drug users which is thought to be the result of communal use of nonsterile needles and syringes.
   c. Keep in mind that many drug users take numerous drugs at one time.
   d. Examine breath for characteristic odour of alcohol, acetone, etc.
   e. Start ECG monitoring if indicated.
6 Try to obtain a history of the drug experiences (from the person accompanying the patient or from the patient himself).
   a. Do not leave the patient alone.

Narcotic Abuse

Examples

Heroin (most frequently involved)
Morphine, codeine, synthetic narcotics (methadone)

Clinical Manifestations

Acute Intoxication

1 Coma.
2 Pinpoint pupils.
3 Cool, damp skin with cyanotic hue.
4 Severe respiratory depression.
5 Fresh needle marks along course of superficial veins; scarred veins.

Emergency Management

1 Maintain respiration.
  a. Give mouth-to-mouth resuscitation; then establish intubation and assisted ventilation.
  b. Have second person listen with stethoscope for breath sounds over both lung fields.
  c. Maintain circulation; use external cardiac compression.
2 Give narcotic antagonist (naloxone hydrochloride [Narcan]) to reverse severe respiratory depression and coma.
3 Continue to monitor the level of responsiveness and respirations, pulse and blood pressure—duration of action of naloxone hydrochloride (Narcan) is shorter than that of heroin, etc., and repeated dose(s) may be necessary.
  Do not leave patient alone—may lapse back into coma rapidly.
4 An intravenous line will be established.
  Patient may be given a bolus of 50% glucose to eliminate possibility of hypoglycaemia.
5 Send urine to laboratory for analysis—opiates can be detected in urine.
6 Secure blood for chemical and toxicologic analysis; also for baseline studies and blood gases.
7 Secure an ECG.

Heroin Withdrawal Syndrome

Clinical Manifestations

1 Lethargy; yawning.
2 Perspiration, lacrimation, runny nose.
3 Dilated pupils, poorly reactive to light.
4 Gooseflesh, muscular aches.
5 Twitching, anorexia, nausea, vomiting, abdominal pain.
6 Chills and fever.

Management

1 Methadone may be ordered if patient is receiving treatment at a methadone centre, or substitution therapy should be given in the hospital centre.
2 Give intravenous fluids since patient is dehydrated from vomiting; may progress to toxic delirium.
3 Assess for concomitant medical problems (hepatitis, pneumonia, severe diarrhoea).
4 Place patient in protected environment under proper medical supervision.

5 Make every effort to enroll patient in a narcotics treatment programme—to intervene in a life-style that fosters addiction.

Hallucinogens or Psychedelic-type Drugs

Common Forms

1 Lysergic acid diethylamide (LSD).
2 Phencyclidine HCl (PCP); called PeaCe, Pill, Hog.

Clinical Manifestations

1 Marked anxiety bordering on panic.
2 Confusion, incoherence, hyperactivity.
3 Hallucinations.
4 Hazardous behaviour (delirium, mania, self-injury).
5 Flashback—recurrence of LSD-like state; may occur weeks or months after drug was taken.
6 Convulsions, coma, circulatory collapse, death.

Emergency Management

1 Determine if patient has ingested hallucinogenic drug or has a toxic psychosis.
2 Try to communicate with the patient—use 'vocal anaesthesia' to reassure him.
   a. 'Talking down' involves understanding the process through which the patient is proceeding and helping him overcome his fears while establishing contact with reality.
   b. Remind the patient that fear is common with this problem.
   c. Reassure the patient that he is not losing his mind; that he is experiencing the effect of drugs and that this will wear off.
   d. Instruct the patient to keep his eyes open—reduces intensity of reaction.
   e. Do not leave the patient alone.
3 Sedate the patient if his hyperactivity cannot be controlled—diazepam (Valium); or a barbiturate may be given.
4 Search for evidences of trauma—hallucinogenic users have a tendency to 'act out' their hallucinations.
5 Manage convulsions; place patient in intensive care unit.
6 Watch patient closely—his behaviour may become hazardous.
7 Monitor for hypertensive crisis if patient has prolonged psychosis due to drug ingestion.
8 Place patient in a protected environment under proper medical supervision to prevent self-inflicted bodily harm.

Amphetamine-type Drugs

Pep pills, 'uppers', 'speed'.

Examples

Amphetamine (Benzedrine)

Dextroamphetamine (Dexedrine)
Methamphetamine (Desoxyn)

Clinical Manifestations

Abrupt or Insidious Development of Behavioural Disturbances

1   Aggressive type of behaviour.
2   Visual misperceptions; auditory hallucinations.
3   Irritability, insomnia.
4   Fearful anxiety/depression; cold, distant hostility.
5   Hyperactivity, stereotyped activities; rapid speech, euphoria.
6   Paranoid suspiciousness.
7   Increasing pulse rate and blood pressure.
8   Hallucinosis; high temperature.
9   Convulsions → coma → death.

Emergency Management

1   Try to communicate with patient—amphetamine paranoid psychosis is frequently seen.
      Patient may have delusions of persecution, ideas of reference, visual and auditory hallucinations, changes in body image, hyperactivity, excitation.
2   Use specific drug therapy to alleviate agitative state.
      a. Usually within 24 hours after last dose of amphetamine patient will begin to spend increasing amounts of time sleeping.
      b. Keep patient relatively quiet and reassured; patient may become aggressive/assaultive and reach a state of panic.
3   Carry out urine checks for amphetamines.
4   Place patient in protective environment—observe for suicidal attempts.
      a. Use techniques of dealing with acutely paranoid individuals; do not move close to patient.
      b. Avoid confined spaces; refer to psychiatric nursing textbook.

Barbiturates—Acute Intoxication

Examples

Pentobarbitone sodium (Nembutal)
Quinalbarbitone sodium (Seconal)
Amylobarbitone sodium (Sodium amytal)

Clinical Manifestations

Barbiturates depress cardiovascular and pulmonary systems.

1   Flushed face.
2   Decreased pulse rate.
3   Increasing nystagmus.
4   Decreasing tendon reflexes.
5   Decreasing mental alertness.

6   Difficulty in speaking.
7   Poor motor co-ordination.
8   Mental confusion.
9   Coma, death.

Emergency Management

1   If patient is not unconscious and is admitted within 4 hours of having ingested barbiturates, attempt gastric lavage.
2   If drowsy, maintain airway and stimulate depressed respirations.
      Consider endotracheal intubation or tracheotomy if there is any doubt about the adequacy of airway exchange.
3   Support cardiovascular and respiratory functions.
4   An intravenous infusion is commenced through large gauge needle or intravenous catheter to support blood pressure—coma and dehydration result in hypotension and respond to infusion of intravenous fluids with elevation of blood pressure.
5   Carry out physical and neurological examinations.
6   Maintain neurological and vital signs and record on observation chart.
7   Blood is taken to estimate serum barbiturate levels.
8   Patient awakening from overdose may demonstrate hostility; this can stimulate automatic angry responses by health personnel.

Barbiturate Withdrawal Syndrome

Clinical Manifestations

1   Shakiness, anxiety, muscular irritability.
2   Orthostatic hypotension (hypotension caused by being in the upright position), tachycardia.
3   Grand mal convulsions, hyperpyrexia.
4   Possible death.

Nursing Alert: Symptoms of barbiturate withdrawal are serious because abrupt withdrawal from the drug may be life-threatening.

Emergency Management

1   Maintain airway and stimulate depressed respiration.
2   Administer phenobarbitone according to level of patient's tolerance.
3   Give oxygen and intravenous fluids as required.
4   Gradually reduce dosage of barbiturates.
5   Watch for excessive agitation, confusion and convulsions.

Nonbarbiturate Sedatives

Examples

Glutethimide (Doriden)
Meprobamate (Equanil)

Chlordiazepoxide (Librium)
Diazepam (Valium)

Clinical Manifestations

1   Decreasing mental alertness.
2   Confusion.
3   Slurred speech.
4   Ataxia.
5   Pulmonary Oedema.
6   Coma, possible death.

Management

On the whole, these drugs do not produce severe side effects.

1   Maintain a clear airway.
2   Allow patient to rest until consciousness returns.

Salicylate Poisoning (Aspirin)

Clinical Manifestations

1   Abdominal pain, haematemesis (early).
2   Late signs and symptoms:
   a. Hyperpnoea (rapid breathing).
   b. Disturbed acid-base balance.
   c. Tinnitus and vertigo.
   d. Mental aberrations.
   e. Hyperventilation.
   f. Convulsions; coma.
   g. Sweating.

Emergency Management

1   Treat respiratory depression.
2   Carry out gastric lavage—will remove significant amounts of salicylates up to 24 hours following ingestion.
3   Give water, milk or activated charcoal—to delay absorption of ingested poison after vomiting or lavage.
4   Blood is taken for plasma salicylate levels, pH and electrolytes.
5   Support patient with intravenous infusions to correct electrolyte imbalance and maintain hydration.
6   Correct acid-base disturbances (sodium bicarbonate or sodium lactate, potassium, etc.).
7   Administer blood transfusion if indicated.
8   Prepare for peritoneal dialysis or haemodialysis for patients with severe intoxication.
9   Give vitamin K for bleeding—salicylates lower plasma prothrombin by interfering with vitamin K utilization in the liver.

ALCOHOLISM

Acute Alcoholism

Clinical Manifestations

Caused by depressant action of alcohol on nervous system.

1 Drowsiness, inco-ordination, slurring of speech—or
2 Belligerency, grandiosity, uninhibited behaviour.
3 Odour of alcohol on breath.
4 Blood alcohol concentration.

Emergency Management

1 Approach the patient in a nonjudgemental manner. (Alcoholic patients have a tendency to stimulate rejecting behaviour in health care personnel.)
   a. Expect patient to use mechanisms of denial and defensiveness.
   b. Adapt a firm, consistent, accepting and reasonable attitude.
   c. Speak calmly.
   d. If patient appears drunk, he is probably drunk even though he denies any alcohol intake.
   e. Take a blood alcohol test as directed.
2 Allow the drowsy patient to 'sleep off' the state of alcoholic intoxication.
   a. Observe for symptoms of respiratory depression.
   b. Protect the airway.
   c. Undress the patient and cover with a blanket.
3 Sedate the belligerant, noisy patient as directed. Monitor the patient carefully.
4 Examine the patient for injuries and organic disease which can easily be masked by alcoholic intoxication; alcoholics suffer more injuries than the general population.
   a. Look for symptoms of head injury. Assess the neurologic status of the patient.
   b. Assess for alcoholic coma—a medical emergency.
   c. Evaluate for pneumonia, which is common in alcoholic individuals.
   d. Watch for hypoglycaemia.
5 Hospitalize if necessary.

Delirium Tremens (Alcoholic Hallucinosis)

Delirium tremens is an acute psychotic state that follows a prolonged bout of steady drinking or diminution or cessation of alcoholic intake.

Clinical Manifestations

1 Anxiety; uncontrollable fear.
2 Tremulousness, restlessness and agitation, irritability, insomnia.
3 Talkativeness; preoccupation.

4   Visual, tactile and auditory hallucinations (usually of a frightening nature).
5   Autonomic overactivity—tachycardia, profuse perspiration, fever.

Nursing Alert: Delirium tremens is a serious complication and poses a threat to the life of the alcoholic patient.

Emergency Management

Objective

To give proper sedation to enable the patient to rest and recover without the danger of injury or exhaustion.

1   Take the blood pressure since the patient's subsequent medication may depend on his blood pressure readings.
2   Carry out physical examination to identify pre-existing or contributing illnesses or injuries (cerebral injury, pneumonia, etc.).
3   Sedate the patient with sufficient dosage of medication to produce adequate sedation—to reduce his agitation, prevent exhaustion and promote sleep.
    a. A variety of drugs and combinations of drugs are used—chloral hydrate, diazepam (Valium), etc.
    b. The dosage may be adjusted according to the patient's blood pressure response.
4   Place the patient in a private room where he can be observed closely.
    a. Keep room lighted—to reduce incidence of visual hallucinations.
    b. Observe patient closely—he may become homicidal or suicidal in response to his hallucinations if he is having alcoholic hallucinations.
    c. Have someone stay with the patient as much as possible—presence of another person has a reassuring and quieting effect.
    d. Explain every procedure done to the patient in detail.
    e. Explain visual misinterpretations (illusions)—strengthens link with reality.
    f. Use restraints if patient is not under direct and constant observation.
5   Maintain electrolyte balance and hydration via oral or intravenous route—fluid losses may be extreme because of profuse perspiration and agitation.
6   Record temperature, pulse, respiration and blood pressure frequently (every 30 min in severe forms of delirium)—in anticipation of peripheral circulatory collapse and/or hyperthermia (the two most common lethal complications).
7   Administer phenytoin sodium (Dilantin) or other anticonvulsant drugs as prescribed to prevent or control alcoholic or epileptic convulsions.
8   Assess respiratory, hepatic and cardiovascular status of patient—pneumonia, liver disease and cardiac failure are complications.
    a. Hypoglycaemia may accompany alcoholic withdrawal because of depletion of liver glycogen stores and possible liver impairment.
    b. Administer parenteral dextrose if liver glycogen is depleted.
9   Give supplemental vitamin therapy and a high protein diet; these patients are usually vitamin deficient.
10 Refer to alcoholic treatment centre for subsequent follow-up and rehabilitation.

PSYCHIATRIC EMERGENCY

Psychiatric emergency is a sudden serious disturbance of behaviour, affect or thought which makes the patient unable to cope with his life situation and interpersonal relationships.

Behavioural Manifestations

Overactive

1 Disturbed, unco-operative, unpredictable paranoid behaviour.
2 Anxiety and panic-like state.
3 Assaultive and destructive impulses and behaviour (patient may be noisy or disturbed from acute alcohol or drug intoxication).
4 Crying, depression, intense nervousness.

Underactive

1 Depression.
2 Fearfulness, detached attitude.
3 Slowing of responses.
4 Sad facial expression.

Suicidal

Emergency Management

Overactive

1 Determine (from family, ambulance driver, etc.) if patient has had past mental illness, hospitalizations, injuries or serious illnesses, uses alcohol or drugs, or has experienced crises in interpersonal relationships or intrapsychic conflicts.
2 Try to gain control of the situation.
   a. Introduce yourself by name to the patient.
   b. Tell him "I am here to help you".
   c. Repeat patient's name from time to time.
   d. Speak in one-thought sentences. Be consistent.
   e. Give the individual space. Let him slow down by himself and allow him to become compliant.
   f. Approach the patient with a calm, confident and firm manner—this attitude is therapeutic and will help calm the patient.
   g. Be interested in and listen to the patient—encourage him to talk of his thoughts and *feelings*.
   h. Offer appropriate explanations. Tell the truth.
3 Give tranquillizer or psychotropic agent for emergency management of functional psychosis. Chlorpromazine (Largactil) or haloperidol (Haldol) acts specifically against psychotic symptoms of thought fragmentation and perceptual and behavioural aberrations.
   a. Initial dosage depends on body weight and severity of symptoms.
   b. Observe patient for 1 hour after initial dose to determine degree of change in psychotic behaviour.

c. Subsequent dosages depend on patient's reaction.
d. If behaviour is caused by hallucinogens (LSD, etc.) psychotropic drugs (exerting an effect on the mind) are not used.
4   Use restraints only as a last resort.
5   Admit to psychiatric unit or arrange for psychiatric outpatient treatment.

Underactive

1   Listen to the patient in a calm, unhurried manner—offer follow-up services.
2   Give antidepressants with antianxiety agents.
3   Attempt to find out if patient has thought about or attempted suicide.
4   Anticipate that the patient may be suicidal.
5   Notify relatives about a seriously depressed patient.
6   Refer patient to hospital psychiatric unit.

Suicidal

Suicide is an act that stems from depression (from illness, loss of a loved one, loss of body integrity or status).

1   Treat the emergency condition brought about by the suicide attempt (gunshot wound, lacerations, overdose, etc.).
2   Prevent further self-injury—a patient who has made a suicidal gesture may do so again.
3   Admit to intensive care unit (if condition warrants) or psychiatric unit.

SEXUAL ASSAULT

Rape is sexual attack on any unwilling victim. The patient should be seen immediately upon entrance into the emergency department.

Emergency Management

Objectives

To give sympathetic support.
To reduce the emotional trauma of the patient.

1   Respect the privacy and sensitivity of the patient; be kind and supportive.
    a. The manner in which the patient is received and treated in the emergency department is important to the future psychological well-being of the patient. Crisis intervention should begin when the patient enters the department.
        (1) Emotional trauma may be present for weeks, months, years. Patient may go through phases of psychologic reactions:
            (a) Phase of disorganization—fear, guilt, humility, anger, self-blame.
            (b) Phase of resolution (putting incident into perspective)—may have sleep disturbances, phobias, sexual fears.
        (2) Reassure patient that anxiety is natural and that appropriate support is available from professional and community resources.
    b. Accept the emotional reactions of patient (hysteria, stoicism, overwhelmed feeling, etc.).

2   Leave clothing undisturbed. The police should be informed if the patient consents. A police surgeon is sent, accompanied by a policewoman.
3   Assist with the physical examination.
   a. Secure informed consent from patient (or parent/guardian if patient is a minor) for examination and for the taking of photographs if necessary—may be used as legal evidence.
   b. Take history *only* if patient has not already talked to police officer, social worker, crisis intervention worker, etc. Do not ask the patient to repeat the history.
   c. Record general appearance of patient—evidence of bruises, lacerations, secretions, torn and bloody clothing.
   d. Record emotional state.
   e. Assist patient to undress. Drape properly. Save clothing; place in plastic bag, label appropriately and give to proper law enforcement authorities. Do not wash the patient until she has been seen by the police surgeon.
   f. Assist with vaginal examination.
      (1) Use water-moistened vaginal speculum for examination; do not use lubricant.
      (2) Assist with securing laboratory specimens:
         (a) Swab from vaginal pool for acid phosphatase, blood group antigen of semen, and precipitin tests against human sperm and blood.
         (b) Secure wet mount of material from fornix—examined immediately for motile sperm.
         (c) Obtain separate smears from vulva.
         (d) Obtain culture of body orifices for gonorrhoea.
         (e) Carry out tests for sexually transmitted disease.
         (f) Conduct test for pregnancy if there is question that patient may be pregnant.
         (g) Collect the following if indicated:
            (1) Oral and rectal swabs and smears.
            (2) Clipped pubic hairs or combings.
            (3) Fingernail scrapings.
            (4) Photographs.
4   Treat associated injuries as indicated.
5   Give patient option of prophylaxis against venereal disease.
   a. Probenecid orally, followed in 30 min by intramuscular penicillin.
   b. Patient with allergy to penicillin may receive alternate therapy which may not be effective in treatment of incubating syphilis; patient should have a serology check in 6 weeks.
6   Offer antipregnancy measures if patient is of childbearing age, is using no contraceptives, and is at high risk in menstrual cycle.
   a. Hormonal therapy—oral stilboestrol or ethyloestradiol if given within 48 hours of coitus for 5 days renders endometrium inhospitable for implantation; usually effective in preventing pregnancy following unprotected intercourse.
   b. Advise patient of possible occurrence of side effects (nausea, vomiting).
   c. Inform patient that if she misses a menstrual period she has the option of having menstrual extraction or abortion.
7   Offer cleansing douche if patient desires.

8   Provide for follow-up services:
    a. Make appointment for follow-up surveillance for pregnancy and venereal disease.
    b. Encourage patient to return to previous level of functioning as soon as possible.
    c. Inform patient of counselling services to prevent long-term psychologic effects.
    d. Patient should be accompanied by family/friend when leaving department.

NURSING IN DISASTER CONDITIONS

A *disaster* is a catastrophe which may be either natural of man-made in origin—produced either accidently or by design.

Nursing Functions in Disasters

Since the nurse is delegated greater responsibilities in emergency and disaster situations, when mass casualties occur, nursing functions at such times may include:

1   Administering first aid such as artificial ventilation, cardiopulmonary resuscitation including defibrillation (if equipment is available), drug administration, intubation, the use of mechanical ventilators, maintenance of a patent airway, intratracheal catheterization and emergency tracheotomy.
2   Controlling haemorrhage.
3   Treating shock.
4   Recognizing trauma to any organ or system.
5   Showing a proficiency in intravenous techniques—in the use of equipment, fluids, medications, and central venous pressure measurements.
6   Properly and adequately cleansing and treating wounds, including closure of uncomplicated wounds.
7   Recognizing common fractures; bandaging and splinting.
8   Administering anaesthetics under medical supervision.
9   Assisting in surgical procedures.
10 Inserting nasogastric tubes for purposes of lavage and feeding.
11 Assessing the presence or absence of physiological and pathological reflexes in determining the degree of trauma to the central nervous system.
12 Catheterizing males and females.
13 Administering immunizing agents as directed.
14 Recognizing life-threatening conditions in their early stages—acute pulmonary oedema, respiratory complications, gastrointestinal bleeding, etc.
15 Managing psychiatric emergencies. Managing psychologically disturbed persons.
16 Managing normal deliveries.

Sorting (triage)

The sorting of casualties (also called *triage*) involves placing patients in categories for treatment on the basis of diagnosis and prognosis.

1 Sorting is a continuous process.
2 The most responsible and able persons of the medical team are assigned sorting responsibilities.

Classification for Priority in Treatment

1 *Minimal treatment*—patients who can be returned to active duty immediately.
2 *Immediate treatment*—patients for whom the available expedient procedures will save life or limb.
3 *Delayed treatment*—patients who, after emergency treatment, will incur little increased risk by having surgery withheld temporarily.
4 *Expectant treatment*—critically injured patients who will be given treatment if time and facilities are available.

Priorities of Treatment

The following is a priority schedule which serves as a guide for establishing the flow of casualties from the disaster area through the first aid station to forward treatment centre and hospital.

First Priority (individuals needing immediate attention to save life)

1 Any wound interfering with airway or causing airway obstruction. (This includes sucking chest wounds, tension pneumothorax and maxillofacial wounds in which asphyxia is present or an impending threat.)
2 Any wound requiring immediate pressure.
3 Shock due to major haemorrhage, to wounds of any organ system, fractures, etc. (some of these conditions may be so urgent that immediate lifesaving measures will have to be taken by the person doing the sorting).

Second Priority (individuals needing early surgery)

1 Visceral injuries, including perforations of the gastrointestinal tract; wounds of the biliary and pancreatic system; wounds of the genitourinary tract; and thoracic wounds without asphyxia.
2 Vascular injuries requiring repair. All injuries which require the use of a tourniquet fall into this group.
3 Closed cerebral injuries with increasing loss of consciousness.

Third Priority (patients who require surgery but can tolerate a delay)

1 Spinal injuries in which decompression is required.
2 Soft-tissue wounds in which debridement is necessary, but in which muscle damage is less than major.
3 Lesser fractures and dislocations.
4 Injuries of the eyes.
5 Maxillofacial injuries without asphyxia.

Identification of Casualties

1 Identification is done by an emergency medical tag.
2 Place the tag directly on the body, perferably the wrist; do not attach to clothing since it may be lost.

3 Tags are written out by a clerk who accompanies the sorting officer; clerk completes admission records, clinical records and emergency tags.
4 The following abbreviations are used on the tag:
  T—tourniquet case (add time of application).
  M—morphine given (add time and date).

FURTHER READING

Books

Bradley, D (1980) Accident and Emergency Nursing, Baillière Tindall
Hardy, R H (1981) Accidents and Emergencies: a practical handbook for personal use, 3rd edition, Oxford University Press
Huckstep, R (1978) A Simple Guide to Trauma, 2nd edition, Churchill Livingstone
Jennett, B (1977) An Introduction to Neurosurgery, 3rd edition, Heinemann
Matthew, H and Lawson, A A H (1979) Treatment of Common Acute Poisonings Churchill Livingstone
Mouzas, G L (1979) A Handbook for the Accident and Emergency Department, Heinemann
Muckle, D S (1978) Injuries in Sport, John Wright
Muir, I P K and Barclay, T L (1974) Burns and Their Treatment, Lloyd Luke
Powley, P (1973) Trauma Surgery, John Wright
Skeet, M (Ed) (1981) Emergency Procedures and First Aid for Nurses, Blackwell Scientific
Vale, J A and Meredith, T J (1981) Poisoning Diagnosis and Treatment, Update Books
Wagner, M M (1981) Care of the Burn–Injured Patient, Croome Helm
Wilson, F (1981) Essential Accident and Emergency Care, MTP

Articles

Bradley, D (1981) A learners pull-out guide to the Accident and Emergency Dept, Nursing Times, 77.
British Medical Journal (1981) Inhaled foreign bodies, British Medical Journal, 282: 1694–1650
Jackson, R H (1981) Pictures in Nursing—accidents can happen, Nursing, 24: 1004–47
Lancet (1981) Overdose—will psychiatrist see please? Lancet, 1: 195–196
Lewis, B and Bradbury, Y (1981) Accident and Emergency. Why patients choose A and E, Health and Social Services Journal, 1137–1142
Practitioner (1979) Accidents
Puxan, M (1982) Rape, Practitioner, 226: 296
Wilton, G (1981) Accident and emergency patching up in Balfast, Health and Social Services Journal, 91: 1143–1147

Chapter 6

COMMUNICABLE DISEASES

Communicable diseases are those which are spread (a) from person to person, either directly or indirectly, (b) from animal to person and (c) from insect to person. A sporadic outbreak of a disease is one which occurs in scattered, isolated cases. An epidemic is an outbreak of many cases of the same illness in one area. A pandemic outbreak is a series of epidemics throughout the world. An endemic illness is one which constantly occurs in one area.

THE INFECTION PROCESS

Causative Agent

1 Bacterial (includes cocci, bacilli and spirilla).
2 Viral.
3 Rickettsial.
4 Protozoal.
5 Fungal.
6 Helminthic (worm infestations).

Reservoir (the environment in which the agent is found)

1 Human—man is the reservoir of diseases that are more dangerous to humans than to other species.
2 Animal—responsible for infestations due to trophozoites and worms, for carrying external parasites.
3 Nonanimal—dust, garden soil.

Mode of Escape from the Reservoir

1 From the respiratory tract (most common in man).
2 From the intestinal tract.
3 From the genitourinary tract.
4 From open lesions.
5 Mechanical escape (includes bites of insects).

Mode of Transmission to the Next Host

1 By contact route.
   a. Direct contact.

    b. Indirect contact.

    c. Droplet spread.

2 By vehicle route.

    a. Contaminated food—salmonella.

    b. Water—shigellosis.

    c. Drugs—pseudomonas infections from ophthalmic ointments and from lotions.

    d. Blood—hepatitis.

3 Airborne.

    a. Residue of evaporated droplets that remain suspended in the air.

    b. Dust particles

4 Vector borne.

      Mosquito—malaria.

Mode of Entry of Organisms into Human Body

1 Respiratory tract.
2 Gastrointestinal tract.
3 Direct infection of mucous membranes.
4 Break in the skin.

Susceptible Host

Illness following entrance of infection into the body depends on:

1   Age of host.
2   Absent or abnormal immunoglobulins.
3   Depletion or impairment of T-lymphocyte function.
4   Presence of leucopenia; efficiency of reticulo-endothelial system.
5   Presence of underlying disease.
6   Administration of steroids, radiation or antibiotics may influence the response of the host to infection.
7   Dosage and virulence of the organisms, also the length of exposure.
8   Inherent susceptibility.
9   Nutritional status, fitness, environmental factors.
10 Individual's general physical, mental and emotional status.

Emerging Problems in Communicable Diseases

1 Increase in number of different organisms that are developing resistance to increasing numbers of available antibiotics.
2 Increasing number of travellers from foreign countries, holdiay makers, business men and also immigrants, who may have been in contact with a disease, which may be incubating, but not producing any signs or symptoms until they reach their home country.
3 Increasing number of persons in a state of immunosuppression. These persons, who have been treated for some forms of cancer, or who have received organ transplants, are now surviving from the illness, but are susceptible to invasion by any type of organism, including those usually considered non-pathogenic.

CONTROL AND MANAGEMENT OF COMMUNICABLE DISEASES

Statutory Notification

1 The majority of communicable diseases are compulsorily notifiable to the 'proper officer', this is a doctor on the staff of the area health authority who has been nominated for this purpose. He may be the District Community Physician, or the Area Specialist in Community Medicine (Environmental Health)

2 The responsibility for notification rests upon the doctor who first diagnoses the illness, either the general practitioner or the hospital medical officer.

3 Weekly returns are made by the Medical Officer of Environmental Health (MOEH) to the Registrar General, who publishes a weekly report.

4 Yearly reports are published by the Chief Medical Officer of the Department of Health and Social Security (DHSS), which include the number of cases notified.

5 Serious communicable diseases must be notified by the MOEH immediately to the Chief Medical Officer at the DHSS by telephone and confirmed by letter. This information would be passed on to the World Health Organization. These diseases include smallpox, plague, cholera, yellow fever, leprosy, malaria or rabies contracted in Britain, lassa fever, viral haemorrhagic fever or Marburg disease.

6 The Communicable Disease Surveillance Centre, Colindale, London, has been set up on behalf of the DHSS and the Welsh Office to help to co-ordinate the investigation and control of communicable diseases in England and Wales.

7 The surveillance activities include:
   a. Providing information about communicable diseases in England and Wales and relevant information from other countries.
   b. Providing information about previous incidence of communicable disease in England and Wales.
   c. Monitoring the information gained from local reports to detect significant changes in the pattern of communicable diseases.

The complete list of notifiable diseases is:

Acute meningitis	Plague
Anthrax	Poliomyelitis (acute)
Cholera	Rabies
Diphtheria	Relapsing fever
Dysentery (amoebic or bacillary)	Scarlet fever
Encephalitis (acute)	Smallpox
Infective jaundice	Tetanus
Lassa fever	Tuberculosis
Leptospirosis	Typhoid and paratyphoid
Leprosy	Typhus
Malaria	Whooping cough
Marburg disease	Viral haemorrhagic diseases
Measles	Yellow fever
Ophthalmia neonatorum	

Several other diseases may be notifiable in certain areas, usually for a limited period of time, e.g., acute rheumatism in children under 16 in some Midland areas, brucellosis in some rural areas, and recently scabies has been made notifiable by 29 local authorities.

Nursing Objectives and Management

To Assist in Identifying the Aetiologic Agent, and Establishing the Diagnosis

1 Obtain specimens of urine, faeces, sputum, throat swabbings, nasal swabbings or pyogenic exudates for bacteriological examination.
2 Assist in obtaining specimens of blood, cerebrospinal fluid, bone marrow, and other body fluids or tissues for cytological, serological and bacteriological tests.
3 Assist in appropriate skin tests for specific diagnostic reactions.

To Control the Infection in the Patient

1 Administer the appropriate antibiotic agents as ordered.
2 Assist in administering specific immune therapy, if available, employing immune antiserum, gamma globulin, antitoxin, toxoid, vaccine or an appropriate mixture of antigen and antibody, depending of the circumstances.
3 Observe the patient carefully for evidences of drug or serum sensitivity.

To Prevent Spread of Infection to Others

1 Carry out isolation techniques according to the disease.
2 Observe asepsis as indicated.
3 Use mask technique as required by the disease.
   a. Change mask frequently—moisture increases the permeability of the mask, promoting bacterial growth.
   b. Refrain from handling the mask while it is being worn.
4 Use gown as required by the patient's disease.
   a. If disposable gowns are used, use once and then discard.
   b. If disposable gowns are not available, the gown must be changed daily, or as soon as it is soiled before then, and hung carefully inside the door of the patient's room.
5 Use gloves when indicated by the patient's disease.
   a. Disposable gloves are preferable.
   b. Use once and discard in the appropriate container.
6 Handle needles and syringes carefully.
   a. Disposable syringes and needles should be placed directly into a special box for incineration.
   b. Nondisposable items should be rinsed and then placed in a special bag before returning to central sterile supplies depot.
7 Wash hands immediately after contact with each patient and after every contact with material that has been contaminated and is potentially infectious, and also after removing gown.
8 Use paper towels to turn off the taps, if the sink is not equipped with elbow or foot operated taps.
9 Carry out concurrent disinfection of fomites as required by the patient's disease.

a. Bed linen should be placed in a special bag before being removed from the patient's room, and then 'double-bagged' before transport from the ward.

b. Disposable plates and cutlery should be used, if available; if not, special arrangements must be made for washing up in a machine, or the patient's cutlery and plates must be kept separately.

10   Control the dissemination of infectious droplets.

a. Encourage the patient to cover his mouth and nose when coughing or sneezing, using disposable paper tissues.

b. Wrap contaminated tissues and other articles in paper before disposal.

11   Control dust.

a. Avoid creating dust currents, e.g., shaking bedclothes.

b. Damp dust furniture and vacuum clean floors.

c. Maintain cleanliness of surroundings and wash contamination from any surface as soon as it is soiled.

d. Reduce to a minimum the activity of personnel in the patient's room.

12   Ventilate the patient's room properly with a system that directs air to the exterior of the building and not on to a corridor. Keep the door to the room closed.

To Protect the Patient who is Immunosuppressed or Immune-incompetent (Leukaemia, Organ Transplants)

1   Use protective isolation units if possible—laminar airflow unit with high efficiency filters.

2   Remember that every article brought into the room is potentially dangerous to the patient unless it has been sterilized beforehand.

3   One nurse should attend to the patient throughout the span of duty, and the changes of personnel should be minimized.

4   Clear instructions must be given to visitors. They may be excluded from the room completely, or limited visiting may be allowed, but gowns and masks must be worn.

General Nursing Care of Patient Suffering from an Infectious Illness

To Provide Physiological Support

1   Ensure adequate hydration in the event of excessive fluid loss because of sweating, diarrhoea, vomiting.

a. Encourage liberal fluid intake.

b. Prepare for the administration of intravenous fluids as required.

2   Reduce the fever when indicated (it is often important to watch the temperature curve).

a. Administer antipyretic drugs as prescribed.

b. Tepid sponge the patient as required.

c. Use electric fans, light bedclothes supported by a bed cradle, and cotton nightclothes.

3   Measure and record body temperature, pulse and respiration at frequent intervals.

4   Measure arterial blood pressure at regular intervals if the patient shows a tendency to vascular collapse.

5   Weigh the patient periodically, preferably at the same hour of the day.

6 Provide a light diet, acceptable to the patient, with a sufficient calorie content.
7 Frequent mouth care is essential.

To Provide Symptomatic Relief

1 Combat generalized aching and malaise.
   a. Use warm applications as required.
   b. Apply cold compresses for headache.
   c. Administer analgesic drugs as ordered.
   d. Provide a restful, relaxed environment.
2 Relieve cough.
   a. Humidify inspired air.
   b. Provide a linctus or an expectorant as ordered.
3 Relieve anxiety and depression.
   a. Recognize the loneliness that may be experienced by an isolated patient.
   b. Lend encouragement to the patient faced with a long convalescence.

To Protect Susceptible Individuals and to Provide Surveillance of the General Population

1 Provide a comprehensive health education programme to include:
   a. Availability and importance of prophylactic immunization.
   b. Manner in which communicable diseases are spread, and the methods of avoiding spread.
   c. Importance of seeking medical advice in the event of a febrile illness or unusual skin eruption.
   d. Importance of environmental cleanliness and personal hygiene.
   e. Means of preventing contamination of food and water supplies.
   (1) Discipline, cleanliness and inspection of food handlers.
   (2) Dangers of 'perishable' foods; the identity of food that tends to promote bacterial growth; the methods of food preservation.
   (3) Significance of milk pasteurization.
   (4) Necessity for adequate length of time of cooking, and reaching required temperature for certain foods, e.g., frozen chickens must be completely thawed before cooking, to ensure all parts reach the required temperature.
   (5) Dangers associated with polluted waterways, and the proper toilet facilities on holiday and residential boats.
   (6) Importance of meat inspection.
2 Obtain medical aid for all suspected cases of communicable diseases.
3 Isolate patients with communicable diseases, as well as known contacts and carriers, if this is necessary for the particular disease.
4 Provide methods of eliminating insect, rodent and other animal vectors and reservoirs of infection.
5 Provide vaccination and immunization facilities (Table 6.1).
   a. Make available, and facilitate whatever vaccination procedures are known to be effective and are indicated for the stimulation of active immunity in exposed and susceptible individuals.
   b. Provide specific immune serum (heterologous or human convalescent), or human gammaglobulin if indicated, to provide passive immunity and temporary protection to contacts who are particularly vulnerable.

Table 6.1.   Schedule of Vaccination and Immunization Procedures (taken from DHSS Revised Schedule 1978)

Age	Vaccine	Interval	Notes
During first year of life	Diphtheria, whooping cough, tetanus Oral poliomyelitis vaccine	Three doses: commencing at 3 months; second dose after an interval of 6–8 weeks; third dose after an interval of 4–6 months	If whooping cough vaccine is contraindicated, or declined by the parent, diphtheria and tetanus vaccine should be given
During second year of life	Measles vaccine	There should be an interval of not less than 3 weeks after any other vaccination	*Contraindication.* Immune deficient states
At school entry or entry to nursery school	Diphtheria, tetanus vaccination Oral poliomyelitis vaccine	Preferably an interval of at least 3 years after completing basic course	
Between 11 and 13 years of age	BCG vaccination	There should be an interval of not less than 3 weeks between BCG and rubella vaccination	For tuberculin negative children For tuberculin negative contacts it may be given at any age
Between 11 and 13 years of age. Girls only	Rubella vaccine		Should be offered to all girls whether or not there is a history of rubella
On leaving school, before employment or entering further education	Reinforcing dose Tetanus Oral poliomyelitis vaccine		
Adult life	Poliomyelitis vaccine for previously unvaccinated adults	Oral vaccine. Three doses: 6–8 weeks between first and second dose; 4–6 months between second and third dose	For travellers to countries where poliomyelitis is endemic
	Rubella vaccine for susceptible women of child bearing age		Adult women of child bearing age should be tested for rubella antibodies.

(continued)

Table 6.1 (*cont.*)

Age	Vaccine	Interval	Notes
			Sero-negative women should be offered rubella vaccination. Pregnancy must be excluded before vaccination. Patient must be warned not to become pregnant for 8 weeks after immunization
	Active immunization against tetanus for previously unvaccinated adults	Three doses: 6–8 weeks between first and second doses; third dose 6 months later	

Immunity

Immunity is the resistance that an individual has against disease.

1   Specific immunity to a particular organism implies that an individual has either generated the appropriate antibody in his own body (active immunity) or received ready made antibodies from another source (passive immunity).
2   Immunity may be natural (not obtained through previous contact with the infectious agent) or acquired.
3   Acquired immunity may be active or passive.

Passive Immunity

Passive immunity to a disease is a state of relative temporary protection produced by the actual injection of serum containing antibodies which have formed in a host other than the individual himself.

There are three types of preparations:

1   Standard human immune serum globulin.
2   Special human immune serum globulin with a known antibody content for specific infections.
3   Animal antiserum or antitoxins.

Active Immunity

Active immunity is an immunity that has been produced by the stimulation of the body to produce its own antibodies.

1   It may be produced by clinical infection (the person gets the disease) or by subclinical infection (by coming in contact with the disease).
2   By the introduction of live or killed organisms or their antigens.

3   The organisms have been treated by heating or by chemical inactivation to destroy their harmful properties without destroying their ability to stimulate antibody protection.

CLASSIFICATION OF COMMUNICABLE DISEASES REQUIRING ISOLATION OR PRECAUTIONS

Strict Isolation

1   Private room is essential, and the door must be kept closed.
2   Gowns must be worn by all people entering the room.
3   Masks must be worn by all people entering the room.
4   Hands must be washed on entering and leaving the room.
5   Gloves must be worn by all people entering the room.
6   'Double-bag' technique for soiled dressings.
7   Needles and syringes must be placed in a special 'Sharps' box, which must be sealed before being removed from the room for incineration.

Diseases Requiring Strict Isolation

Pulmonary anthrax	Melioidosis
Burns infected with staphylococcus or Group A streptococcus	Plague
Diphtheria	Staphylococcal pneumonia
Staphylococcal enteritis	Rabies
Hepatitis A and B	Congenital rubella
	Generalized vaccinia

NOTE: All patients admitted with pyrexia of unknown origin who have recently returned from tropical countries, or have been in contact with people who have returned from the tropics, should be isolated with strict precautions until a firm diagnosis is made.

Patients suffering from lassa fever, Marburg disease or smallpox will be transferred to a special hospital. Those in London and the home counties will be taken to Coppetts Wood Hospital, Muswell Hill, London. One hospital is provided by the other regional hospital boards.

Respiratory Isolation

1   Private room is necessary, and the door must be kept closed.
2   Gowns are not necessary.
3   Masks must be worn by all people entering the room who are susceptible tthe disease.
4   Hands must be washed on entering and leaving the room.
5   Gloves are not necessary.
6   The patient should cough or spit into a disposable tissue held close to his mouth, and then discard this into an impervious bag, which must be sealed before being removed for incineration.
7   Special provision must be made for washing up cutlery and crockery, if disposable articles are not available.

Diseases Requiring Respiratory Isolation

Measles
Meningococcal meningitis
Mumps
Whooping cough (pertussis)
Adult rubella

Herpes zoster
Open pulmonary tuberculosis
Chicken pox
Venezuelan equine encephalomyelitis

Enteric Precautions

1 Private room necessary for children only.
2 Gowns must be worn by all people having direct contact with the patient.
3 Masks are not necessary.
4 Hands must be washed on entering and leaving the room.
5 Gloves must be worn by all people having direct contact with the patient or with articles contaminated with faecal material.
6 Disposable urinals, bedpans and potties should be used and should be macerated in the machine immediately after use.

Diseases Requiring Enteric Precautions

Cholera
Staphylococcal entercolitis
Gastroenteritis caused by entero-
  pathogenic or enterotoxic *E. Coli*
Salmonella
Shigella

Hepatitis, viral, type A, B, or type
  non-A, non-B.
Typhoid fever (special precautions may
  be necessary to the disposal of
  faeces)

Wound and Skin Precautions

1 Private room is desirable but not essential.
2 Gowns must be worn by all people having direct contact with the patient.
3 Masks are not necessary except during wound dressing.
4 Hands must be washed on entering and leaving the room.
5 Gloves must be worn by all persons having direct contact with the infected area.
6 Special precautions are necessary for instruments, dressings and linen.

Diseases Requiring Wound and Skin Precautions

1 Burns that are infected, except those infected with *Straphylococcus aureus* or group A streptococcus that are not covered or not adequately contained by dressings (see Strict Isolation).
2 Gas gangrene (due to *Clostridium perfringens*).
3 Herpes zoster, localized.
4 Melioidosis, extrapulmonary with draining sinuses.
5 Plague, bubonic.
6 Puerperal sepsis—group A streptococcus, vaginal discharge.
7 Wound and skin infections that are not covered by dressings or that have copious purulent drainage that is not contained by dressings, except those infected with *S. aureus* or group A streptococcus, which require strict isolation.
8 Wound and skin infections that are covered by dressings so that the discharge is

adequately contained, including those infected with *S. aureus* or group A streptococcus; minor wound infections, such as stitch abscesses, need only secretion precautions.

Discharge Precautions

Secretion Precautions—Lesions

1   Use a 'no-touch' dressing technique (do not touch the wound or dressings with the hands) when changing dressings on these lesions.
2   Employ proper handwashing procedures.
3   Wash hands before and after patient contact; use sterile equipment when changing dressings; double-bag soiled dressing and equipment.
4   These precautions apply only with lesions from which there is a discharge.

Diseases; duration of precautions

1   Actinomycosis, draining lesions—for duration of drainage.
2   Anthrax, cutaneous—until culture-negative.
3   Brucellosis, draining lesions—for duration of drainage.
4   Burn, skin and wound infections, minor—for duration of drainage.
5   Candidiasis, mucocutaneous—for duration of illness.
6   Coccidioidomycosis, draining lesion—for duration of drainage.
7   Conjunctivitis, acute bacterial (including gonococcal)—until 24 hours after start of effective therapy.
8   Conjunctivitis, viral—for duration of illness.
9   Gonococcal ophthalmia neonatorum—until 24 hours after start of effective therapy.
10   Gonorrhea—until 24 hours after start of effective therapy.
11   Granuloma inguinale—for duration of illness.
12   *Herpesvirus hominis* (herpes simplex), except disseminated neonatal disease—for duration of illness. For disseminated neonatal disease, see Strict Isolation; for oral *H. hominis* disease, see Secretion Precautions, Oral.
13   Keratoconjunctivitis, infectious—for duration of illness.
14   Listeriosis—for duration of illness.
15   Lymphogranuloma venereum—for duration of illness.
16   Nocardiosis, draining lesions—for duration of illness.
17   Orf—for duration of illness.
18   Syphilis, mucocutaneous—until 24 hours after start of effective therapy.
19   Trachoma, acute—for duration of illness.
20   Tuberculosis, extrapulmonary draining lesion—for duration of drainage.
21   Tularaemia, draining lesion—for duration of drainage.

Secretion Precautions—Oral

1   The diseases listed in this section can be spread to susceptible persons by contact with oral secretions.
2   Attention should be given to the proper disposal of oral secretions to prevent spread of infection.
3   Instruct the patient to cough or spit into disposable tissues held close to the mouth; discard tissues in an impervious (impenetrable) bag at the bedside.

4   If the patient has nasotracheal suction or tracheotomy, the suction catheter and gloves should be placed in an impervious bag for disposal.
5   Seal the bag before discarding for incineration.

Diseases; duration of precautions

1   Herpangina—for duration of hospitalization.
2   Herpes oralis—for duration of illness.
3   Infectious mononucleosis—for duration of illness.
4   Melioidosis, pulmonary—for duration of illness.
5   Mycoplasma pneumonia—for duration of illness.
6   Pneumonia, bacterial, if not covered elsewhere—for duration of illness.
7   Psittacosis—for duration of illness. (It may be desirable to place patient with acute psittacosis who is coughing and raising sputum in respiratory isolation.)
8   Q fever—for duration of illness.
9   Respiratory infectious disease, acute (if not covered elsewhere)—for duration of illness.
10   Scarlet fever—until 24 hours after start of effective therapy.
11   Streptococcal pharyngitis—until 24 hours after start of effective therapy.

Excretion Precautions

1   The diseases listed in this section can be spread to susceptible persons through the oral route by contact with faecal excretions from a person infected with the organism.
2   Strict attention should be paid to careful handwashing following any patient contact and especially following contact with excretions.
3   Instruct the patient on the necessity of careful handwashing after defaecation.
4   Make sure there is proper sanitary disposal of excretions; a standard sewage system is adequate.

Diseases; duration of precautions

1   Amoebiasis—for duration of illness.
2   *C. perfringens (C. welchii)* food-poisoning—for duration of illness.
3   Enterobiasis—for duration of illness.
4   Giardiasis—for duration of illness.
5   Hand, foot and mouth disease—for duration of hospitalization.
6   Herpangina—for duration of hospitalization.
7   Infectious lymphocytosis—for duration of hospitalization.
8   Leptospirosis (urine only)—for duration of hospitalization.
9   Meningitis, aseptic—for duration of hospitalization.
10   Pleurodynia—for duration of hospitalization.
11   Poliomyelitis—for duration of hospitalization.
12   Staphylococcal food poisoning—for duration of symptoms.
13   Tapeworm disease (only with *Hymenolepsis nana* and *Taenia solium* [pork])—for duration of illness.
14   Viral diseases, other (ECHO or Coxsackie gastroenteritis, pericarditis, myocarditis, meningitis)—for duration of hospitalization.

Blood Precautions

1   The diseases in this category are associated with circulation of the aetiologic agent in blood; be aware of the route of transmission.
2   Blood precautions should be taken for the duration of clincial disease or for as long as the aetiologic agent can be demonstrated in the blood. Blood precautions should be taken with anyone who is HBs Ag-positive.
3   Disposable needles and syringe should be used for patients in isolation. They must not be reused.
4   Used needles need not be recapped; they should be placed in a prominently labelled, impervious, puncture-resistant container designated for this purpose. Needles should not be purposefully bent, because accidental needle puncture may occur.
5   Used syringes should be placed in an impervious bag. Both needle and syringe bags should be incinerated or autoclaved before discarding.
6   Rinse reusable needles and syringes thoroughly in cold water after use; place the needle in a puncture-resistant rigid container; wrap syringes and needles using double-bag technique and return to proper department for decontamination and sterilization.
7   These specifications pertain to needle and syringe precautions and to labelling of blood specimens. Also label blood specimens with patient's diagnosis so that necessary precautions will be taken.

Diseases; duration of precautions

1   Arthropod-borne viral fever (dengue, etc.)—for duration of hospitalization.
2   Hepatitis, viral, type A, B, type non-A, non-B—for duration of hospitalization.
3   Malaria—for duration of hospitalization.

Protective Isolation

1   Private room is necessary, door must be kept closed.
2   Gowns should be sterile and must be worn by all people entering the room.
3   Masks must be worn by all people entering the room.
4   Hands must be washed on entering and leaving the room.
5   Gloves to be used routinely by all personnel having direct contact with the patient.
6   Caps and overshoes may be necessary.
7   Transportation of the patient should be strictly curtailed to avoid possible exposure to infection.

Diseases that Require Protective Isolation

Agranulocytosis
Extensive noninfected burns
Extensive sterile dermatitis
Immune deficiency; immunosuppressive drugs
Leukaemia
Lymphoma

Epidemiology, Therapy and Control of Communicable Infections—see Table 6.2

BACTERIAL DISEASES

Tetanus (Lockjaw)

Tetanus is an acute disease caused by *Clostridium tetani* (tetanus bacillus), spores of which are introduced into the body when an injury becomes contaminated with soil, street dust or animal or human faeces. The bacillus is an anaerobe (cannot live in presence of oxygen).

Clinical Manifestations

Caused by potent neurotoxins elaborated by *C. tetani* which have a special affinity for nervous tissue.

1 Rigidity of muscles; muscle spasms of both flexor and extensor muscle groups.
   a. Trismus—painful spasms of masticatory muscles; difficulty in opening the mouth (lockjaw).
   b. Risus sardonicus—grinning expression produced by spasm of facial muscles.
   c. Recurrent tetanic spasms of almost every muscle group in body—involvement of respiratory muscles may lead to respiratory failure.
2 Hyperirritability; restlessness, headache, low-grade fever.
3 Hyperactive reflexes.

Treatment and Nursing Management

Objective

To prevent the disease from developing.

1 Consider every break in the skin as a potential portal of entry for *C. tetani*.
   a. Tetanus-prone wounds—compound fractures; gunshot injuries; burns; foreign bodies; wounds contaminated with soil or faeces; wounds neglected for more than 24 hours; puncture wounds; wounds infected with other microorganisms; wounds from induced abortions; wounds made by dirty hypodermic needles (drug addicts).

Nursing Alert: Tetanus-prone wounds are those in which there has been an invasion of soil or faeces or those involving a severe traumatic injury. Tetanus may develop from an insignificant wound contaminated by soil.

   b. Wash and clean the wound thoroughly.
2 Treatment depends on the immunization status of the patient. Consider nature and age of wound and conditions under which it occurred.
   a. For previously immunized patient:
      (1) Tetanus toxoid (adsorbed) according to manufacturer's directions.
      (2) Tetanus immune globulin (human) (TIG), as directed.
          Tetanus toxoid and TIG given with separate syringes at different sites.
      (3) Immediate debridement of the wound.
      (4) Antibiotic therapy, usually penicillin.
   b. For patient with no previous immunization (or if immunization is in doubt):
      (1) Tetanus toxoid—course of three injections.

Table 6.2.   Epidemiology, Therapy and Control of Communicable Infections

Disease	Infective Organism	Infectious Sources	Entry Site	Method of Spread
Amoebiasis	*Entamoeba histolytica*	Contaminated water and food	Gastrointestinal tract	Patients and carriers; faecal/ oral route
Bacillary dysentery	*Shigella* group	Contaminated water and food	Gastrointestinal tract	Patients and carriers; faecal/ oral route
Brucellosis	*Brucella melitensis* and related organisms	Milk, meat, tissues, blood, absorbed foetuses and placentas from infected cattle, goats horses, pigs	Gastrointestinal tract	Ingestion of or contact with i fective materi
Chancroid	Ducrey bacillus	Human cases and carriers	Genitalia	Direct sexual contact
Chickenpox (varicella)	Virus	Human cases	Probably nasopharynx	Probably respir tory droplets
Diphtheria	*Corynebacterium diphtheriae*	Human cases and carriers; fomites; raw milk	Nasopharynx	Nasal and oral cretions; resp ratory drople
Encephalitis, epidemic (eastern and western equine)	Viruses	Chicken and wildbird mites; horses; hibernating garter snakes	Skin	Mosquitoes
Gonorrhoea	*Neisseria gonorrhoeae*	Urethral and vaginal secretions	Urethral or vaginal mucosa; pharynx; rectum	Sexual activity
Granuloma inguinale	Donovan body (bacillus)	Infectious exudate	External genitalia; cervix	Sexual intercou
Type A hepatitis	Hepatitis A virus	Person-to-person contact; contaminated food or water; faeces; blood; urine	Gastrointestinal tract; skin	Faecal/oral rou ingestion of parenteral ir oculation wi infected bloo blood produ

* Research developments produce changes in drug therapy. The reader is referred to drug brochure digests to keep abreast of changing dosages and uses.

ncubation Period	Chemotherapy*	Prophylaxis
table	Metronidazole; emetine; chloroquine; diiodohydroxy-quin; chlortetracycline	Detection of carriers and their removal from food handling; plumbing safeguards
48 hours	Ampicillin; chloramphenicol; tetracycline	Detection and control of carriers; inspection of food handlers; decontamination of water supplies
4 days	Tetracycline and streptomycin	Milk pasteurization; control of infection in animals
days	Sulfonamides; streptomycin; tetracycline	Effective case-finding and treatment of infection
6 days	None	Zoster immune globulin (ZIG) (an investigational drug) provided by Centre for Disease Control to high-risk susceptible children exposed to varicella zoster within 72 hours
days	Diphtheria antitoxin; penicillin; erythromycin	Active immunization with diphtheria toxoid
able	None	Eastern equine encephalitis vaccine, dried (available from Centre for Disease Control)
days	Penicillin G, preceded by probenecid	Chemotherapy of carriers and contacts; case-finding and treatment of patients
nown, presumably 80 days	Tetracyclines; erythromycin	Chemotherapy of carriers and contacts; case-finding and treatment of patients
weeks	None	Enteric and blood precautions for infected cases; immunization with gamma globulin

(continued)

Table 6.2 (*cont.*)

Disease	Infective Organism	Infectious Sources	Entry Site	Method of Spread
Type B hepatitis	Hepatitis B virus	Infected blood donor; contaminated injection equipment	Skin	Parenteral injection of human blood, plasm thrombin, fibogen, packed cells, and oth blood produ from an infe person; cont nated needle and syringes venereal con
Infectious mononucleosis	E-B virus	Human cases and carriers	Mouth	Probably oral-pharyngeal route; via bl transfusion i susceptible recipients
Influenza	Virus (types A and B)	Human cases; animal reservoir	Respiratory tract	Respiratory
Lymphogranuloma venereum	*Chlamydia trachomatis*	Human cases	External genitalia; urethral or vaginal mucosa	Sexual interco indirect con with contam nated article clothing
Malaria	*Plasmodium vivax, falciparum, malariae,* and *ovale*	Human cases	Skin	Mosquitoes (anopheles)
Measles	Virus	Human cases	Respiratory mucosa	Nasopharynge secretions
Meningococcal meningitis	*Neisseria meningitidis*	Human cases and carriers	Nasopharynx; tonsils	Respiratory droplets
Mumps	Virus	Human cases (early)	Upper respiratory tract	Respiratory droplets
Paratyphoid fever	*Salmonella paratyphi A* and *B* and related organisms	Contaminated food, milk, water; rectal tubes; barium enemas	Gastrointestinal tract	Infected urine and faeces
Pneumococcal pneumonia	*Streptococcus pneumoniae*	Human carriers; patient's own pharynx	Respiratory mucosa	Respiratory droplets

ncubation Period	Chemotherapy*	Prophylaxis
eeks to months	None	Screening of blood donors; avoidance of unnecessary use of blood and blood derivatives
weeks	None	None
72 hours	None	Specific virus vaccine
days	Tetracyclines	Case-finding and treatment of infection
able, pending strain	Chloroquine; primaquine; amodiaquine; quinine; proguanil	Co-ordinated measures for wide-scale mosquito control; prompt detection and effective treatment of cases; suppressive drugs in malarious areas
days	None	Measles vaccine
days	Penicillin; chloramphenicol	Meningococcal polysaccharide vaccine to persons at risk; rifampin for carriers or contacts
6 (av.) days	None	Live mumps vaccine
days	Chloramphenicol; ampicillin; sulfa-trimethoprim	Control of public water sources, food vendors, food handlers, treatment of carriers
able	Penicillin	Control of upper respiratory infections; avoidance of alcoholic intoxication

(continued)

Table 6.2 (*cont.*)

Disease	Infective Organism	Infectious Sources	Entry Site	Method of Spread
Poliomyelitis	Polioviruses (Types I, II, III)	Human cases and carriers	Gastrointestinal tract	Infected faeces; pharyngeal secretions
Rocky Mountain spotted fever	*Rickettsia rickettsii*	Infected wild rodents, dogs, wood ticks, dog ticks	Skin	Tick bites
Rubella (German measles)	Virus	Human case	Respiratory mucosa	Nasopharyngeal secretions
Scarlet fever	*Streptococcus haemolyticus*	Human cases; infected food	Pharynx	Nasal and oral secretions
Syphilis	*Treponema pallidum*	Infected exudate or blood	External genitalia; cervix; mucosal surfaces; placenta	Sexual activity; contact with open lesions; blood transfusion; transplacental inoculation
Tetanus	*Clostridium tetani*	Contaminated soil	Penetrating and crush wounds	Horse and cattle faeces
Trichinosis	*Trichinella spiralis*	Infected pigs	Gastrointestinal tract	Ingestion of infected pork, undercooked
Tuberculosis	*Mycobacterium tuberculosis*	Sputum from human cases; milk from infected cows (rare in UK)	Respiratory mucosa	Sputum; respiratory droplets
Tularaemia	*Pasteurella tularensis*	Wild rodents and rabbits	Eyes; skin; gastrointestinal tract	Handling infected animals; ingestion of undercooked infected meat; drinking contaminated water; bites from infected flies, ticks

ncubation Period	Chemotherapy*	Prophylaxis
2 days	None	Wide-scale application of parenteral (Salk) and oral (Sabin) poliovirus vaccines; case isolation
0 days	Tetracyclines; chloramphenicol	Avoidance of tick-infested areas, or wearing of protective clothing in such areas; frequent search for and prompt removal of ticks from body; specific vaccination of exposed persons
-21 days	None	Rubella virus vaccine; immune serum globulin (human) given to contacts of rubella. Rubella in early stages of pregnancy legally recognized as indication for abortion
days	Penicillin	Case isolation; prophylactic chemotherapy with penicillin; asepsis during obstetrical procedures; specific chemoprophylaxis for persons with rheumatic fever
70 days	Penicillin; erythromycin; tetracycline	Case-finding by means of routine serologic testing and other methods; adequate treatment of infected individuals
1 days av. 10 ays)	Tetanus immune globulin (human) [TIG]	Wound debridement; toxoid booster injections for patients previously immunized; tetanus toxoid and tetanus immune globulin (separates sites and separate syringes) for nonimmune persons
8 days	None	Regulation of hog breeders; adequate meat inspection; thorough cooking of pork
iable	Isoniazid; ethambutol; rifampin; streptomycin	Early discovery and adequate treatment of active cases; milk pasteurization
0 days	Streptomycin; tetracyclines; chloramphenicol	Use of rubber gloves when skinning/handling potentially infectious wild animals; avoidance of contact with potentially infected rodents; adequate cooking of wild rabbit dishes; vaccination of hunters, butchers, laboratory workers risking heavy exposure

(continued)

Table 6.2   (*cont.*)

Disease	Infective Organism	Infectious Sources	Entry Site	Method of Spread
Typhoid fever	*Salmonella typhi*	Contaminated food and water	Gastrointestinal tract	Infected urine and faeces
Typhus, endemic	*Rickettsia typhi (mooseri)*	Infected rodents	Skin	Flea bites
Whooping cough (pertussis)	*Bordatella pertussis*	Human cases	Respiratory tract	Infected bronch secretions

(2) TIG or antitoxin as directed.
(3) Immediate debridement of wound.
(4) Antibiotic therapy—tetanus organism sensitive to tetracycline and penicillin.
  c. Equine or bovine antitoxin is usually *not* given because of high incidence of allergic and anaphylactic reactions. *If used, its administration must be preceded by careful screening for sensitivity according to manufacturer's directions.*

Treatment of Tetanus

Objective

To prevent respiratory and cardiovascular complications.

1   Maintain an adequate airway—tetanic spasm of larynx, pharynx and respiratory muscles usually occurs during convulsions and may lead to asphyxia and death.
  a. Prepare for insertion of a cuffed endotracheal tube—laryngeal spasms cause airway obstruction, inadequate pulmonary ventilation, hypoxia, cyanosis and death.
  b. Prepare patient for tracheotomy—relieves laryngeal dyspnoea, reduces risk of aspiration, and permits speedy application of controlled ventilation.
  c. Maintain patient on mechanical ventilation.
  d. Aspirate secretions as necessary—observe aspirate and keep a record of its appearance to assess for signs of pulmonary infection (e.g., sputum becomes coloured).
  e. Curariform drugs (with mechanical ventilation) may be needed to maintain an adequate airway.

Nursing Alert: The hearing of the patient with respiratory paralysis may be acute. Do not make unguarded comments in his presence.

2   Give TIG (human) in an effort to neutralize the toxins and to ensure that appropriate circulating levels will be present when the wound is debrided.
3   Carry out effective wound care; debride all necrotic tissue—necrotic tissue favours growth of tetanus bacillus.

ncubation Period	Chemotherapy*	Prophylaxis
weeks	Chloramphenicol; ampicillin; sulfa-trimethoprim	Decontamination of water sources; milk pasteurization; individual vaccination of high risk persons; control of carriers
weeks	Tetracyclines; chloramphenicol	Delousing procedures; case quarantine
nmonly days	Erythromycin, ampicillin	Active immunization with vaccine; case isolation

4 Give antibiotics (penicillin)—to eradicate persisting *C. tetani* and other pathogens form the wound.
5 Maintain the fluid and electrolyte balance.
6 Support the patient during tetanic spasm and convulsions—due to the action of toxins in the cells of central nervous system; mortality rate of patients with frequent and severe spasms is high.
7 Provide for continuing observation of the patient.
   a. Plan nursing management for minimal patient disturbance—tactile stimulation may promote spasms.
       (1) Place patient in a quiet room.
       (2) Avoid sudden stimuli and light—slightest stimulation may trigger paroxysmal spasms.
       (3) Be alert for the development of fractures of the vertebral bodies, which may occur with severe spasm.
       (4) Give muscle relaxants, sedatives, anticonvulsants—to treat muscle rigidity and convulsions.
       (5) Keep vein open—for infusions and in the event of cardiac/respiratory arrest.
   b. See Volume 3, Chapter 1, Conditions of the Nervous System, for management of the patient with convulsive seizures and for management of the unconscious patient.
8 After recovery the patient should receive the primary immunization series (for tetanus) plus booster dose every 10 years.

Nursing Isolation Procedure

No isolation or precautions are required but a side room is normally used for quietness.

Gas Gangrene

Gas gangrene is a severe infection caused by gram-positive clostridia which may complicate compound fractures and contused or lacerated wounds. Several species of clostridia (*C. welchii, C. perfringens, C. septicum, C. novyi, C. histolyticum, C.*

sporogenes) and others may produce gas gangrene. These organisms are anaerobes and spore-formers and are normally found in the intestinal tract of man and in soil.

Altered Physiology

Injury → bacteria (clostridia) invade devitalized tissue, especially where blood supply is compromised → bacteria multiply and produce toxins → toxins cause haemolysis, vessel thrombosis, and damage to myocardium, liver and kidneys.

Clinical Manifestations

1 Sudden and severe pain at site of injury—caused by gas and oedema in the tissues.
2 Rapid, feeble pulse progressing to circulatory collapse—death from toxaemia is frequent.
3 Anaemia (from haemolysis); prostration; apprehension.
4 Delirium and stupor.
5 Appearance of wound:
   a. Skin is white and tense intially; colour then progresses to a dusky hue.
   b. Crepitus (crackling)—produced by gas in the tissue.
   c. Vesicles appear; are filled with red, watery fluid.
   d. Muscle is dark red and oedematous; contains red, watery, foul-smelling fluid.
   e. Gas bubbles seen emanating from tissues—toxins ferment muscle sugar; produce acid and gas, which digest muscle protein. (Obvious gangrene is present.)

Treatment and Nursing Management

1 Prepare patient for surgical removal and debridement of necrotic tissue—this is preventive as well as curative.
   a. Early excision of all devitalized and infected tissue with wide incisions will render wound unsuitable for growth of clostridium.
   b. Extensive incisions (once infection has developed) in affected part allow air to inhibit growth of anaerobic organisms.
2 Place patient in hyperbaric oxygen chamber if available—increases the dissolved oxygen in the arterial system by increasing the partial pressure of the oxygen breathed by the patient; may interrupt toxin formation and microbial replication (reproduction).
3 Give antibiotic therapy (penicillin; tetracyclines; chloramphenicol)—may prevent spread of infection.
4 Support the patient with toxaemic manifestations—gas bacillus infection produces an intense toxaemia.
   a. Monitor central venous pressure and urinary output.
   b. Give intravenous fluids to support cardiovascular system; maintain fluid and electrolyte balance.
5 Antiserum may be of value.

Isolation Nursing Procedure

Use wound and skin precautions until the wound stops draining.

Staphylococcal Disease

Staphylococci are responsible for a wide variety of infections. They cause most superficial infections, but they also produce serious infections of the lungs, pleural space, bones, kidneys and surgical wounds.

Examples of Staphylococcal Disease

1 *Skin infections*—furuncles (boils), impetigo, carbuncles, abcesses, infected lacerations.
2 *Invasion of lymphatics*—axillary, cervical, mediastinal, retroperitoneal or subdiaphragmatic abscesses.
3 *Invasion of bloodstream*—acute bacterial endocarditis, staphylococcal pneumonia, empyema, perinephritic abscess, hepatic abscess, staphylococcal enteritis, pyogenic arthritis, meningitis, osteomyelitis, generalized sepsis.

Infectious Agent

Various strains of coagulase-positive staphylococci (*Staphylococcus aureus*).

Modes of Transmission

1 Nasal secretions, draining wound, asymptomatic nasal carrier.
2 Aerosolization during dressing changes.
3 Intravenous needles (drug abusers).

Hospital Staphylococcal Infections

Include all of the above infections.

Susceptible Hospital Patients

1 Chronically ill or debilitated patients.
2 Patients receiving systemic steroids or antimetabolite therapy.
3 Patients undergoing major or prolonged surgery.
4 Infants in the nursery.

Prevention and Control

1 All hospitals and nursing homes should enforce aseptic techniques supervised by infection control committee of the individual hospital.
2 Personnel with staphylococcal lesions should not work in the hospital until healing has occurred or cultures have become negative after treatment.
3 Patients with staphylococcal infections should be placed under strict isolation precautions until antibiotic treatment has rendered cultures negative for staphylococci.
4 Reduce cross traffic between hospital areas housing infected patients and those in which noninfected patients are quartered.

Specific Therapy for Staphylococcal Infections (Systemic)

1 Penicillinase-resistant penicillins and cephalosporins—flucloxacillin, cloxacillin, methicillin, vancomycin, cephalothin.

2   Intravenous administration usually selected because of large doses of drug required.

Nursing Isolation Procedures Required for Staphylococcal Disease (*S. aureus*)

1   Burns—strict isolation, wound and skin precautions or secretion precautions, depending on extent of infection, for duration of illness (wounds or lesions: until they stop draining).
2   Enterocolitis—enteric precautions until patient is off antibiotics and is culture-negative.
3   Gastroenteritis—excretion precautions for duration of illness.
4   Lung abscess, draining—strict isolation for duration of illness (until drainage stops).
5   Pneumonia—strict isolation for duration of illness.
6   Skin infection—strict isolation, wound and skin precautions, or secretion precautions for duration of illness (depending on extent of infection).
7   Wound infection—strict isolation, wound and skin precautions, or secretion precautions (depending on extent of infection) for duration of illness.

Preventive Measures and Health Teaching

1   Public should be educated concerning personal hygiene.
2   Persons with draining lesions should be isolated from their group and treated.

Streptococcal Infections

Most *streptococcal infections* in man are caused by group A beta haemolytic streptococci. Beta haemolytic streptococci gain entrance to the body primarily through the upper respiratory tract or skin; transmitted by persons with streptococcal infections or by those who are asymptomatic carriers.

Beta Haemolytic Streptococcal Infections

1   Streptococcal sore throat ('strep' pharyngitis).
2   Scarlet fever (streptococcal throat with a rash which occurs if infectious agent produces erythrogenic toxin to which patient is not immune).
3   Sinusitis, otitis media, mastoiditis, peritonsillar abscess.
4   Pericarditis, arthritis, peritonitis, meningitis.
5   Pneumonia and empyema.
6   Wound and skin infections—impetigo, puerperal infections, erysipelas.

Poststreptococcal Diseases (sequel of Haemolytic Streptococci)

1   Rheumatic fever.
2   Acute glomerulonephritis.

Diagnosis

1   Throat culture and sensitivity test.
2   Culture from wounds.

Treatment

1   Penicillin is the drug of choice in streptococcal infections (except enterococcal streptococci); several forms are available.
    a. Therapy should be continued for at least 10 days—to eliminate the organism, to reduce frequency of suppurative complications, to prevent the majority of cases of rheumatic fever and to help prevent further spread of streptococci.
    b. Cephalosporins or erythromycin may be used for penicillin-sensitive patients.
2   Make sure the patient understands the importance of completing the course of antibiotic treatment.

Nursing Isolation procedures

Streptococcal disease (group A)

1   Burns—strict isolation, wound and skin precautions or secretion precautions (depending on extent of infection) until wounds or lesions stop draining.
2   Endometritis (puerperal sepsis)—wound and skin precautions until 24 hours after initiation of effective therapy.
3   Pharyngitis—secretion precautions until 24 hours after initiation of effective therapy.
4   Pneumonia—strict isolation until 24 hours after initiation of effective therapy.
5   Scarlet fever—secretion precautions until 24 hours after initiation of effective therapy.
6   Skin infection—strict isolation, wound and skin precautions or secretion precautions (depending of extent of infection) until wounds or lesions stop draining.
7   Wound infection—strict isolation, wound and skin precautions or secretion precautions (depending on the extent of infection) until wound stops draining.
8   Streptococcal disease (not group A) unless covered elsewhere—none.

Preventive Measures and Health Teaching

1   Public should be educated concerning the relationship of streptococcal infections to heart disease and glomerulonephritis.
2   Pasteurize milk.
3   Food handlers should be instructed about hygienic procedures.
4   Obstetrical patients should be protected from personnel or visitors with respiratory or skin infections.
5   Long-term penicillin prophylaxis may be used for high-risk individuals (rheumatic heart disease).

Gram-negative Infection

Gram-negative infections are bacterial infections caused most frequently by *Escherichia coli*, *Enterobacter* species, *Klebsiella pneumoniae*, *Pseudomonas aeruginosa*, and the *Proteus* species.

Related Terms

Septic shock—circulatory shock occurring as a complication of a severe infection (usually by gram-negative enteric bacilli, although gram-positive cocci can cause bacterial shock).
Bacteraemia—bacterial invasion of the bloodstream.

Predisposing Events

1   Most gram-negative bacilli are not invasive in normal hosts; they are opportunistic bacteria that become invasive in persons with diminishing defence mechanisms.
2   Diagnostic and treatment procedures (tubes, catheters, etc.) result in disruption of usual protective barriers normally provided by the skin and mucous membranes.
3   The advent of potent immunosuppressive drugs, cytoxic drugs, steroids, ratiation, etc., contribute to diminishing the defence mechanisms of the patient.
4   The following contribute to the development of gram-negative infections:
   a. Genitourinary tract—indwelling catheters, instrumentation, urinary obstruction.
   b. Gastrointestinal tract—from obstruction, perforation, neoplasia, abscesses, diverticuli.
   c. Biliary tract—cholangitis, obstruction (stones), surgical procedures.
   d. Reproductive system—abortion, instrumentation, postpartum period.
   e. Vascular system—venous cutdowns, intravenous catheters, intracardiac pacemakers, total parenteral nutrition, pressure-monitoring devices, surgical procedures.
   f. Skin—leukaemia, agranulocytosis, immunosuppressive and cancer chemotherapeutic agents.
   g. Respiratory tract—tracheotomy, mechanical ventilation, aspiration.

Prevention

1   Handwashing by personnel and patient—fundamental to the control of all infections.
2   Protective isolation for patients receiving large doses of immunosuppressive drugs.
3   Strict aseptic technique for all diagnostic/therapeutic procedures—wounds, tracheotomies, tube drainage, catheters, intravenous therapy, cardiac pacing, ventilatory equipment.
4   Use of nursing surveillance to prevent cross-infection.
5   Monitoring of sterilization procedures and cleaning practices.
6   Obtaining of environmental and patient cultures as indicated.
7   Try to avoid housing two patients with indwelling catheters in the same room.

Clinical Manifestations

1   Shaking chill and rapid rise in temperature.
2   Warm, dry skin (during early stage).

3 Alteration in personality (inappropriate behaviour)—due to reduction in cerebral blood flow.
4 *Hypotension.*
   a. Tachycardia/tachypnoea.
   b. Cool, clammy skin.
   c. Peripheral cyanosis.
   d. Oliguria.
   e. Vascular collapse—death may occur as a result of vascular collapse.

Treatment and Nursing Management

Objectives

To recognize and treat the development of bacteraemia.
To improve perfusion to the vital organs.

1 Examine patient carefully to identify source of sepsis.
   a. Assist with collection of blood culture—to identify aetiologic agent and for sensitivity testing.
   b. Obtain other smears and cultures as indicated.
2 Administer appropriate antibiotic agent—give promptly when patient is too ill to await result of culture.
   a. Most severe infections leading to septic shock are caused by a relatively small number of organisms. Therapy is usually started before bacteriological diagnosis is made because of seriousness of illness.
   b. Drugs in common use in the treatment of gram-negative infections include cephalosporins, aminoglycosides (gentamicin, tobramycin), chloramphenicol, and carbenicillin.
3 Remove any foreign source of possible infection (when possible)—venous or bladder catheters.
4 Assist with surgical drainage of localized infection.
5 Prevent and treat shock and other complications.
   a. Monitor the state of responsiveness; skin temperature, moisture, colour, turgor; appearance of mucous membranes and nails; pulse and respiration; input and output; blood pressure.
   b. Administer adequate volume of fluid and blood.
      (1) Insert two or three large intravenous catheters—for rapid fluid and blood replacement.
      (2) Administer blood, plasma, low molecular weight dextran, or saline as directed for volume expansion and to combat vascular collapse.
      (3) Follow central venous pressure measurements—provides gauge for restoration of volume replacement (rate and amount).
      (4) Follow measurements of left ventricular filling pressures (Swan-Ganz).
   c. Administer oxygen to keep arterial Po_2 at desired level.
      (1) Follow blood gas and pH measurements to assess patient's need for assisted ventilation. Inadequate respiratory exchange is a frequent cause of death in gram-negative shock.
      (2) Patient is usually hypoxic from increased arteriovenous shunting and from hypermetabolism from high fever.
   d. Monitor serum electrolytes every several hours.

e. Administer sodium bicarbonate if severe acidosis exists.
f. Administer vasoactive drugs, digitalis, diuretics and other pharmacologic agents as directed.
g. Treat disseminated intravascular coagulation.

Typhoid Fever

Typhoid fever is a bacterial infection transmitted by contaminated water, milk, shellfish or other foods. It is caused by *Salmonella typhi*, which is harboured in human excreta. Today it is spread chiefly by carriers, patients who have recovered from the fever, but whose stools or urine may spread these bacilli for years.

Its characteristic lesion consists of ulcers which form in the ileum and colon, and its distinctive clinical features consist of long-continued fever, rose-spot rash, enlarged spleen, slow pulse and leucopenia.

Altered Physiology

Organism enters body by gastrointestinal tract; it invades the walls of gastrointestinal tract, leading to bacteraemia which localizes in mesenteric lymph nodes, in the masses of lymphatic tissue in the mucous membrane of the intestinal wall (Peyer's patches), and in small, solitary lymph follicles in the ileum and colon; ulceration of the intestines may ensue.

Clinical Manifestations

Gradual Onset

1 Severe headache, malaise, muscle pains, nonproductive cough.
2 Chills and fever; temperature rises slowly, reaching highest level in 3–7 days (40–41°C (104–105°F)).
3 Pulse is full and slow in comparison to height of fever; may have distinct dicrotic wave.
4 Skin eruption—irregularly spaced small rose spots on abdomen, chest, back. Each spot fades over a period of 3–4 days.
5 Epistaxis may occur.

Second Week

1 Fever remains consistently high.
2 Abdominal distension and tenderness; constipation or diarrhoea.
3 Delirium in severe infections—from severe toxaemia.

Third Week

Gradual decline in fever and subsidence of symptoms.

Diagnosis

1 White blood count—leucopenia is a distinctive haematologic feature, but is not always present.
2 Blood culture—positive for organism after first week.

3 Stool culture—positive for organism after first week.
4 Urine culture—organism may or may not be present.
5 Blood serum agglutination test usually becomes positive by end of second
   week.

Treatment and Nursing Management

Objectives

To give supportive care.
To observe for haemorrhage and perforation.

1 Give specific treatment for typhoid.
   a. Chloramphenicol as directed. Monitor blood count to detect chloramphenicol
   toxicity.
   b. Combination of sulfamethoxazole and trimethoprim (Septrin) may be given
   for chloramphenicol-resistant strains of typhoid.
   c. Ampicillin or amoxicillin are also in use.
2 Give supportive care—typhoid fever is a nursing challenge.
   a. Support patient during period of toxaemia—patient may be drowsy, partially
   incontinent or delirious.
   b. Give steroids if ordered for toxic or delirious patients.
   c. Prepare for blood transfusions if indicated.
   d. Take rectal temperature every 2–4 hours.
      (1) Give tepid sponge for temperature of 40°C (104°F) or more.
      (2) Encourage a high fluid intake.
   e. Watch for bladder distension—patient may lose urge to micturate during toxic
   state. Keep input and output record.
   f. Observe for retention of faeces.
      (1) Enemas are given under *low* pressure to diminish chance of intestinal
      perforation.
      (2) Relieve distension with rectal tube, inserted for a short time.
   g. Give a high calorie, low residue diet during febrile stage.
3 Watch for complications which can occur after an apparent clinical cure.
   a. *Intestinal haemorrhage*—from erosion of blood vessel in ulcerated small
   intestine (occurs in 10% of patients).
      (1) Clinical manifestations:
         (a) Apprehension, sweating, pallor.
         (b) Weak, rapid pulse; narrowing pulse pressure.
         (c) Hypotension
         (d) Bloody or tarry stools.
      (2) Treatment:
         (a) Withhold food.
         (b) Give blood transfusions.
   b. *Perforation of intestine*—from erosion of one of the ulcers; most common
   during third week.
      (1) Symptoms:
         (a) Sudden, sharp abdominal pain—may stop suddenly.
         (b) Abdominal rigidity.
         (c) Shock.

(2) Treatment:
Prepare for intestinal decompression procedure, intravenous fluids and surgical intervention if conservative measures do not produce clinical improvement.

Isolation Nursing Procedure

Use enteric precautions until three successive cultures of faeces taken after cessation of antibiotics are negative for *S. typhi*. Disposable bedpans may be used. Nondisposable bedpans should be disinfected in a steam sterilizer.

Prevention and Health Teaching

1   Prevention: typhoid vaccine, one subcutaneous injection followed by second injection 4 or more weeks later; booster injection every 3 years.
2   Maintain environmental hygiene.
    a. Protect and purify water supplies.
    b. Employ sanitary waste disposal techniques.
    c. Pasteurize milk and dairy products; refrigerate while transporting.
    d. Supervise foods served, especially raw foods.
    e. Ensure that food handlers use handwashing facilities.
3   Patient must be followed with routine stool culture after recovery to detect the development of the carrier state—approximately 2–5% of typhoid patients become permanent carriers, harbouring the organism and excreting it in their urine and stools.
    a. Carriers may be given ampicillin—to attempt to abolish carrier state (there is evidence that treating certain patients with salmonella in their stools may prolong the carrier state).
    b. Positive stool culture after 6–12 months indicates a carrier.
    c. Carriers must not become food or milk handlers.
4   Education of the patient is essential. The MOEH will usually visit the home.

Salmonella Infections (Salmonellosis)

Salmonellosis is a form of food poisoning characterized by acute gastroenteritis; it is caused by certain species of the genus *Salmonella*. The patient is infected via the oral route by contaminated food or drink.

Infectious agent—1500 known serotypes of salmonella—most common in the UK are *S typhimurium*, *S. enteritidis*, *S. agona*, *S. heidelberg* and *S. hadar*.

Nursing Alert: Common food offenders causing salmonella infections include commercially processed meat pies, poultry (especially turkey), sausage (lightly cooked), foods containing egg or egg products and unpasteurized milk or dairy products.

Clinical Manifestations

1   Diarrhoea—sudden onset of frequent, bulky stools followed by profuse, watery diarrhoea; may lead to marked dehydration.
2   Abdominal pain.

3   Nausea and vomiting.
4   Fever.
5   Other manifestations due to infectious agent localizing in any body tissue—abscesses, cholecystitis, arthritis, endocarditis, meningitis, pericarditis, pneumonia, pyelonephritis.

Diagnosis

Culture of faeces, blood and urine.

Treatment

Objective

To prevent dehydration and electrolyte imbalance.
Treatment is supportive:

1   Restrict food until nausea and vomiting subside.
2   Offer clear liquids as tolerated.
3   Correct fluid and electrolyte depletion with intravenous infusions.
4   Give antispasmodics as directed.
5   Treatment is similar to that for typhoid fever if patient has focal (abscess) or systemic infection.

Nursing Isolation Procedure

Use enteric precautions for duration of illness.

Preventive Measures and Health Teaching

1   Food service workers should have training courses and on-going in-service training in facts about food-borne illnesses, avoidance of food contamination, food storage methods, cleaning of food preparation and service areas, and maintenance of good personal hygiene.
2   Raw eggs or egg drinks should not be eaten, nor should cracked or dirty eggs be used.
3   All foods from animal sources, especially fowl, egg products and meat dishes, should be thoroughly cooked.
4   Foods should be refrigerated during storage and should be protected against insects/rodents.
5   Any person handling food should be instructed to wash hands after toilet use, before and after food preparation.
6   Chicks, ducklings and turtles (as well as other domestic animals and pets) are sources of infection.
7   The patient must wash his hands after toilet use, particularly during illness and carrier state (2–4 weeks)—to prevent infection of others.
8   Diarrhoea in infants should be investigated immediately, since salmonellae play an important role, particularly in infants less than 1 year old.

Shigellosis (Bacillary Dysentery)

Shigellosis, an acute bacterial disease of the intestinal tract, includes a group of enteric infections caused by bacilli of the *Shigella* group of which there are four types: *S. sonnei*, most common in the UK, *S. dysenteria*, *S. boydii*, *S. flexneri*. The source of infection is faeces from an infected person. The route of spread is faecal/oral.

Clinical Manifestations

1   Fever and headache.
2   Abdominal cramps.
3   Severe prostration.
4   Persistent diarrhoea—passage of varying amounts of blood, mucus and pus.

Diagnosis

Isolation of *Shigella* from faeces or rectal swabs.

Treatment and Nursing Management

Objectives

To provide aggressive treatment for the patient.
To prevent the spread of shigellosis to the patient's contacts, i.e., to eliminate the carrier state.

1   Determine the type of shigella—organism is recovered from patient's stool.
2   Do sensitivity testing for selection of antibiotic—multiresistance to antibiotics is common.
3   Give antibiotics which are absorbed from intestinal tract (neomycin, tetracyclines, chloramphenicol)—may shorten duration of illness.
4   Maintain fluid and electrolyte balance—to prevent profound dehydration owing to an excessively great loss of salts in the diarrhoeic stools.
   a. Assess weight loss, skin turgor, dryness of mucous membranes, urinary volume, vital signs.
   b. Weigh daily and measure urinary volume.
5   Offer clear fluids during acute stage of illness.
6   Carry out epidemiology studies of every patient in whom the organism is found.
   a. Ask if patient has been recent traveller to Middle or Far East or has had contacts with travellers from these countries.
   b. Notify local authorities.

Nursing Isolation Procedure

Use enteric precautions until three consecutive cultures of faeces taken 24 hours apart after cessation of antibiotic therapy are negative for infecting strain.

Preventive Measures and Health Teaching

1   See Health Teaching for typhoid fever, p. 238.
2   Programme of fly control.

3 Surveillance of water sanitation; adequate sewage disposal.
4 Detection and treatment of carriers.
5 Handwashing after defaecation.

Botulism

Botulism is a type of poisoning which affects the central nervous system; it is caused by eating food in which *Clostridium botulinum* has grown and produced toxins. The organism is widely distributed in soil. Human intoxication usually follows ingestion of contaminated foods preserved in jars and tins. It is very rare in the UK.

Clinical Manifestations

1 Nausea and vomiting.
2 Blurred vision; diplopia.
3 Dizziness.
4 Severe dryness of mouth and throat.
5 Difficulty in speaking and swallowing.
6 Respiratory paralysis with progressive muscle paralysis; botulinal toxins may diminish release of acetylcholine at the neuromuscular junction—extraocular, pharyngeal and extremity paralysis follow.

Course

1 Variable; illness may be prolonged, with a high risk of superinfection and fatal outcome.
2 Recovery in survivors may be prolonged.

Clinical Evaluation

1 Electromyography—to differentiate botulism from atypical Guillain–Barré syndrome.
2 Mouse-toxin neutralization test—for detection of botulinal toxin; patient's serum sent to laboratory that has capacity for performing this test.
3 Examination of faecal samples—examined for botulinal toxin.

Treatment and Nursing Management

Objectives

To prevent respiratory failure.
To eliminate the toxin and *C. botulinum* from the gastrointestinal tract.

1 Give intensive respiratory support—death is frequently due to onset of respiratory failure.
   a. Prepare for tracheotomy, mechanical ventilation.
   b. Carry out blood gas determinations as necessary.
2 Give cathartics, enemas and gastric lavage (when these can be safely administered)—to eliminate unabsorbed toxin and *C. botulinum* from the gastrointestinal tract.

3   Administer trivalent ABE botulinal antitoxin as directed (has a high reaction rate).
    a. Determine if there is a history of allergy, asthma, hay fever.
    b. Perform a skin test for sensitivity.
    c. Have ventilatory equipment and emergency drugs ready in event of life-threatening reaction.
4   Guanidine hydrochloride may be administered—enhances the release of acetylcholine from the nerve terminals; not as effective in overcoming respiratory paralysis as it is in combating paralysis of extremities and extraocular muscles.
5   Treat superimposed infections with antibiotics if necessary.

Prevention and Health Teaching

1   Home canners should be taught how to prevent botulism.
2   Home-canned foods should be inspected before being eaten—foods contaminated with *C. botulinum* look soft, contain gas bubbles and give off an odour of decay. However, this is not always certain.
3   Canned foods should be boiled 10–20 min and stirred thoroughly before serving—toxin is heat-labile and is destroyed by proper cooking of foods.
4   Be careful in preparing food for canning at high altitudes since it is difficult to provide a temperature high enough to destroy the spores of *C. botulinum*. Use pressure cooker method of canning at high altitudes.

Nursing Isolation Procedure

No precautions are necessary. Botulism is an intoxication, not an infection.

Gonorrhoea

Gonorrhoea is an infection involving the mucous membrane of the genitourinary tract; it is caused by the gonococcus *Neisseria gonorrhoeae*. It is an infectious disease which is transmitted sexually, the exception being gonococcal ophthalmia of the newborn. It may be acquired by sexual intercourse, orogenital, and/or anogenital contacts between members of the opposite sexes as well as members of the same sex.

Epidemiology

1   Changes in sexual behaviour; liberalization of attitudes.
2   Sexual contact at earlier ages.
3   Greater personal mobility.

Clinical Problems

1   Gonorrhoea is increasing in the UK. There were 43 835 new cases in England in 1968, and 68 676 in 1976.
2   Gonorrhoea has a short incubation period which permits rapid spread; a high percentage of infected females are symptom-free.
3   Syphilis and gonorrhoea are frequently observed in the same patient.
4   Gonorrhoea is becoming increasingly resistant to penicillin in some countries.

Complications

1 Sterility in women; pelvic infection.
2 Secondary foci of infection may develop in any organ system—disseminated gonorrhoea, gonococcal arthritis, tenosynovitis, bursitis, endocarditis, pelvic infection, meningitis, lesions of the skin, severe proctitis, postgonococcal urethritis (male).

Clinical Manifestations

Nursing Alert: 80% of women who have the disease may be asymptomatic and unaware that they are infected. There is a fairly high incidence of asymptomatic males with gonorrhoea.

Women (small percentage)

Vaginal discharge.
Urinary frequency and pain.
Pelvic infection, when gonococcus spreads through fallopian tubes (salpingitis).
  Fever
  Nausea and vomiting
  Lower abdominal pain
Gonococcal septicaemia.

Men (incubation period 3–4 days or longer)

Painful urination; mucopurulent urethral discharge.
Spread of infection to posterior urethra, prostate, seminal vesicles and epididymis.
Prostatitis.
Pelvic pain and fever.
Epididymitis.
  Severe pain, tenderness, and swelling
Postgonococcal urethritis and urethral stricture become major problems in male.

Anal Manifestations

1 Anal itching and irritation—erythema and oedema of anal crypts.
2 Painful defaecation.
3 Sensation of rectal fullness; anal discharge.

Oral Manifestations

May be affected by gonorrhoeal process directly (direct contact of oral cavity with infecting organisms) or indirectly (secondary to infection elsewhere in the body).
  The majority of pharyngeal infections are asymptomatic.

1 Sore throat/pharyngeal inflammation.
2 Lips—may show intensely painful ulcerative inflammation.
3 Gingiva—erythematous, spongy and tender.
4 Tongue—red and dry with ulcerations or swollen and glazed with eroded areas.
5 Soft palate and uvula—reddened and oedematous.
6 Oropharynx—may be covered with vesicles.

Diagnosis

Women

Culture specimen obtained from the cervix and anal canal and inoculated on separate Modified Thayer–Martin (MTM) culture plates.

Men

1 Smear of urethral exudate for microscopic examination.
2 In homosexuals: additional culture specimens obtained from anal canal and pharynx and inoculated on Modified Thayer–Martin culture plates.
3 Culture of oral cavity with Thayer–Martin Medium (sugar fermentation required) if indicated.

Treatment

Objective

To eradicate the organism.

1 Uncomplicated gonococcal infection.
   a. Penicillin G (drug of choice) intramuscularly, 1.2 megaunits. This is preceded by 0.5 g Probenecid, given by mouth, ½ hour before the injection. In cases where penicillin resistance may be present, 2.4 or 3.6 megaunits may be given.
      (1) Have patient wait in clinic 20–30 min after penicillin injection—in case of anaphylactoid reaction.
      (2) Have adrenalin, intravenous fluids and ventilatory equipment available.
2 Alternative regimens.
   a. Oral therapy: Ampicillin by mouth together with probenecid
   b. Therapy for patients allergic to penicillin or probenecid or with history of previous anaphylactic reactions.
      (1) Tetracycline hydrochloride by mouth on a 4-day schedule—or
      (2) Spectinomycin hydrochloride intramuscularly in a single injection.
3 Treatment of sexual contacts: Same treatment as for gonorrhoea.
4 Follow-up—imperative due to a higher resistance of *Neisseria* gonococci to antibiotics.
   Culture should be obtained from appropriate sites 7–14 days after completion of treatment.
5 Secure serologic test for syphilis at time of diagnosis.
6 Patients with gonorrhoea who also have syphilis must be given additional treatment depending on stage of syphilis.
7 Treatment of complications of gonorrhoea (endocarditis, bacteraemia, arthritis, etc.) is individualized.

Nursing Isolation Procedure

Use secretion precautions for duration of illness (until lesions stop draining).

Principles of Control

1 Gonorrhoea is not a reportable disease; careful records are kept by venereal disease (VD) clinics, and contacts are traced by specially trained personnel.

2   Each patient should be interviewed for names of contacts. Conduct interview and record history in nonjudgemental, empathetic manner.
3   Contacts of known gonorrhoea cases should be investigated; known contacts should be treated.
4   The patient should be instructed to avoid reinfection by sexual activity with untreated previous sexual partners until they have been tested and treated.

Health Teaching

1   VD is acquired by sexual contact (vaginal sexual intercourse, anal intercourse, oral intercourse) and by close and direct contact with an infected person.
2   A person who thinks that he or she may have VD or who has been exposed to someone who might have it should have a checkup. Immediate treatment should be sought if symptoms develop.
3   Anyone who is sexually active with a number of sexual partners should have regular checkups.
4   Washing the sex organs (before and after sexual contact) and the use of a condom may give limited protection against VD.
5   Birth control pills and intrauterine devices give no protection against VD.
6   Gonorrhoea and syphilis are different diseases, caused by different germs; they attack the body in different ways but are spread in the same manner. A person may have both gonorrhoea and syphilis at the same time.
7   There appears to be no natural or acquired immunity to gonorrhoea and syphilis. A person can get gonorrhoea and syphilis again and again.
8   Pregnant women may pass infection of syphilis to unborn child. Pregnant women may pass gonorrhoea to baby during the birth process.
9   Bacteria from gonorrhoea may enter the bloodstream and affect joints, joint linings, heart valves, etc.

Meningococcal Meningitis (Cerebrospinal Fever)

Meningitis—inflammation of the meninges, or coverings of the brain; may be caused by bacterial, mycobacterial or viral agents.

Meningococcal meningitis is an acute bacterial infectious disease caused by the meningococcus, *Neisseria meningitidis*. It starts as an infection of the nasopharynx or the tonsils and is followed by menigococcal septicaemia, which extends to the meninges of the brain and the upper region of the spinal cord. There are several distinct immunologic strains of the meningococcus, but the groups A, B and C are the most important.

Clinical Manifestations

Symptoms result first from infection and then from increased intracranial pressure.
1   High fever.
2   Nausea and vomiting.
3   Headache, irritability, confusion, delirium, convulsions.
4   Neck, shoulder and back stiffness.

5 Appearance of petechiae (usually on legs); may progress to large ecchymotic or purpuric lesions.
6 Resistance to neck flexion.
   a. *Positive Kernig's sign*—when lying with the thigh flexed on the abdomen, patient cannot completely extend his leg (a sign of meningeal irritation).
   b. *Positive Brudzinski's sign*—when the patient's neck is flexed on the chest, flexion of the knees and hips is produced. When passive flexion of the lower extremity on one side is made, a similar movement will be seen on the contralateral (opposite) extremity.

Source of Infection

Human cases and carriers.

Method of Spread

By contact or droplet infection.

Diagnosis

Organism usually demonstrated by smear and culture of cerebrospinal fluid, oropharynx and blood.

Clinical Features

1 Meningococcus may localize in the brain, skin or joint synovia.
2 Predisposing factors include otitis media, mastoiditis, sickle cell anaemia (or other haemoglobinopathies), recent neurosurgical procedures, head trauma, respiratory infection, immunologic defects.
3 The disease occurs in winter and spring months; epidemics are most apt to occur when people live in crowded quarters.

Treatment and Nursing Management

Objective

To observe and treat for vasomotor shock and collapse.

1 Support patient undergoing diagnostic lumbar puncture—cerebrospinal fluid will usually be cloudy with elevated pressure.
2 Give specific drug therapy, depending of culture and sensitivity results—initially by intravenous route; therapy continued for minimum of 10 days.
   a. Penicillin G (drug of choice); chloramphenicol for patients allergic to penicillin.
   b. Most antibiotics enter cerebrospinal fluid and central nervous system inefficiently.
3 Maintain a clear airway—altered consciousness may lead to airway obstruction.
   a. Carry out arterial blood gas determinations.
   b. Provide oral airway or cuffed endotracheal tube or tracheotomy as patient's condition indicates.
   c. Administer oxygen to maintain arterial Po_2 at desired levels.

Tuberculosis

Tuberculosis is an infectious disease caused by the tubercle bacillus, *Mycobacterium tuberculosis*. It usually invades the lungs, but it also involves, and sometimes produces gross lesions in other isolated organs, or it may be widespread. The incidence of tuberculosis notifications has decreased from over 80 000 in 1912 to 10 000 in 1975.

Transmission

1   The term *mycobacterium* is descriptive of the organism, which is a bacterium that resembles a fungus. The organisms multiply slowly and are characterized as acid-fast aerobic organisms which can be killed by heat, sunshine, drying and ultraviolet light.
2   Tuberculosis is an airborne disease transmitted by droplet nuclei, usually within the respiratory tract of a person with active ulcerative lesions who expels them during coughing, talking, sneezing or singing.
3   When an uninfected person inhales the droplet-containing air, the organism is carried into the lung to the pulmonary alveoli.

Pathology

1   A primary complex consists of the original site of the infection, together with the reaction occurring in the regional lymph nodes. When the primary focus is in the lungs, the hilar glands are those which are affected.
2   These changes occur within about 6 weeks and may be asymptomatic.
3   The primary lesion in the lungs usually heals. A systemic reaction occurs and this includes the development of a degree of immunity, and of a positive reaction to a tuberculin test, e.g., Mantoux test.
4   The lung lesion may become smaller and calcify. It may be evident on chest x-ray when it is completely quiescent. It may proceed to necrosis of tissue, causing caseation and cavitation.
5   The initial lesion may progress:
    a. By invasion of adjacent tissues.
    b. By invasion of the bloodstream.
    c. Via the bronchial tree.
6   In children the hilar nodes may cause compression of the lobar bronchi, which may result in a collapsed lobe, and the subsequent development of bronchiectasis.
7   Postprimary infection refers to any development of tuberculosis after the first few weeks of the original infection. It may occur about 2 years after the original infection, but may be many years later.

Conditions Contributing to the Development of Tuberculosis

1   General physical debilitation.
2   Constant exposure to active tubercle bacilli.
3   Lowered resistance because of:
    a. Presence of other disease (diabetes, silicosis, etc.).
    b. Age; over 30.

4   Immune deficiency diseases.
5   Recent gastrointestinal surgery.
6   Steroid therapy.
7   Alcoholism.
8   Pregnancy.

Clinical Manifestations

Patient may be asymptomatic or may have insidious symptoms that are ignored.

1   Generalized systemic signs and symptoms:
    a. Fatigue, anorexia, loss of weight and strength, low grade fever, irregular menses.
    b. Some patients have acute febrile illness, chills, generalized influenza-like symptoms.
2   Pulmonary signs and symptoms.
    a. Cough (imperceptible onset) progressing in frequency and producing mucoid or mucopurulent sputum.
    b. Haemoptysis; chest pain.

Diagnosis

1   Sputum smear and culture—diagnosis made by finding the acid fast bacilli in sputum obtained by coughing and expectoration. If little sputum is present, gastric aspiration should be carried out first thing in the morning, to obtain sputum which has been swallowed during the night. The culture involves incubation on a plate of Dover's medium for 3–7 weeks.
2   Tuberculin skin test—inoculation of tubercle bacillus extract (tuberculin) into the intradermal layer of the inner aspect of the forearm.
3   Multiple puncture tests—introduction of tuberculin into the skin by multiple puncture.
4   Chest x-ray.
5   Biopsy of pulmonary nodules.
6   Culture of aspirate of pleural effusion if this is present.

Treatment

Objective

To eliminate all viable tubercle bacilli.

1   Administer prescribed antituberculosis drugs (Table 6.3).
    a. A combination of drugs is given to reduce viable microbial organisms as rapidly as possible and to minimize the chance of persistence of drug-resistant organisms.
    b. Chemotherapy is prolonged to eliminate all organisms, since the tubercle bacillus multiplies slowly.
    c. There are 11 antituberculosis drugs currently on the market; isoniazid (INH), ethambutol (EMB), rifampin and streptomycin (SM) are the drugs most commonly used for initial treatment (first line drugs).
    d. Intensive triple drug regimen for initial therapy:

Streptomycin (intramuscularly) with oral administration of isoniazid and ethambutol (for 30–90 days)—followed by maintenance therapy with isoniazid and ethambutol for a minimum of 24 months after sputum cultures have been converted from positive to negative.

e. A variety of combinations of antituberculosis drugs have been used with success.

2   Majority of patients improve rapidly after antituberculosis therapy is begun; symptoms abate and number of acid-fast bacilli on sputum smear decreases.

Nursing Isolation Procedure

Respiratory isolation for patients with open pulmonary tuberculosis.

Prevention of Spread of Infection

Objectives

To identify, notify and effectively treat infected patients.
To trace the source of the infection of newly notified cases.
To screen the families and close contacts of newly notified cases, by means of chest x-rays and Mantoux tests.

1   Promote a vaccination programme for all schoolchildren at the age of 13 years (see Schedule of Vaccination and Immunization).
2   Vaccinate new born babies if either parent has pulmonary tuberculosis.
3   Screen immigrants coming from countries where there is known to be a high rate of tuberculosis.
4   Teach the patient and the family about the disease.
a. Teach the patient to cover nose and mouth when coughing or sneezing with disposable tissues, which should be burnt after use.
b. Teach the patient and family about the principles of nutrition. Ensure that there is sufficient financial income for a good diet to be provided.
5   A number of patients suffering from tuberculosis may have associated medical or social problems. Alcoholism should be treated at the appropriate specialist clinic. Patients with psychiatric or social problems often need prolonged help.

Patients whose housing and social conditions are satisfactory, may be admitted to hospital for 4–8 weeks, so that assessment of the effectiveness of drug therapy is possible, following the initial diagnostic procedures. Those with alcoholic, psychiatric or social problems may be in hospital for several months.

ACTINOMYCOSIS

Actinomycosis is a chronic, suppurating, granulomatous disease. The usual pathogen in man is an anaerobic gram-positive branching filamentous bacterium,*

---

* Actinomycosis has traditionally been classified as a mycotic or fungal disease because it characteristically resembles the deep mycoses, but the actinomycetes are now classified as bacteria.

Table 6.3. Drug Therapy of Tuberculosis*

Drugs and Dosage	Excretion	Relatively Common Reactions	Less Common Reactions	Mode of Action
1 Isoniazid 5 mg/kg/body wt. p.o. (usually 300 mg QD as single dose)	Renal Hepatic	Peripheral neuritis Hepatic dysfunction	Central nervous system effects: insomnia, headache, restlessness, psychosis, increased reflexes, muscle twitching, paresthesias, convulsions (high dosage), drowsiness, excitement, delay in micturition Optic neuritis and optic atrophy Constipation, dryness of mouth, allergic reactions, hepatitis, agranulocytosis, exfoliative dermatitis, rheumatic symptoms	Interferes with DNA synthesis and intermediary metabolism
2 Ethambutol 15 mg/kg p.o. (usually given as single dose)	Renal	Optic neuritis	Anaphylactoid reaction, dermatitis, pruritus, joint pain, anorexia, fever, headache, dizziness, mental symptoms, peripheral neuritis, elevated uric acid, liver damage	Inhibits RNA synthesis and phosphate metabolism
3 Rifampin 600 mg/day p.o.	Hepatic	Gastrointestinal upset	Headache, drowsiness, ataxia, mental symptoms, visual disturbances, weakness, fever, pain in extremities, numbness, hypersensitivity, urticaria, rash, eosinophilia, sore mouth, hepatitis, thrombocytopenia, leucopenia, anaemia, immunosuppression, renal damage, elevated uric acid	Inhibits RNA polymerase, blocking DNA-directed RNA synthesis
4 Streptomycin 1 g/day or 2–3	Renal	Eighth nerve toxicity, vertigo, tinnitus, dizziness, deafness	Pyrexia, headache, dermatitis, pruritus, renal insufficiency, transient dermal anaesthesia	Inhibits protein synthesis by direct action

No.	Drug and dose	Excretion/metabolism	Toxicity	Toxicity	Mode of action
	...g t.i.d., p.o. (sodium salt should be 5 g t.i.d., p.o.)		nausea, vomiting, anorexia, diarrhoea	prothrombinaemia, dermatitis, hypothyroidism, renal insufficiency, anaphylactoid reaction, hepatitis	Inhibits protein synthesis
6	Ethionamide 0.5 g or 1 g p.o. daily in one dose	Rapidly inactivated site? Little free drug excreted in urine	Gastrointestinal toxicity; anorexia, nausea, vomiting, diarrhoea	Hepatotoxicity, purpura, gynecomastia, impotence, peripheral neuropathy, psychic depression, drowsiness, asthenia, acne, allergic skin rash, difficulty in diabetic control, renal impairment	
7	Pyrazinamide 0.5–1.0 g t.i.d., p.o.	Renal	Hepatotoxicity Uric acid retention	Gout, arthralgia, anorexia, nausea and vomiting, dysuria, malaise, fever	Unknown
8	Kanamycin 1.0 g i.m. 3–5 times weekly	Renal	Eighth nerve toxicity; dizziness, tinnitus, deafness Renal irritation; albuminuria, cells and casts Local irritation and pain	Renal damage, eosinophilia, allergic dermatitis, fever, headache, paresthesias	Inhibits protein synthesis
9	Cycloserine 250 or 500 mg q 12 h p.o.	Renal	Central nervous system toxicity; headache, vertigo, lethargy, tremor, dysarthria, apraxia, coma, behavioural changes, psychotic episodes, convulsions Allergic dermatitis		May inhibit cell wall synthesis
10	Capreomycin 15 mg/kg/day, usually 1 g	Renal	Renal damage, vestibular damage, local pain, eosinophilia, rash, fever	Anaphylaxis	Inhibits protein synthesis
11	Viomycin 1 g q 12 h 2 days/week i.m.	Renal	Renal impairment: albuminuria, cells and casts Eighth nerve toxicity: dizziness, tinnitus, deafness Allergic reactions with eosinophilia (skin, fever, etc.)	Fluid retention with oedema, renal damage, electrocardiographic abnormalities, electrolyte pattern disturbances	Inhibits protein synthesis

* From Mayock, R L and Macgregor, R R, Diagnosis, Prevention and Early Therapy of Tuberculosis, in Dowling, H F (Ed) (1976) Disease-a-Month, May. Copyright © 1976 by Year Book Medical Publishers, Inc., Chicago. Used by permission.

Actinomyces israelii, that may be found in the tonsillar crypts of apparently healthy individuals, from scrapings of teeth and gums, and in the gastrointestinal tract (appendix and anorectal regions). Minor trauma, aspiration or surgical manipulation may initiate the infectious process.

Pathology

1 The characteristic lesions are firmly indurated granulomas which spread slowly to adjacent tissues and break down focally to form multiple sinus tracts which penetrate to the surface.
2 The exudate from the sinus tracts contains the characteristic sulfur granules which are visible masses of the organisms.

Clinical Manifestations

Actinomycosis involves three major forms of infection:

1 *Cervicofacial type*—swelling about the teeth, submaxillary region and neck producing a flat, hard, painless tumour mass which is fixed firmly to the jawbone. Granuloma ultimately breaks down and becomes riddled with abscesses which perforate externally.
2 *Abdominal type*—affects any visceral organ, especially the caecum and appendix, ovaries and tubes. Tumour mass, resembling carcinoma, develops. By extension it may involve the abdominal wall, discharging externally through open sinuses.
3 *Thoracic type*—acute and chronic inflammatory reaction may involve lungs, pleura, mediastinum or chest wall, producing chest pain, fever, cough and haemoptysis.

Diagnosis

Biopsy of cutaneous lesion—may demonstrate the sulfur granules.

Treatment

1 Give penicillin (drug of choice)—therapy should be continued for weeks to months to prevent recurrence.
2 Patients with penicillin sensitivity may be given tetracycline, erythromycin, lincomycin or clindamycin.
3 Surgical drainage, rejection of damaged tissue and excision of sinuses and fistulous tracts are necessary adjuncts to antibiotic therapy.

Nursing Isolation Procedures

Secretion precautions until wounds or lesions stop draining.

Health Teaching

1 Encourage good dental hygiene to reduce infection around teeth.
2 There is a possibility of *Actinomyces* infection associated with the use of an intrauterine device, especially when other pelvic infection is present.

SPIROCHETAL INFECTIONS

Syphilis (Lues)

Syphilis is a chronic infectious multisystem disease caused by *Å Treponema palidum* (a spirochete). It is acquired by sexual contact or may be congenital in origin.

Incidence

Most prevalent in teenagers and young adults.
More prevalent in males than females.
More prevalent in large urban centres.
Promiscuity and indiscretion are factors.

Epidemiology

Tracing the source and spread of infections by interviewing known patients for sex contacts.

1   Interviewing and re-interviewing every reported patient with syphilis for sex contacts.
2   Rapid investigation to identify contacts for examination within a minimal time period.
3   Identifying and conducting blood tests of other persons who by definition (suspect or associate) are possibly involved sexually in an infectious chain (cluster procedure). (Promiscuous persons have somewhat similar sexual behaviour patterns.)
4   Epidemiologic (preventive or prophylactic) treatment of sexual contacts and infectious syphilis cases.
5   All pregnant women are screened for syphilis as a routine.

Clinical Manifestations

Syphilis is capable of destroying tissue in almost any organ in the body; it thus produces a wide variety of clinical manifestations.

Stages of Untreated Syphilis

Incubation period

1   10–90 days; average 21 days.
2   No symptoms or lesions.
3   Spirochetaemia is present; patient's blood is infective.

Primary (early) syphilis

1   Most infectious stage; lasting 1–6 weeks.
2   Manifestations include:
     a. Chancre or primary sore—appears at the site where the treponema enters the body (glans penis, scrotum, cervix, labia, anus, lips, mouth, tonsils, eyelids, nipple).

Chancre remains for short time and heals without treatment (3–6 weeks), leaving a thin atrophic scar.

b. Enlargement of regional lymph nodes.

Secondary syphilis

1   Lesion appears 6–8 weeks after onset of primary lesion; may involve any cutaneous or mucosal surface of the body as well as any organ.
2   Skin lesions—bilaterally symmetrical in distribution, polymorphous (macular, papular, follicular, pustular).
   a. Moist papules occur most frequently in anogenital region (condylomata) and in mouth.
   b. Lesions of mouth, throat and cervix (mucous patches) frequently occur in secondary stage.
   c. Generalized patchy hair loss on scalp.
3   Generalized lymphadenopathy.
4   Arthritic and bone pain.
5   Acute iritis.
6   Hoarseness, chronic sore throat.

Late syphilis (clinically destructive stage after latent period)

1   Manifestations may occur 10–30 years after exposure; recovery unpredictable.
2   Syphilis will mainly affect cardiovascular system (aneurysm of ascending aorta, aortic insufficiency), central nervous system and skeletal system.

Diagnosis

There are two types of serologic tests:

Nontreponemal or Reagin Tests

To detect antibody-like substances, called reagin, found in serum of infected patient; these tests are not always specific and there may be false-positive reactions.

1   Flocculation tests—a reaction in which a suspension of antibody particles when added to serum, plasma or spinal fluid containing antibody will form small, usually visible clumps, or floccules.
   a. Venereal disease research laboratory (VDRL).
   b. Kline.
   c. Kahn.
   d. Hinton.
   e. Mazzini.
2   Complement fixation tests—involves bringing together an active complement, an antigen and its antibody under proper temperature and time conditions.
   a. Kolmer.
   b. Wasserman.
3   Rapid reagin tests—specific-purpose tests using flocculation procedures on plasma or serum; used as a rough screening guide.

Treponemal Tests

Test for detection of treponemal antibody produced in response to syphilitic infection.

1   Treponema pallidum immobilization test (TPI).
2   Fluorescent treponemal antibody test (FTA).
3   Fluorescent treponemal antibody absorption test (FTA-ABS)—the standard test in most state health laboratories.

Treatment (for early syphilis)

1   Give Benzathine penicillin G (intramuscularly)—drug of choice because it provides effective treatment in a single visit or aqueous procaine penicillin G (intramuscularly) for 8 days.
    a. Screen for history of previous reaction to penicillin; reaction can occur in patient with negative history.
    b. Patient should be detained 30 min after administration of parenteral penicillin in case of development of anaphylactoid reaction.
2   Patients who are allergic to penicillin may be given tetracycline or erythromycin.
3   Post-treatment follow-up is essential—treatment failures do occur and retreatment is required, followed by quantitative VDRL at 1, 3, 6 and 12 months.
4   Jarisch–Herxheimer reaction—a reaction appearing within hours after initiating treatment of syphilis (particularly in the secondary stage) and subsiding within 24 hours; consists of transient fever and flu-like symptoms of malaise, chills, headache and myalgia. It may involve release of endotoxin-killed treponemes or from an allergic phenomenon.
    a. Managed by bed rest and aspirin.
    b. Warn patient that this reaction may be expected.

Nursing Isolation Procedures

Secretion precautions for mucocutaneous manifestations until 24 hours after initiation of effective therapy.

Prevention and Health Teaching

1   All patients known to have been exposed to syphilitic lesion should be treated.
2   Preventive treatment should be given before or after exposure.
3   Programme of public health and sex education should be conducted.
4   Patient should be instructed to refrain from sexual intercourse with previous partners not under treatment.
5   Mass serologic examinations of special groups with known high incidence of venereal disease should be conducted.

VIRAL INFECTIONS

Influenza

Influenza is an acute infectious disease caused by an RNA-containing myxovirus. It is characterized by respiratory and constitutional symptoms. Epidemics of influenza develop rapidly; there is a fairly high mortality rate among the elderly and those debilitated by chronic disease.

Aetiology

1 The primary factor in the aetiology of influenza is a filtrable virus of which three major strains have been isolated; designated types A, B and C.
2 The numerous variants within a given type are called subtypes.
3 Group A appears to be the most virulent and is responsible for the most recent epidemics.
4 Influenza appears to become epidemic when antibody levels wane or when the antigens of prevalent influenza viruses have changed enough to render the population susceptible.
5 Transmission is by close contact or by droplets from the respiratory tract of an infected person.

Clinical Course

1 The virus is airborne and multiplies in the upper respiratory tract—selected invasion of nasal, tracheal and bronchial mucosal cells.
2 Influenza virus damages the ciliated epithelium of the tracheobronchial tree, rendering the patient vulnerable to the development of secondary invaders such as pneumococci or staphylococci, *Haemophilus influenzae*, streptococci and other organisms.

Clinical Manifestations

1 Fever: 39–40°C (102–104°F).
2 Headache and profound malaise.
3 Respiratory features—dry cough, sore throat, nasal obstruction and discharge.
4 Muscular aches—especially in back and legs.

Treatment and Nursing Management

Objectives

To offer the patient supportive therapy.
To prevent and treat complications (respiratory, cardiac, neurological).

1 Give aspirin or aspirin compounds every 4 hours for fever, headache and myalgia.
2 Offer cough syrup for dry, hacking cough.
3 Use a vaporizer—to reduce irritation to respiratory mucosa.
4 Give liberal fluid intake.
5 Watch for dyspnoea in early course of influenza—points to bronchopneumonia, which is a potentially life-threatening disease.
   a. Pneumonia may also be of viral, mixed viral or bacterial origin.
   b. Treat pneumonia.
      (1) Obtain cultures of throat, blood and sputum immediately.
      (2) Give antibiotic therapy as required—usually penicillin G or erythromycin.
      (3) Assess for vasomotor collapse.
      (4) Observe for acute respiratory failure.

(5) Initiate tracheal suctioning, tracheal intubation and assisted ventilation as required.
6 Assess for neurologic complications—from direct invasion of the nervous system or by autoimmune response (hypersensitivity) in the nervous system.
7 Watch for development of myocarditis.

Prevention

1 *Vaccination.*
   a. Active immunization consists of a single dose of vaccine (influenza virus vaccine, bivalent) for either primary or annual booster vaccination.
   b. Dose volumes are specified in manufacturer's labelling.
   c. Influenza vaccine should be given by mid-November.
2 Vaccination is recommended for persons who have such chronic conditions as:
   a. Heart disease of any aetiology, particularly with mitral stenosis or cardiac insufficiency.
   b. Chronic bronchopulmonary diseases, such as asthma, chronic bronchitis, bronchiectasis, tuberculosis and emphysema.
   c. Chronic renal disease.
   d. Diabetes mellitus and other chronic metabolic disorders.
3 Vaccination recommended for older persons (over 65)—excess mortality in older age groups.
4 Selective use of antiviral agents.
   a. Amantadine hydrochloride has been used for prevention and modification of influenza caused by type A influenza viruses.
   b. To be effective, amantadine should be given prior to and for the duration of exposure to type A influenza virus.
   c. Patients with high priority for antiviral therapy include:
      (1) Patients with chronic respiratory, cardiovascular, etc., disease.
      (2) Patients hospitalized for treatment of other illnesses.
      (3) Elderly persons residing in nursing homes or other institutions.
5 Vaccination should be repeated when a new strain of virus appears.

Nursing Isolation Procedures

Usually none. There may be some instances when respiratory isolation of patients with influenza is indicated, especially if the diagnosis can be made on or soon after admission.

Health Teaching

1 The risk of developing influenza is related to crowding and close contacts of groups of individuals.
2 Restrict visiting privileges within health care facilities during epidemics—to minimize chance of introducing influenza.
3 It appears wise to humidify home and office air and to discourage cigarette smoking for high risk persons.

Infectious Mononucleosis

Infectious mononucleosis ('mono'; glandular fever) is an acute infectious disease of the lymphatic system caused by the Epstein–Barr virus, a member of the herpes group. Cytomegalovirus infection can produce a clinical picture closely resembling infectious mononucleosis.

Incidence and Transmission

1   Occurs mainly between ages of 14 and 30; high frequency of occurrence in college students and military population.
2   The virus is excreted in saliva of patients with active disease or of those who are carriers, and is spread by intimate personal contact. It can also be transmitted by blood transfusion.

Clinical Manifestations

May be vague and masquerade as those of leukaemia, hepatitis, drug rash.

1   Fever
2   Sore throat.
3   Skin rash—faint erythematous or maculopapular eruption on trunk and proximal extremities.
4   Lymphadenopathy.
5   Bilateral periorbital oedema.
6   Enlargement of the spleen.

Diagnosis

1   Blood smears—show lymphocytosis and atypical lymphocytes.
2   Heterophil antibody agglutination test—increase in titre.
3   Rising EBV antibody (Epstein–Barr virus titre).
4   Abnormal liver function tests.

Treatment

1   The treatment is symptomatic and supportive.
    a. Encourage patient to obtain additional rest and a nutritious diet.
    b. Give aspirin for headache, muscle pains and chills.
2   Observe for complications—rupture of spleen, Guillain–Barré syndrome causing respiratory failure, glottic oedema and hepatic failure.
3   Steroids may be helpful in severe cases.

Health Teaching

1   Patient is to avoid strenuous exercise—exertion or trauma may cause rupture of spleen. (Competitive sports should be avoided until full recovery.)
2   Observe for upper quadrant pain radiating to shoulder with signs of peritoneal irritation—evidence of splenic rupture.
3   Prepare for exploratory laparotomy.

Nursing Isolation Procedures

Secretion precautions for duration of the illness.

Arthropod-borne Viral Encephalitis

Encephalitis (inflammation of the brain) may be caused by a number of agents, including viruses, bacteria and chemicals. The viral encephalitides comprise a group of acute infections that affect predominantly the nervous system (brain, spinal cord and meninges). Each variety is caused by a specific virus. For each of these viruses there exists a particular animal reservoir, and each finds its access to man through the bite of a particular species of blood-sucking arthropod, e.g., mosquitoes, ticks.

Occurrence

1   In the UK, the only form due to organism of this group is benign lymphocytic meningitis.
2   Travellers from tropical or subtropical countries may have different types, e.g., St. Louis encephalitis from the USA, Murray Valley encephalitis from Australia.

Mode of Transmission

Bite of infective mosquitoes.

Clinical Manifestations (variable)

Acute onset:
   High fever.
   Severe headache.
   Signs of meningeal and spinal cord irritation.
   Disorientation; coma—convulsions in infants.

Diagnosis

1   Lumbar puncture—reveals lymphocytosis in cerebrospinal fluid.
2   Rising titre of complement-fixing or neutralizing antibodies.

Treatment

1   There is no specific therapy for arthropod-borne viral encephalitis.
2   Reduce intracranial pressure.
   a. Assist patient undergoing repeated lumbar punctures if cerebrospinal fluid pressure is elevated.
   b. Give intravenous mannitol or a urea-invert sugar preparation to reduce intracranial pressure.
3   Maintain the airway—use mechanical ventilation as required.
4   Control convulsive seizures.
5   Support patient during periods of prolonged coma.

6   Ensure adequate nutrition.
   a. Give intravenous nutrition for 48–72 hours if patient is comatose.
   b. Feed via nasogastric tube if patient remains in coma.

Health Teaching

1   Control mosquitoes.
2   Give passive protection (human or animal serum) to accidentally exposed workers.

Nursing Isolation Procedures

No isolation or precautions are necessary.

Rabies

Rabies is an acute severe viral infection affecting the central nervous system, which is transmitted to humans from the saliva of an infected animal, usually through a bite, but it can also occur through mucous membrane, but not intact skin. Animals most likely to be affected are dogs, cats, foxes and bats. No cases of rabies originating in England and Wales have been reported since 1902, but there have been 12 cases of imported rabies since 1946. In 1976, there were 11 552 cases of animal rabies in France and West Germany, and rabies has spread throughout Europe.

Incubation Period

1   In humans, the incubation period varies from 2–9 weeks, but may occasionally be shorter or very much longer.
2   The incubation period tends to be shorter if the bite is on the face or neck and also tends to be shorter in children than in adults.

Clinical Manifestations

Prodromal Stage

1   Headache and nausea.
2   Fever.
3   Malaise, loss of appetite, mental depression.
4   Pain and paraesthesia in the bitten area, and an abnormal sensation radiating proximally from the site of the wound.

The disease may then develop in one of two forms:

Stage of Excitement

1   Intermittent episodes of excitement, alternating with periods of alert calm.
2   Hydrophobia.
3   Hallucinations.
4   Severe spasms of throat and respiratory muscles.
5   Paralysis, coma and death may supervene.

Paralytic Stage

1   Signs of ascending flaccid paralysis with sphincter involvement and sensory disturbances.
2   Death results from respiratory and bulbar paralysis.

Diagnosis

1   History of exposure and development of characteristic symptoms.
2   Demonstration of rabies antigen in corneal smears and skin biopsy material.
3   Isolation of rabies virus from specimens of saliva, cerebrospinal fluid and other secretions. These specimens should be sent to Virus Reference Laboratory, Colindale.

Prophylaxis: Mangement of Patient After a Bite.

Reproduced from *Memorandum on Rabies*, DHSS, 1977, HMSO.

Guide for Post-exposure Treatment

WHO Expert Committee on Rabies (1973)

The recommendations given here are intended only as a guide. It is recognized that in special situations modifications of the procedures laid down may be warranted. Such special situations include exposure of young children and other circumstances where a reliable history cannot be obtained, particularly in areas where rabies is known to be endemic, even though the animal is considered to be healthy at the time of exposure. Such cases justify immediate treatment, but of a modified nature, for example, local treatment of the wound as described below, followed by administration of a single dose of serum or three doses of vaccine daily; provided that the animal stays healthy for 10 days following exposure, no further vaccine need be given. Modification of the recommended procedures would also be indicated in a rabies-free area where animal bites are frequently encountered. In areas where rabies is endemic, adequate laboratory and field experience indicating no infection in the species involved may justify local health authorities in recommending no specific antirabies treatment.

Practice varies concerning the volume of vaccine per dose and the number of doses recommended in a given situation. In general, the equivalent of 2 ml of a 5% brain-tissue vaccine, or the dose recommended by the producer of a particular vaccine, should be given daily for 14 consecutive days. To ensure the production and maintenance of high levels of serum-neutralizing antibodies, booster doses should be given at 10, 20 and 90 days following the last daily dose of vaccine in *all* cases.

Combined serum-vaccine treatment is considered by the Committee as the *best* specific treatment available for the post-exposure prophylaxis of rabies in man. Experience indicates that vaccine alone is sufficient for minor exposures. Serum should be given in a single dose of 40 i.u./kg of body weight for heterologous serum and 20 i.u./kg of body weight for human antirabies immunoglobulin; the first dose of vaccine is inoculated at the same time as the serum but at another site. Sensitivity to heterologous serum must be determined before its administration.

Treatment should be started as early as possible after exposure but in no case should it be denied to exposed persons whatever time interval has elapsed.

In areas where antirabies serum is not available full vaccine therapy including three booster inoculations should be administered.

A. LOCAL TREATMENT OF WOUNDS INVOLVING POSSIBLE EXPOSURE TO RABIES

(1)   *Recommended in all exposures*

(a) First-aid treatment

Since elimination of rabies virus at the site of infection by chemical or physical means is the most effective mechanism of protection, immediate washing and flushing with soap and water, detergent or water alone is imperative (recommended procedure in all bite wounds including those unrelated to possible exposure to rabies). Then apply either 40–70% alcohol, tincture or aqueous solutions of iodine, or 0·1% quaternary ammonium compounds.*

(b) Treatment by or under direction of a doctor

(1)   Treat as (a) above and then:
(2)   apply antirabies serum by careful instillation in the depth of the wound and by infiltration around the wound;
(3)   postpone suturing of wound; if suturing is necessary use antiserum locally as stated above;
(4)   where indicated, institute antitetanus procedures and administer antibiotics and drugs to control infections other than rabies.

Public Health Laboratories Holding Stocks of Rabies Vaccines and Antisera

The Central Public Health Laboratory, Colindale Avenue, London NW9 5HT (tel. 01–205 7041).

The Regional Public Health Laboratory, Fazakerley Hospital, Lower Lane, Liverpool L9 7AL (tel. 051–525 2323).

The Regional Public Health Laboratory, Institute of Pathology, Newcastle General Hospital, Westgate Road, Newcastle upon Tyne NE4 6BE (tel. 0632–38811).

The Regional Public Health Laboratory, East Birmingham Hospital, Bordesley Green East, Birmingham B9 5ST (tel. 021–772 4311), ext. 4080).

Public Health Laboratory, Church Lane, Heavitree, Exeter EX2 5AD (tel. 0392 77833).

The Regional Public Health Laboratory, Bridle Path, York Road, Leeds LS15 7TR (tel. 0532 645011).

The Regional Public Health Laboratory, University Hospital of Wales, Heath Park, Cardiff CF4 4XW (tel. 0222–755 954).

---

* Where soap has been used to clean wounds, all traces of it should be removed before the application of quaternary ammonium compounds because soap neutralizes the activity of such compounds.

B. SPECIFIC SYSTEMATIC TREATMENT

Nature of Exposure	Status of Biting Animal Irrespective of Previous Vaccination		Recommended Treatment
	At Time of Exposure	During 10 days*	
I Contact, but no lesions; indirect contact; no contact	Rabid	—	None
II Licks of the skin; scratches or abrasions; minor bites (covered areas of arms, trunk and legs)	(a) Suspected as rabid†	Healthy	Start vaccine. Stop treatment if animal remains healthy for 5 days*‡
		Rabid	Start vaccine; administer serum upon positive diagnosis and complete the course of vaccine
	(b) Rabid; wild animal,§ or animal unavailable for observation		Serum + vaccine
III Licks of mucosa; major bites (multiple or on face, head, finger or neck)	Suspect† or rabid domestic or wild§ animal, or animal unavailable for observation		Serum + vaccine. Stop treatment if animal remains healthy for 5 days*‡

* Observation period in this chart applies only to dogs and cats.
† All unprovoked bites in endemic areas should be considered suspect unless proved negative by laboratory examination (brain FA).
‡ Or if its brain is found negative by FA examination.
§ In general, exposure to rodents and rabbits seldom, if ever, requires specific antirabies treatment.

RICKETTSIAL INFECTIONS

Q Fever

Q fever is an influenzal-like illness with signs of atypical pneumonia. It is spread by infected livestock, and possibly by unpasteurized milk.

Aetiology

1 The organism responsible for Q fever is the *Coxiella burneti*, and was originally isolated in Australia in 1937.

2   Although infected cattle are the main source, the organism has also been isolated from pigeons, domestic poultry and migrating wild birds.

Occurrence

1   Mainly confined to agricultural countries with the exception of Scandinavia and New Zealand.
2   About 100 human cases are confirmed annually in the UK, mostly among farm workers, abattoir workers and veterinary surgeons.

Clinical Manifestations

1   Incubation period of about 19 days.
2   Sudden onset of headache, shivering, pains in the legs and anorexia.
3   Dry cough.
4   Sometimes, appearance on x-ray resembling an atypical pneumonia. Lung lesions may vary considerably.
5   Intermittent or remittent fever lasting from 2 days to 3 weeks.

Diagnosis

1   Patient's history.
2   Positive complement fixation test.

Treatment

1   Chloramphenicol or tetracyclines for 7–10 days, according to the time for the pyrexia to subside.
2   Give analgesics as required for pain in legs or chest.
3   Maintain upright posture in bed, physiotherapy as required.
4   Convalescence is usually uneventful, and the mortality rate is low.

Prevention

1   Pasteurization of milk.
2   Wearing of gloves during calving or lambing, especially for those who handle the placenta.

PROTOZOAN DISEASES

Malaria

Malaria is an acute infectious disease caused by protozoa which strongly resemble leucocytes. Transmission is by way of an intermediate host (the bite of an infective female Anopheles mosquito). Malaria has also been transmitted via blood transfusions and from the use of shared needles and syringes by narcotic addicts.

Aetiology

Four species of malaria parasites—grouped under generic name *Plasmodium*, each causing a different type of malaria. The parasite has a complicated life cycle. Not all patients demonstrate classical cycles of fever and chills.

1 *P. vivax*—causes benign tertian malaria with a 36–48-hour cycle of chills and fever.
2 *P. falciparum*—causes falciparum or malignant tertian malaria (36–48-hour cycle)
   a. This is the most serious type of malaria because of development of high parasitic densities in the blood.
   b. Infected red cells tend to agglutinate and form microemboli.
3 *P. malariae*—causes quartan malaria with fever and chills every third day.
4 *P. ovale*—less common form of malaria.

Clinical Manifestations

1 Paroxysms of shaking chills; rapidly rising fever.
2 Profuse sweating; headache.
3 Splenomegaly, hepatomegaly, orthostatic hypotension, anaemia.
4 Paroxysms may last about 12 hours after which cycle may be repeated daily, every other day or every third day.

Diagnosis

1 Demonstration of malaria parasites in blood films by microscopic examination—microscopic examination confirms presence, species and density of parasites.
2 Residence in or travel from an endemic area important diagnostic clue.

Clinical Problems

1 Malaria causes more disability and a heavier economic burden than any other parasitic disease.
2 In much of Southeast Asia, *P. falciparum* infections are increasingly drug-resistant.
3 Mosquitoes evolve resistance, against insecticides.
4 The use of antimalarial drugs depends on the stage of the life cycle of the parasite which is affected; malarial parasites can evolve drug-resistant forms.
5 The number of imported cases into the UK is rising. In 1967, there were 111 notifications in England and Wales, and in 1977, this had risen to 1477.

Treatment and Nursing Management

Objectives

To destroy the blood trophozoites and schizonts that cause the signs, symptoms and the pathological effects that characterize the disease.

1 Determine the species of parasite infecting the patient by obtaining a blood film. The most favourable time for discovery of the parasite is during, or 12–18 hours after, a chill.

2   Give specific therapy.
    a. *P. vivax* (mostly from India and SE Asia)—Choraquine; primaquine; or a combination of these two drugs.
    b. *P. falciparum* (from SE Asia and the Far East). There is a problem because of drug resistance, therefore a combination of drugs is used.
        (1) Quinine sulphate
            Pyramethamine (Daraprim)
            Sulphadiazine, or
        (2) Quinine sulphate
            Tetracycline
    Also sulformethoxine with pyrimethamine (Sulphadoxine).
3   Give supportive nursing care.
    a. Record regular observations of the patient.
    b. Keep fluid balance charts to identify signs of:
        (1) Pulmonary oedema.
        (2) Renal symptoms.
    c. Arrange for daily blood tests for estimating serum quinine, bilirubin, blood urea nitrogen concentrations, parasitic count and packed red cells.
    d. If there are any signs of respiratory or renal involvement, arrange for blood gases and plasma electrolytes.
    e. Consider a patient with severe falciparum malaria as a medical emergency.
        (1) Prepare for intermittent intravenous infusions of quinine.
        (2) Watch for neurological toxicity from quinine—twitching, delirium, confusion, convulsions and coma.
        (3) Oxygen may be necessary if tissue anoxia is present.
        (4) Watch for jaundice—this is related to the density of the malarial parasites in the blood; also, abnormality of hepatic function is common in falciparum malaria.
4   Evaluate the degree of anaemia—this is related to the severity of the infection.
5   Watch for abnormal bleeding—nose bleeds, oozing from venepuncture sites, passage of blood in the stools. This may be due to either decreased production of clotting factors by a damaged liver or to disseminated intravascular coagulation.

Nursing Isolation Precautions

1   Blood precautions for duration of hospitalization.
2   Screened rooms in tropical climates.

Preventative Measures and Health Teaching

1   In tropical areas, mosquito bites should be prevented.
    a. Effective repellents should be used.
    b. Houses should be sprayed with insecticide.
    c. Use bed netting.
    d. Install wire mesh screens across all windows.
2   Control and destroy mosquitoes.
    a. Drain and fill breeding places.

b. Control mosquitoes in an epidemic area by aerial or ground ultra low volume applications of insecticides such as malathion or naled.

3   Give malaria prophylaxis to people residing in or travelling to endemic areas. (chemoprophylaxis). It is important that the malarial parasite is not resistant to the particular drug, and that the drug is taken regularly during exposure and for 4 weeks afterwards. The following drugs may be used: chloroquine 2 tablets (300 mg) once weekly; proquanil (Paludrine) 100 mg daily; pyramethamine (Daraprim) 1–2 tablets (25–50 mg) once weekly; mepacrine 1 tablet (100 mg) daily, commencing 14 days before exposure so as to build up a blood concentration to an effective level; quinine 1 tablet (250–300 mg) daily.

4   Treat all new cases of malaria.

PARASITIC INFECTION

Amoebiasis (Amoebic Dysentery)

Amoebiasis is a worldwide parasitic disease which is responsible for multiple medical-surgical problems. It is caused by the protozoa *Entamoeba histolytica* and is acquired by ingestion of the cyst stage of *E. histolytica* in food or water contaminated by infected human faeces.

Incidence

1   Occurs as an endemic infection of man in most regions of the world.
2   In the UK it only occurs in travellers from tropical areas.

Pathological Insights

1   *E. histolytica* lives in the large intestine and feeds mainly on bacteria.
2   Amoeba may be located in the bowel lumen and intestinal wall or outside the gastrointestinal tract.
   a. Trophozoites develop from viable cysts in small intestine.
   b. Trophozoites may erode intestinal mucosa, invade the bloodstream and travel to the liver via the portal circulation.
   c. Amoebas can produce abscesses and other serious complications.

Clinical Manifestations

1   Diarrhoea—watery, foul-smelling stools, often containing blood-streaked mucus.
2   Abdominal discomfort.

Diagnosis

1   Stool specimen for *E. histolytica*. (Trophozoites or cysts may be found in the faeces.)
   a. Several stool specimens should be collected daily.
   b. Stool specimen should be examined *immediately* for trophozoites.

2 Positive serological tests (indirect haemagglutination test and indirect fluorescent antibody test.
3 Examination of exudate from liver abscess for trophozoites.

Complications

1 Liver abscess
2 Lung suppuration.
3 Meningoencephalitis.
4 Intestinal obstruction, rupture of colon; peritonitis.
5 Amoeboma (amoebic granuloma found in caecum, rectum, transverse colon, sigmoid).

Treatment

Objectives

To give specific therapy.
To support the patient's general condition.

1 Specific therapy—metronidazole (Flagyl) produces cessation of diarrhoea and discharge of parasite from stools.
   Serial follow-up of stools is necessary.
2 Keep patient on bed rest if diarrhoea is acute.
3 Prepare for aspiration of liver abscess.
   Dehydroemetine or emetine plus chloroquine phosphate may be given for hepatic abscess.
4 Offer nonirritating, low residue bland foods—weak tea, broth, rice, toast, soft-cooked eggs.
5 Give intravenous infusions as indicated to correct fluid and electrolyte imbalance resulting from severe diarrhoea.

Nursing Isolation Procedures

Excretion precautions (p. 219) for the duration of illness.

Health Teaching

1 Provide sanitation and safe water supplies. Water should be boiled or chlorinated.
2 Control the fly population in homes.

FUNGAL INFECTIONS

Mycoses and Histoplasmosis

Fungi are primitive organisms that take their nourishment from living plants and animals and from decaying organic material. The three main types of mycoses (fungal infections), determined by the tissue level at which the fungus settles, are:

1 Systemic or deep mycoses—primarily involve the internal organs, usually centring in the lungs.
2 Subcutaneous mycoses—involve the skin, subcutaneous tissue and sometimes the bone.
3 Superficial or cutaneous mycoses—grow in outer layer of skin (epidermis), in hair and in nails.

Histoplasmosis is a chronic systemic fungus infection caused by a spore-bearing mould called *Histoplasma capsulatum*. This highly infectious mycosis is transmitted by airborne dust which contains *H. capsulatum* spores. (Partially decayed droppings of pigeons, chickens and birds offer an excellent medium for growth of this fungus.)
    In the UK the most important fungal infections are:

1 *Candida albicans* which may cause a comparatively mild problem, but which may be very troublesome in debilitated patients or those receiving chemotherapy.
2 Ringworm which is usually passed on from infected household pets. Griseofulvin is the usual treatment for this.
3 Tinea pedis (athlete's foot) which is widespread among schoolchildren and others visiting communal swimming baths.
4 Cryptococcus neoformans which causes a form of meningitis. It is an infection associated with pigeon's nests and pigeon's droppings.

HELMINTHIC INFESTATIONS

Trichinosis

Trichinosis is infestation by the parasite *Trichinella spiralis*, one of the roundworms. It is acquired by consuming infected meat, usually pork.

Clinical Course

1 Tiny embryos of the parasite *T. spiralis* become encysted in the muscle fibres of an infected pig.
2 These calcified cysts appear in meat (chiefly pork); resemble tiny grains of sand.
3 If insufficiently cooked pork is eaten, the embryos are set free by the gastric juice and develop in the intestine during the following week, becoming adult worms 3–4 mm long.
4 These worms make their way into the mucous membranes and there produce myriad embryos (larvae) (period of invasion).
5 The larvae, carried by the bloodstream and their own activity, migrate to all parts of the body (period of migration).
6 The larvae gradually become encysted in striated skeletal muscle.

Clinical Manifestations

Intestinal Stage

1 Malaise.
2 Gastrointestinal complaints, diarrhoea.

3   Mild fever—progresses to high and spiking by third week.
4   Nausea and vomiting.

Muscular Invasion (symptoms derive from inflammatory process developing in the muscles)

1   Oedema of the eyelids; scleral haemorrhages; pain on eye motion.
2   Generalized pain and soreness in the muscles (myalgia).
3   Cardiac irregularities (occasional)—from trichinae in the heart muscle; may be fatal.
4   Difficulty in breathing, masticating, swallowing, speaking.

Diagnosis

1   Biopsy specimen of muscle—reveals larvae. (Deltoid, biceps, gastrocnemius muscles are sites of biopsy.)
2   Positive serologic tests (precipitin, complement-fixation, bentonite-flocculation, fluorescent-antibody)—demonstrable titres 3–4 weeks after infection.
3   Rising eosinophil count—appears in second week.
4   Positive skin test.

Treatment

The treatment is symptomatic; there is no satisfactory treatment.

1   Thiabendazole (Mintezol)—may produce clinical improvement and prevent or minimize effects of illness.
        Adverse effects—nausea, vertigo, vomiting, rash.
2   Corticosteroid agents may be given to relieve symptoms in the acute stage.
3   Keep the patient on bed rest until he experiences some relief of symptoms.
4   Give analgesics to relieve muscle pain.
5   Carry out ECG evaluations to determine evidence of myocarditis.

Nursing Isolation Procedures

None required.

Prevention and Health Teaching

1   The public should be educated regarding the importance of thoroughly cooking all pork and pork products, especially sausage. There should be no trace of pink in cooked pork.
2   Smoking, pickling, seasoning and spicing do not make pork safe unless it is cooked (especially homemade sausage).
3   Minced beef may be contaminated by a meat grinder that has been used for pork.
4   Garbage intended for feed for pigs should be cooked.
5   Pork should be inspected to determine if disease is present.
6   This disease was more prevalent in the USA than in the UK, but now the numbers of cases are diminishing. This is thought to be due to the increasing use of freezers, as the cysts are readily destroyed by low temperatures.

Hookworm Disease

Hookworm disease (ancylostomiasis; 'ground itch') is the result of infestation of the small intestine by one of two quite similar roundworms about 1.2 cm (0.5 in) long. Two species are parasitic in the human intestinal tract:

Necator americanus (predominant species in the USA).

Ancylostoma duodenale.

The infection is usually contracted by penetration of the skin by infected larvae in the soil.

Incidence

This is a common problem in the tropics, particularly among barefoot workers. Estimates suggest that about one-sixth of the world's population may be affected, about 500 000 000 people. In a 2-year study of immigrant schoolchildren in Birmingham in 1968–70, 37% were found to be infected.

Clinical Course

1 Hookworm eggs are passed in human faeces onto the ground (indiscriminate defaecation habits). Eggs develop into infective larvae.
2 The larvae enter through the mouth if the individual eats with dirty hands, or they *bore through the skin of bare feet* ('ground itch').
3 After gaining access to the blood or lymph vessels, they are carried via the blood to the lungs, migrate from the pulmonary capillaries into the alveoli, reach the pharynx and are swallowed, maturing to adult forms in the bowel.

Clinical Manifestations

1 Dermatitis ('ground itch')—occurs at site where larvae penetrate skin.
2 *Gastrointestinal symptoms*—maturation of worms in the intestine is usually marked by onset of diarrhoea and other gastrointestinal symptoms.
   a. Nausea and vomiting.
   b. Flatulence, diarrhoea or constipation.
3 Low-grade fever.
4 *Severe anaemia* and hypoalbuminaemia—the worms attach to intestinal mucosa and suck blood; a single adult worm can extract 0.05 ml of blood daily. The patient's iron stores become depleted. A low serum protein often develops (protein malnutrition).
   Severe anaemia may produce:
   a. Symptoms of heart failure.
   b. Tachycardia.
   c. Poor growth and development.
5 *Dry cough and dyspnoea*—from rupture of larvae through the capillary bed and their dissemination throughout bronchial tree.

Diagnosis

1 History of anaemia and malnutrition.
2 Recovery and identification of the eggs in faeces.

Treatment

1   Specific therapy—one of the following drugs:
   a. Bephenium hydroxynaphthoate (Alcopara).
   b. Pyrantel pamoate (Antiminth).
   c. Tetrachloroethylene.
2   Ensure that the patient is eating a nutritious diet—hookworm disease occurs in persons suffering from malnutrition.
   a. Correct anaemia prior to therapy for worms in patients with severe anaemia.
   b. Give protein and iron supplementation—to aid in correction of anaemia.

Nursing Isolation Procedures

None required.

Prevention and Health Teaching

1   Dispose of excreta in a sanitary manner; this is an important facet of health education.
2   Instruct the patient to wear shoes at all times.
3   Night soil (human excrement used as fertilizer) and sewage effluents should not be used for fertilizer.

Ascariasis (Roundworm Infestation)

Ascariasis is an infection caused by *Ascaris lumbricoides* (intestinal roundworm). It is characterized by an early pulmonary invasion from larval migration and a later more prolonged intestinal phase.

Incidence

Although this is more common in the tropics, the distribution is worldwide, and infections occur in western Europe.

Clinical Course

1   Indiscriminate defaecation in streets, fields and doorways provides a major source of infective eggs.
2   Infection may be contracted from eating raw vegetables when night soil is used for fertilizer; water pollution may cause water transmission.
3   Eggs are swallowed and pass into intestine where they hatch into larvae.
4   Larvae penetrate the intestinal mucosa and enter lymphatics and blood vessels.
5   After reaching the lungs, they pierce the capillary wall, crawl up the trachea, are swallowed and are returned to the small intestine where they grow, mature and mate.

Clinical Manifestations

1   *Pulmonary Phase*—cough, fever and blood-tinged sputum.
2   *Intestinal Phase*—masses of worms cause gastrointestinal discomfort, colicky and epigastric pain.

Nursing Alert: Large masses of worms may migrate into various organs of the body and cause obstruction (to trachea, bronchi, bile duct, appendix, pancreatic duct).

Diagnosis

1 Stool specimen—for detection of ova and worms in stool.
2 Patient occasionally vomits a worm.

Treatment

One of the following may be given:

1 Piperazine citrate, bephenium hydroxynaphthoate, tetramisole.
2 Follow-up stool examination should be done 1–2 weeks after treatment.

Nursing Isolation Procedures

None required.

Preventive Measures and Health Teaching

1 All patients with infestations should be treated.
2 Adequate toilet facilities should be provided.
3 The importance of personal hygiene should be explained.

Oxyuris Vermicularis (Threadworm)

The threadworm (*Oxyuris vermicularis*) causes the most common form of intestinal roundworm infestation in the UK and is most prevalent in children.

Clinical Problems

1 One may produce 5000–15 000 eggs.
2 Ingested eggs hatch in the small intestine; embryos reach adulthood in the caecum.
3 The gravid female worm migrates down the large intestine and deposits eggs on the skin of the perianal area.
4 The eggs that survive are ingested and reach maturity in 2–6 weeks in the gastrointestinal tract.
5 Scratching leads to contamination of the hands and nails; hand to mouth contact results in reinfection.
6 Infective eggs may contaminate food and drink, bed linen, dust, etc.

Clinical Manifestations

Threadworm infected person may be asymptomatic.

1 Intense itching (nocturnal) above the anus—from nocturnal migration of gravid females from anus and deposition of eggs in perianal folds of skin.
2 Restlessness; nervousness.
3 Vaginitis—from threadworm migration into the vagina.

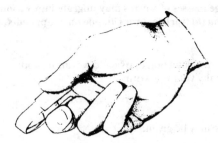

Figure 6.1. Most suitable method of finding eggs in perianal areas. Bend sellotape back over index finger with sticky side out. (Courtesy of 'Forum on Infection'.) Prepared slides are also available.

Diagnosis

1   Anal impressions on sellotape taken in morning before going to toilet or bathing, so that ova deposited during the night will not be removed (Fig. 6.1).
   a. A family member may be taught the method so that the test may be carried out first thing in the morning.
   b. Wash hands thoroughly.
2   Detection (inspection) of characteristic eggs about the anus.

Treatment

Drugs include:

1   Piperazine citrate (Antepar)—requires multiple doses.
2   Thiabendazole (Mintezol).
3   Mebendazole (Vermox).

Prevention of Reinfection; Health Teaching

1   All members of the family should be treated, or reinfection is apt to occur. Treat on the same day to eliminate cross-infection.
2   To prevent reinfection:
   a. Cut fingernails short—eggs may be obtained from beneath the nails of infected person.
      (1) Avoid nail biting.
      (2) Wash hands frequently during treatment period.
      (3) Scrub nails with a brush, especially before going to bed.
   b. Wash hands with soap and water after using toilet and before meals.
   c. Wash around anal area upon rising (after diagnostic test).
   d. Apply salve or ointment to anal area—to prevent despersal of eggs.
   e. Infected child should wear snug fitting cotton pants—to discourage contact of hands with perianal region and contamination of bed linen.
   f. See that infected person sleeps alone.
   g. Handle bedding and nightwear carefully—there are large numbers of infective eggs in a contaminated house that cause reinfection.
   h. Clean sleeping quarters frequently.

i. Reassure mother and family members that pinworms are not a sign of poor hygiene or housekeeping.

Nursing Isolation Procedures

Excretion precaution (p. 219) for duration of illness.

FURTHER READING

Books

Brewis, R A L (1980) Lecture Notes on Respiratory Disease, Blackwell Scientific Publications

Dick, G (1978) Immunization, Update Publications

Gillies, R R (1978) Lecture Notes on Medical Microbiology, Blackwell Scientific Publications

Hare, R and Cook, M (1975) Bacteriology and Immunity for Nurses, Churchill Livingstone

Hoeprich, P D (Ed) (1972) Infectious Diseases, Harper and Row

Meredith Davies, B (1979) Community Health, Preventive Medicine and Social Services, Ballière Tindall

Muir Gray, J A (1979) Man Against Disease, Oxford University Press

Parry, W H (1979) Communicable Diseases, Unibooks, Hodder and Stoughton

DHSS (1977) Memorandum on Rabies, HMSO

Articles

Ayton, M (1981) National surveillance of communicable diseases, Nursing: 1st series, No. 29, 1248–1251

Collins, B J (1981) The spread of infection, Nursing: 1st series, No 29, 1252–1254

Keay, E (1981) Coppetts Wood—an infectious disease unit, Nursing: 1st series, No 29, 1273–1277

Iveson-Iveson, J (1979) Prevention and how to stay healthy, Nursing Mirror: 149 (19) 18

Iveson-Iveson, J (1980) Students' forum, infectious diseases, Nursing Mirror: 151 (8) 26–28

Maunder, J W (1981) Parisitology, Nursing: 1st series, No 29, 1290–1291

Miller, G (1978) Ten years of measles vaccinations, Nursing Times: 74 (50) 2059–2060

Strange, J L (1980) Hospitals should do the sick no harm, Nursing Times: 76 (51) Suppl. 1–4

Tedder, R S (1981) Hepatitis B, Nursing: 1st series, No 29, 1284–1288

Chapter 7

CARE OF THE PATIENT WITH CANCER

GENERAL CONSIDERATIONS

The Optimistic Side of Cancer

1 One-third of all cancer patients are cured.
2 Improved treatment modalities enable patients with cancer to live longer, more comfortably and more productively.
3 Most cancer patients spend almost all their time away from hospitals and only come to the hospital intermittently for treatment.
4 More intense efforts at patient rehabilitation are proving effective.
5 Research continues unabated, and, as findings accumulate, prospects for specific cures are encouraging.

Cancer's Warning Signals

C hange in bowel or bladder habits
A sore that does not heal
U nusual bleeding or discharge
T hickening or lump in breast or elsewhere
I ndigestion or difficulty in swallowing
O bvious change in wart or mole
N agging cough or hoarseness

Benign and Malignant Tumours

	Benign	Malignant
Type of cell	Adult	Young
Nature	Closely resembles parent tissue	Tends to be anaplastic (reverting to primitive cells)
Growth	Slow	Rapid, usually
Encapsulated	Often	Never
Effect on surrounding tissue	Never invades	Invades widely
Localization	Remains at original site	Nonlocalized—forms secondary growths by metastasis
Recurrence after removal	Does not tend to recur	Tends to recur

Metastasis

1   Direct invasion—tumours do not just expand, but may infiltrate between the surrounding tissue cells, causing disorganization and destruction.
2   Lymphatic spread—malignant cells may invade the lymphatic system and grow as a column or be broken off and carried as the embolus to the draining lymph node.
3   Blood spread—tumour cells may enter the blood stream from the lymphatics or invade blood cells directly.
4   Cavity spread—a tumour may spread from one structure to another across cavities, often in a fluid medium such as pleural or peritoneal fluid, urine or cerebrospinal fluid.

Incidence

1   The annual death toll from malignancy in the UK is over 100 000.
2   Cancer is the second commonest cause of death in the UK.
3   Cancer occurs at any age. Although rare in the young, it remains the second largest killer of children and young people. It strikes with increasing frequency as age advances.
4   There will be about 200 000 new cases of cancer diagnosed this year.
5   No organ in the body is exempt.
6   The commonest tumours in males are lung (30%) and digestive tract (20%), and in females breast (25%) and digestive tract (20%).

Diagnosis

Many techniques may be used to diagnose tumours, depending upon their site. These include:

1   Full physical examination.
2   Haematology, e.g., full blood count, urea and electrolytes, biochemical tests.
3   Radiology, e.g., straight x-rays, lymphography, arteriography, mammography, tomography.
4   Radioisotopes, e.g., radioactive iodine scans.

5 Computerized tomography (CT scanning).
6 Ultrasound.
7 Endoscopy and biopsy.
8 Cytology, e.g., cervical smear.

Staging

Various staging systems available which indicate the extent of the tumour. TNM system is the most common:

T = primary tumour, scale 1–4 indicates size.
N = regional nodes, scale 1–4 indicates extent of local spread.
M = distant metastases. 0 = none, 1 = exist.

Treatment

1 Modalities of treatment include surgery, radiotherapy, radioactive substances (including radioisotopes), various drugs (pharmaceuticals and hormones) and immunotherapy. (See pp. 296–297.)
2 Method of treatment will depend on the type of malignancy, stage, localization or spread, condition of patient, and the doctor; a single method or combination of methods may be required.

Surgery

1 *Biopsy*—a piece of tissue is cut out surgically from the questionable area and sent to pathology laboratory for diagnostic verification.
2 *Preventive or prophylactic surgery*—removal of lesions which, if left in the body, are apt to develop into cancer. Example: polyps in rectum may lead to cancer of colon.
3 *Palliative surgery*—a type of surgery which attempts to relieve the complications of cancer, e.g., obstruction of the gastrointestinal tract, pain produced by tumour extension into surrounding nerves.
4 *Curative surgery*—the removal of the primary site of malignancy and any lymph nodes to which the neoplasm has extended. Such surgery may be all that is required.
5 *Surgery combined with radiation, chemotherapy or immunotherapy*—combinations of treatment required to halt the spread of a malignancy.

NOTE: Details of surgical treatment are given in the sections relating to specific disease entities.

CHEMOTHERAPY FOR CANCER

Value of chemotherapy in treating a malignancy.

1 As yet no *one* drug is available to cure all malignant tumours.
2 Chemotherapeutic agents are most useful in the treatment of leukaemias, Hodgkin's disease, lymphomas, Ewing's tumour, Wilm's tumour, testicular tumours and retinoblastomas.
3 Recent work has demonstrated the value of using chemotherapeutic agents in

combination with surgery and/or radiotherapy in tumours where the recurrence risk is high.

4   Chemotherapy may also be used to relieve symptoms in those patients in whom surgery or radiotherapy is no longer beneficial.

5   Combinations of chemotherapeutic agents are often more effective and no more toxic than single agents.

6   Precise timing in administering these drugs is vital to achieve the optimum effect.

7   Some chemotherapeutic agents have unpleasant systemic effects. It is imperative that the nurse knows what these are and how to minimize them.

Pharmacologic Action (Table 7.1)

1   These drugs are capable of destroying young, rapidly multiplying cells, such as malignant cells.

2   They interfere with manufacture of nucleic acids (inhibit the chain of synthesis or function of DNA and RNA) so that cellular growth and reproduction are inhibited.

3   Since many normal cells in the body also grow rapidly and have short life spans (e.g., bone marrow, gastrointestinal tract lining, hair follicles), many chemotherapeutic agents directly attack these normal cells. Herein lies the challenge.

Method of Administration

Drugs may be given orally, subcutaneously, intravenously, intramuscularly, intra-arterially or intrathecally depending on the drug.

Intravenous Administration.

1   See Principles of Intravenous Therapy. Additional specific concerns related to administration of chemotherapeutic agents include the following:

a. In general, avoid venepuncture in an arm where:

(1) Dissection of the axillary nodes has been performed.

(2) Radiotherapy has caused marked fibrosis in the axillary area.

b. Avoid areas of sclerosis, thrombosis or scar formation.

c. Avoid prolonged tourniquet application in order to prevent cutaneous haemorrhage.

2   If a small focal haematoma develops during insertion of needle into a vein, do not use this avenue for administration of toxic chemotherapeutic agents because of the danger of extravasation.

3   Maintain constant supervision during administration of potentially locally toxic chemotherapeutic agents.

4   If any doubt exists regarding vein patency or safety of drug administration, discontinue administration.

5   It is better to prevent *extravasation* than to treat it.

a. Symptoms:

Pain (severe enough to cause patient to cry out); area may appear red, mottled and/or swollen—often leading to necrosis.

b. Treatment:

(1) Apply ice compresses to slow down local tissue metabolism.

Table 7.1.   Commercially Available Anticancer Drugs

Drug	Toxicity	Nursing Action
Alkylating Agents		
Busulphan (Myloran)	1 Bone marrow depression	Observe for infection, bleeding, anaemia
	2 Gynaecomastia Amenorrhoea Impotence	Inform patient and give psychological support
	3 Skin pigmentation	Inform patient
	4 Pulmonary fibrosis	Steroids usually given
Chlorambucil (Leukeran)	1 Bone marrow depression	Observe for infection, bleeding, anaemia
	2 Nausea and vomiting	Dietary control. Encourage fluids. Give antiemetics
	3 Dermatitis	Apply calamine lotion or steroid creams
Cyclophosphamide (Endoxana)	1 Bone marrow depression	Observe for infection, bleeding, anaemia
	2 Nausea and vomiting	Dietary control. Encourage fluids. Give antiemetics
	3 Stomatitis	Oral hygiene. Bland diet
	4 Alopecia	Inform patient. Arrange wig
	5 Alteration in taste	Use of flavourings
	6 Chemical cystitis	Maintain adequate fluid intake
Dacarbazine (DTIC, DIC)	1 Bone marrow depression	Observe for infection, bleeding, anaemia
	2 Nausea and vomiting	Dietary control. Encourage fluids. Give antiemetics
	3 Alopecia	Inform patient. Arrange wig
	4 Flu-like syndrome	Observe for symptoms
	5 Renal impairment	Observe for symptoms
	6 Liver damage	
		Avoid extravasation
Melphalan	1 Bone marrow depression	Observe for infection, bleeding, anaemia
	2 Nausea and vomiting	Dietary control. Encourage fluids. Give antiemetics
	3 Alopecia	Inform patient. Arrange wig
Nitrogen mustard (Mustine)	1 Bone marrow depression	Observe for infection, bleeding, anaemia
	2 Nausea and vomiting	Dietary control. Encourage fluids. Give antiemetics *Protect eyes and skin of person administering drugs. Avoid extravasation*
Triethylene triphosphamide (Thiotepa)	1 Bone marrow depression	Observe for infection, bleeding, anaemia

(continued)

Table 7.1   (*cont.*)

Drug	Toxicity	Nursing Action
	2 Nausea and vomiting	Dietary control. Encourage fluids. Give antiemetics
	3 Allergic reaction	Regular observations
	4 Gastrointestinal perforation	Observe for abdominal pain
	5 Mild anaemia	Encourage adequate rest
Antimetabolites		
Cyclohexyl cyclorotheyl nitrosurea (CCNU)	1 Delayed bone marrow depression (4–6 weeks)	Maintain awareness
	2 Nausea and vomiting	Dietary control. Encourage fluids. Give antiemetics
	3 Stomatitis	Oral hygiene
	4 Alopecia	Inform patient. Arrange wig
Cytosine arabinoside (Ara-C) (Cytosar) (Cytarbarine)	1 Bone marrow depression	Observe for infection, bleeding, anaemia
	2 Nausea and vomiting	Dietary control. Encourage fluids. Give antiemetics
	3 Stomatitis	Oral hygiene
	4 Hyperuricaemia	Observe urinary output
5 Fluorouracil (5–FU)	1 Bone marrow depression	Observe for infection, bleeding, anaemia
	2 Nausea and vomiting	Dietary control. Encourage fluids. Give antiemetics
	3 Stomatitis	Oral hygiene
	4 Diarrhoea	Dietary control. Encourage fluids. Antidiarrhoea drugs
	5 Alopecia	Inform patient. Arrange wig
6–Mercaptopurine (6MP)	1 Bone marrow depression	Observe for infection, bleeding, anaemia
	2 Nausea and vomiting	Dietary control. Encourage fluids. Give antiemetics
	3 Stomatitis	Oral hygiene. Bland diet
	4 Diarrhoea	Dietary control. Encourage fluids. Antidiarrhoea drugs
	5 Liver dysfunction	Observe for jaundice. Test for bilirubin in urine
Methotrexate	1 Bone marrow depression	Observe for infection, bleeding, anaemia
	2 Nausea and vomiting	Dietary control. Encourage fluids. Give antiemetics
	3 Stomatitis	Oral hygiene. Bland diet
	4 Diarrhoea	Dietary control. Encourage fluids. Antidiarrhoea drugs

(*continued*)

Table 7.1   (*cont.*)

Drug	Toxicity	Nursing Action
	5 Skin rash	Calamine lotion or steroid cream
	6 Cystitis	Encourage fluids. Observe urinary output
Thioguanine (6TG)	1 Bone marrow depression	Observe for infection, bleeding, anaemia
	2 Nausea and vomiting	Dietary control. Encourage fluids. Give antiemetics
Natural Products		
Bleomycin	1 Nausea and vomiting	Dietary control. Encourage fluids. Give antiemetics
	2 Stomatitis	Oral hygiene. Bland diet
	3 Alopecia	Inform patient. Arrange wig
	4 Tumour pain	Give analgesics
	5 Anaphylaxis	Emergency equipment to hand. Close observations
	6 Pulmonary fibrosis	Weekly chest x-ray
		Protect eyes and skin of person administering drug. Avoid extravasation
Dactinomycin (Actinomycin D) (Cosmegen)	1 Bone marrow depression	Observe for infection, bleeding, anaemia
	2 Nausea and vomiting	Dietary control. Encourage fluids. Give antiemetics
	3 Stomatitis	Oral hygiene. Bland diet
	4 Diarrhoea	Dietary control. Encourage fluids. Antidiarrhoea drugs
	5 Alopecia	Inform patient. Arrange wig
	6 Anorexia	Small appetizing meals
	7 Skin pigmentation	Inform patient
	8 Mental depression	Psychological support
		Avoid extravasation
Doxyrubicin (Adriamycin)	1 Bone marrow depression	Observe for infection, bleeding, anaemia
	2 Nausea and vomiting	Dietary control. Encourage fluids. Give antiemetics
	3 Stomatitis	Oral hygiene. Bland diet
	4 Diarrhoea	Dietary control. Encourage fluids. Antidiarrhoea drugs
	5 Alopecia	Inform patient. Arrange wig
	6 Fever	
	7 Red urine (up to 12 days)	Inform patient
	8 Cardiotoxicity	ECG essential predose. Observation of pulse
		Avoid extravasation

(continued)

Table 7.1   (*cont.*)

Drug	Toxicity	Nursing Action
Mithramycin	1 Nausea and vomiting	Dietary control. Encourage fluids. Give antiemetics
	2 Stomatitis	Oral hygiene. Bland diet
	3 Diarrhoea	Dietary control. Encourage fluids. Antidiarrhoea drugs
	4 Haemorrhagic epistaxis	Stop bleeding. Apply ice packs, etc.
	5 Hypocalcaemia	Observe for increased neural and muscular excitability
	6 Headache, depression, drowsiness	Inform patient. Careful observation
Mitomycin C	1 Bone marrow depression	Observe for infection, bleeding, anaemia
	2 Nausea and vomiting	Dietary control. Encourage fluids. Give antiemetics
	3 Stomatitis	Oral hygiene. Bland diet
	4 Alopecia	Inform patient. Arrange wig
	5 Paraesthesia	Observe carefully
	6 Pruritis	Apply antipruritic cream
Rubidomycin (Daunorubicin)	1 Bone marrow depression	Observe for infection, bleeding, anaemia
	2 Nausea and vomiting	Dietary control. Encourage fluids. Give antiemetics
	3 Stomatitis	Oral hygiene. Bland diet
	4 Alopecia	Inform patient. Arrange wig
	5 Red urine	Inform patient
	6 Abdominal pain	
	7 Congestive cardiac failure	ECG essential predose. Observe and report symptoms *Avoid extravasation*
Vinblastine (Velbe) (Velban)	1 Bone marrow depression	Observe for infection, bleeding, anaemia
	2 Nausea and vomiting	Dietary control. Encourage fluids. Give antiemetics
	3 Alopecia	Inform patient. Arrange wig
	4 Peripheral neuritis	Report symptoms. Observe for numbness, ataxia
	5 Headache, dizziness	Observe carefully. Give analgesics
	6 Constipation	Give mild aperients
L-asparaginase	1 Nausea and vomiting	Dietary control. Encourage fluids. Give antiemetics
	2 Malaise	Psychological support

(*continued*)

Table 7.1   (*cont.*)

Drug	Toxicity	Nursing Action
	3 Anaphylaxis	Emergency equipment ready. Hydrocortisone and piriton ready
	4 Hypoglycaemia	Collection of specimens
	5 Hypoalbuminaemia	Collection of specimens
Vincristine (Oncovin)	1 Nausea and vomiting	Dietary control. Encourage fluids. Give antiemetics
	2 Stomatitis	Oral hygiene. Bland diet
	3 Alopecia	Inform patient. Arrange wig
	4 Peripheral neuritis	Report symptoms. Observe for numbness, ataxia
	5 Constipation	Give mild aperients
	6 Dysuria, polyuria	Observe urinary output
Platinum	1 Bone marrow depression	Observe for infection, bleeding, anaemia
	2 Severe nausea and vomiting	Dietary control. Encourage fluids. Give antiemetics
	3 Diarrhoea	Dietary control. Encourage fluids. Antidiarrhoea drugs
	4 Renal failure	Forced diuresis. Observe urea and creatinine

Other Agents

Drug	Toxicity	Nursing Action
Hydroxyurea	1 Bone marrow depression	Observe for infection, bleeding, anaemia
	2 Nausea and vomiting	Dietary control. Encourage fluids. Give antiemetics
	3 Stomatitis	Oral hygiene. Bland diet
	4 Anorexia	Small, appetizing meals
	5 Alopecia	Inform patient. Arrange wig
	6 Erythema, rash, pruritis	No perfumed soap. Encourage skin cleanliness
Procarbazine (Natulan)	1 Bone marrow depression	Observe for infection, bleeding, anaemia
	2 Nausea and vomiting	Dietary control. Encourage fluids. Give antiemetics
	3 Alopecia	Inform patient. Arrange wig
	4 Mild CNS toxicity	Observe and report
	5 MAO inhibitor	No alcohol, cheese, Marmite, yoghurt, sedatives, narcotics, tricyclic antidepressants or antihistamines

(*continued*)

Table 7.1 (cont.)

Drug	Toxicity	Nursing Action
Hormones		
Oestrogens		
Diethylstilbestrol (DES)	1 Nausea and vomiting	Dietary control. Encourage fluids. Give antiemetics
Ethinylestradiol		
Stilboestrol	2 Fluid retention	Avoid salt and salty foods.
		Encourage movement. Avoid injections
	3 Feminization	Inform patient. Give psychological support
	4 Hypercalcaemia	Rehydration with forced diuresis
	5 Uterine bleeding	Inform patient
Anti-oestrogens		
Tamoxifen (Nolvadex)	1 Nausea and vomiting	Dietary control. Encourage fluids. Give antiemetics
	2 Fluid retention	Avoid salt and salty foods. Encourage movement. Avoid injections
	3 Hypercalcaemia	Rehydration with forced diuresis
	4 Photosensitivity of skin	Avoid exposure to sunlight
Androgens		
Nandrolone	1 Coarse facial hair	Remove with depilatory cream. Avoid shaving
Phenyl propionate		
(Durabolin)	2 Thinning of scalp hair	Inform patient
Drostanolone (Masteril)	3 Hoarse, deep voice	Inform patient
	4 Oily skin, acne	Strict cleansing. Use astringent
	5 Increased libido	Inform patient
Progesterones		
Hydroxyprogesterone	1 Nausea	Inform patient
(Primolut-depot)	2 Headache	Give analgesics
Medroxyprogesterone	3 Fluid retention	Avoid salt and salty foods. Encourage movement. Avoid injections
(Provera)		
Norethisterone	4 Hypercalcaemia	Rehydration with forced diuresis
Corticosteroids		
Prednisone	1 Local oedema, 'moon face'	Inform patient
Prednisolone	2 Fluid retention	Avoid salt and salty foods. Encourage movement. Avoid injections

(continued)

Table 7.1   (*cont.*)

Drug	Toxicity	Nursing Action
	3 Hypertension	Regular blood pressure recording
	4 Osteoporosis	High calcium, high protein diet
	5 Impaired hearing	Inform patient. Discuss safety measures
	6 Gastrointestinal disturbance	Give antacids. Observe for haematemesis and melaena
	7 Diabetes mellitus	Observe for polyuria and polydipsia. Routine urine testing
	8 Changes in mood	Careful observation
	9 Susceptibility to infection	Strict attention to hygiene

    (2) Some individuals recommend local infiltration of the involved area with an anti-inflammatory agent, i.e., hydrocortisone.

    (3) Late, warm compresses may be applied; local management as indicated.

  c. If only a small amount of drug is extravasated and frank necrosis does not occur, phlebitis may still result, causing pain for several days and/or induration at the site that may last for weeks or months.

6   Observe for occurrences other than extravasation:

  a. Intraluminal

    (1) Symptoms:

       (a) Patient may describe sensations of pain, stretching or pressure within the vessel, originating near venepuncture site or 7·5–12·5 cm (3–5 in) along vein course.

       (b) Discolouration—deep blue or purple 5–10 cm (2–4 in) proximal to venepuncture site.

    (2) Treatment:

       Wait and observe; change puncture site or discontinue administration of drug.

  b. Subcutaneous tissue

    (1) Symptoms:

       Itching, muscle cramp, pressure within arm, possible urticaria.

    (2) Treatment:

       (a) Wait and observe; change puncture site, or discontinue administration of drug.

       (b) Notify doctor if systemic effects are observed.

Isolated Perfusion

A seldom-used technique whereby large doses of cytotoxic drugs are administered to an isolated extremity, organ or region of the body (excluding systemic circulation).

Intra-arterial Infusion

The introduction percutaneously of a catheter into a major artery followed by the continuous administration (by means of a pump) of a chemotherapeutic agent. Treatment may be continued over several days.

Nursing Care of Patients Receiving Chemotherapeutic Agents for Neoplastic Disease

1   Be aware of the drugs, their route of administration, their mode of action and the expected effect, both toxic and therapeutic.
2   Be aware of the interaction of drugs and their stability in solution. Know how they should be stored and how they should be diluted.
3   Provide the patient with encouragement and enough information to become a participant in his own care.
4   Give emotional support. Treatment with chemotherapy can be prolonged and the patient may become depressed.
5   Be alert for manifestations of gastrointestinal tract disturbances:
    a. Anorexia—offer small, attractive meals at regular intervals. Encourage relatives to bring home-made treats.
    b. Nausea and vomiting—keep the environment free of the sights, sounds and smells that cause nausea. Encourage fluids and keep an accurate fluid balance chart. Antiemetics may be given prophylactically.
    c. Diarrhoea—encourage fluids and give a bland, low residue diet. Antidiarrhoea drugs may be given. Recognize that patient's nutritional state may be jeopardized. Be aware of patient's fluid and electrolyte balance.
6   Note the manifestations of bone marrow depression:
    a. Be aware of the patient's blood count.
    b. Observe for evidence of infection or bleeding—examine the skin, throat and mouth daily.
    c. Record the patient's temperature every 4 hours.
    d. Avoid intramuscular injections. If they must be given, apply firm site pressure afterwards.
    e. Warn the patient to avoid cuts, e.g., suggest the use of an electric razor.
7   Assess status of oral mucosa and utilize measures to minimize mucosal trauma.
    a. Encourage regular mouth care with a soft toothbrush.
    b. Inspect the mouth regularly.
    c. Avoid highly spiced and highly seasoned food.
8   Promote patient comfort and offer analgesics if he is experiencing pain.
9   Maintain adequate nutritional levels.
10   Take special care of the skin and hair:
    a. Encourage movement. If the patient is confined to bed he should be turned every 2 hours. The use of sheepskins and other aids may be helpful.
    b. If there is alopecia, the patient can be reassured that the hair will grow back again. Arrange for a wig to be fitted before treatment starts.
11   If the patient is receiving vinca-alkaloids, avoid constipation by giving mild aperients prophylactically.
12   Attend to the psychological needs of the patient.
    a. Provide diversional and recreational therapy.
    b. Provide rest periods as part of the care plan.

c. Promote self-esteem by allowing the patient to be an active participant in his care.

d. Encourage the patient's family and friends to share in the caring.

e. Be honest with the patient about all aspects of his therapy and condition.

RADIATION DIAGNOSIS AND THERAPY

Radiation is frequently used in diagnosing and treating cancer.

Sources of Radiation

1 Naturally occurring radioactivity, e.g., radium.
2 Artificially produced radioactivity—radioisotopes.
  a. X-ray machines.
  b. Teletherapy using solid sources, e.g., ^{60}Co.
  c. Implants and applicators, e.g., ^{137}Ce.
  d. Unsealed radioactive sources, e.g., ^{131}I.

Definitions

1 *Nuclide*—any atomic entity capable of existing for a measurable lifetime, usually more than 10^{-9} seconds.
2 *Radionuclide* (radioactive nuclide)—one that disintegrates with the emission of particular or electromagnetic radiations.
3 *Radioactivity*—the disintegration of the atom which gives up energy in the form of rays or particles.
4 *Isotope*—an element whose nucleus contains a fixed number of protons but has a differing number of neutrons, thereby changing its weight.
  a. Optimal ratio between proton and neutrons is stable.
  b. By using nuclear reactors, it is possible to bombard a stable isotope with additional free neutrons.
  c. Most radioisotopes emit:
    (1) Particulate radiation—small fragments of the nucleus having mass and size (alpha and beta particles).
    (2) Electromagnetic radiations—rays that have no mass (x-rays).
5 *Radioactive decay or disintegration.*
  a. The rate of decay varies from isotope to isotope.
  b. 'Half-life' or decay rate is the time required to reduce a particular radioactive substance by one-half of its atoms, thereby reducing it to half of its initial activity.
    Example: Radium-225—half-life of over 1600 years.
  c. A radioisotope administered to a patient in unsealed form has a relatively short life and is essentially inactive after therapeutic use has been completed.
    Example: ^{131}I—half-life about 8 days.
  d. Longer lasting isotopes are implanted temporarily in the patient in a sealed container.
    Example: ^{60}Co—half-life about 5 years.

6   *Units of measurement (activity):*
    a. Curie (Ci)—basic unit for measuring amount of activity in a radioactive sample.
    b. Millicurie (mCi)—one-thousandth of a curie.
    c. Microcurie (μCi)—one-millionth of a curie.
7   *Units for measuring radiation exposure or absorption:*
    a. Roentgen (r.)—a standard unit of exposure (usually applied to x-rays or gamma rays).
    b. Rad—a unit to measure absorbed dose (1 rad = amount of radiation required to deposit 100 ergs of energy per gramme of irradiated material).
    c. Rem—a unit of measure of radiation-dose equivalent which relates to biological effectiveness (roentgen equivalent man).

Biological Aspects and Clinical Application

Nature and Indications for Use

1   Individualized to produce effective ionization within a tumour while avoiding unnecessary irradiation of normal structures.
2   Low voltage—KeV (thousand electron volts).
    Super voltage—MeV (million electron volts).
3   Tissues most likely to respond to radiation exposure—those originating from reticulo-endothelial tissues (leukaemia, lymphomas) and those from embryonal tissues (teratomas).
4   Tissues least likely to respond—bone and muscle.

Factors Affecting the Benefit of Radiation Exposure vs. Risk of Tissue Damage

1   *Dose rate*—a prescribed dose causes less tissue destruction if given in small amounts over a long period of time rather than given all at once.
2   *Area of body exposure*—the larger the area exposed, the greater the effect.
3   *Cell susceptibility.*
    Greater susceptibility—rapidly dividing cells with no specialized function (e.g., lympocytes and germ cells).
    Lesser susceptibility—nondividing cells and highly differentiated cells (e.g., nerve or muscle cells).
4   *Biological variability*—individual differences play a role in human susceptibility. Examples:
    a. Healthy person more responsive than malnourished individual.
    b. Skin is especially vulnerable to radiation injury.
    c. Bone marrow is very radiosensitive; therefore, such damage is potentially the most lethal.
    d. Radiation cataracts result from excessive eye exposure.
    e. Lung fibrosis occurs following injudicious radiation of chest.

Symptoms of Radiation Syndrome—High Level

Major portion of body exposed to large doses of irradiation (*over 100 rems*) in a short period of time.

1   Prodromal—nausea, vomiting, malaise.

2 Latent—symptoms subside.
3 Illness—general malaise, epilation (hair loss), haemorrhage (petechiae, nose-bleed), pallor, diarrhoea, inflammation of mouth and throat, leucopenia.
4 Recovery or death.

Symptoms of Radiation Syndrome—Low Level

Low levels of radiation over a long period of time.
Examples:

1 Radiologists—may acquire leukaemia.
2 Clock dial painters—may develop sarcomas (from radium-containing luminizing paint).
3 Gonad exposure to radiation—may affect progeny.

Radiological Precautions During Radiography or Radiotherapy

1 No one is permitted in the room where a patient is undergoing radiography or radiotherapy.
2 Fail safe mechanisms must be provided to avoid accidental exposure to radiation.
3 Appropriate lead shielding should be used to protect the patient's most vulnerable areas, e.g. lungs, gonads.

Nursing Support and Action in Radiation Therapy

Physical and Psychological Preparation of the Patient

1 Provide psychological support to this patient because radiation therapy is associated with fears:
   a. Of being burned.
   b. Of being disfigured.
   c. Of death and dying.
   d. Of inability to perform normal bodily functions.
   e. Of pain.
   f. Of sterility and loss of sexual function.
2 Recognize systemic responses to fear:
   a. Mouth dryness, pupillary dilatation.
   b. Hand tremor, vomiting, severe palpitations.
3 If above signs are noted, initiate open discussion, since this often relieves anxiety.
4 Remove all opaque objects such as pins, buttons and hairpins, and replace clothing with a gown for body x-rays.
5 Have patient remain perfectly still; maintain position with use of sandbags, etc., if required.
6 Tell patient that there will be no sensation or pain accompanying either picture taking or penetration of x-rays.
7 Advise him that he will be alone in the room for the protection of the technician but that he will be in voice contact.
8 Determine from the doctor what he has told the patient about radiotherapy, particularly in the case of the patient with advanced cancer.

9 If a series of treatments is to be given, include the patient in the planning phase.
10 Give special attention to diet and medications; administer antinauseants, analgesics, specific for diarrhoea, proctitis and cystitis.
11 Explain the need for routine blood counts.

Skin Manifestations

1 Inform the patient that some skin reaction can be expected but that it varies from patient to patient. Example: dry erythema, desquamation, moist erythema, healing, epilation, tanning, telangiectasis.
2 Apply no lotions, ointments, cosmetics, etc., to the site of radiation, unless prescribed by the doctor. Avoid talcum powder because it contains heavy metals which increase the effect of radiation on the skin. Baby products can be safely used.
3 Discourage vigorous rubbing, friction or scratching, because it can destroy skin cells.
4 Take precautions against irritation from friction, exposure to sunlight and extremes in temperature.
5 Do not apply adhesive or sellotape to the skin.

Mucous Membrane Damage

1 Oral mucosa.
   a. There may be a change in or loss of taste.
   b. There may be various degrees of soreness and inability to swallow.
   c. Avoid irritants such as smoking, spicy food, alcoholic beverages.
   d. Use mild cleansing agents in the mouth.
2 Digestive tract.
   a. Diarrhoea is a common symptom if large areas are irradiated or if colon is significantly affected.
   b. Treat diarrhoea with simple measures such as Kaolin or opiate-like agents (Lomotil); it may be necessary to suspend treatment for a few days.

Dietary Disturbances

1 Provide dietary restrictions to relieve symptoms of chronic radiation enteritis. It may be necessary to administer diet free of gluten, protein, lactose to overcome or avoid absorptive problems resulting from atrophy of intestinal villi.
2 Maintain high level of nutrition but eliminate those foods that irritate the mucous membrane; this may preclude the need for nasogastric feeding.

Systemic Reactions

Nausea, vomiting, fever, loss of appetite, malaise.

1 Administer sedatives for greater comfort.
2 Select fluids and foods that will not induce or aggravate nausea.
3 Provide small, frequent meals rather than three larger meals.
4 Suggest time for rest and relaxation; avoid noise, confusion.
5 Recognize that the patient needs encouragement and understanding.

RADIOISOTOPE THERAPY

Types of Radioisotope Therapy

Teletherapy

Utilizes gamma rays from a radioactive source which is kept in a shielded unit placed at a distance from the patient.

1 Radioisotope Cobalt-60 (^{60}Co) and Cesium-137 (^{137}Ce) deliver radiation similar to that produced by supervoltage x-ray apparatus.
2 Cobalt therapy unit requires extra shielding because rays are being emitted constantly. Because gamma rays cannot be entirely absorbed, personnel are advised to spend minimum time in this room.
3 *Advantages of cobalt over conventional x-ray:*
   a. Skin problems are significantly reduced.
   b. Bone or cartilage involvement is lessened.
   c. Electronic circuits are not required.
4 *Disadvantages of cobalt*
   a. Because it has a half-life of 5 years, it is necessary to replace the cobalt.
   b. Radiation energy cannot be varied.
   c. Cost of room shielding is high.

Plesiotherapy

1 *External Moulds*—a packaged and screened container in which a radioisotope can be placed and applied directly to the skin surface.
   Examples:
   a. Cobalt can be applied in this manner to small areas, as in the treatment of carcinoma of the lip, larynx, ear, etc.
   b. ^{182}Ta (radioactive tantalum) can be applied in a flexible wire mould (e.g., to the external surface of a retinoblastoma involving eyeball and optic nerve, to the bladder wall).
   c. ^{90}Sr (radioactive strontium) and ^{90}Y (yttrium) as in external moulds used for shallow irradiation of eye neoplasms.
2 *Intracavity Isotope Therapy*
   Examples:
   a. Liquid radioisotopes—^{198}Au (radioactive colloidal gold) introduced into the pleural cavity to treat malignant ascites.
   b. Solid sources—^{137}Ce introduced into the cervix or uterus to treat gynaecological tumours.
3 *Interstitial Isotope Therapy*
   Examples:
   a. Radioactive needles, seeds, tubes or wires can be implanted directly into tumour tissue: ^{60}Co, ^{137}Ce, ^{198}Au, ^{222}Rn, ^{182}Ta.
   b. Implants may be temporary or permanent; they may be supplementary to surgery or to external beam irradiation.
   c. Radioactive solutions may be injected directly into the tumour or surrounding tissue. Colloidal solution of radioactive colloidal gold (^{198}Au) is one of the most commonly used solutions.

4   *Internal Irradiation*
     Example:
     Oral ingestion of radioiodine (^{131}I)—used in the treatment of carcinoma of the thyroid. In this instance the target tissue has an affinity for the therapeutic agent.

Nursing Management of Patients Receiving Radioisotopes

Identification of the Patient as a Radiation Source

1   Place a radioactive symbol at the end of the bed or outside his room.
2   Identify the chart cover, doctor's and nurse's order sheets and special radiation instruction sheet with the radioactive symbol.
3   For patients receiving the most minute quantities of tracer radioisotopes, such identification (see above) is not necessary.
4   Personnel who may be exposed to penetrating radiation (x-rays or gamma rays) should wear film badges on front of the body.

Radiation Instruction Sheet

1   Type of radioactivity used.
2   Time of insertion.
3   Anticipated time of removal.
4   Precautions to follow.
5   Whom to notify when in doubt or in an emergency.

Factors Affecting the Amount of Radiation

1   *Amount* of radioactivity present, 10, 20, 30 mCi, etc.
2   The *distance* of the nurse from the patient.

NOTE: The inverse square law applies: doubling the distance from a radiation source cuts intensity received to one-fourth.

3   Amount of *time* spent in actual contact with patient.
4   Degree of *shielding* utilized.
     Chosen according to type of radiation—alpha, beta, gamma (see Fig. 7.1).
5   Amount of *body area exposed* to radiation.

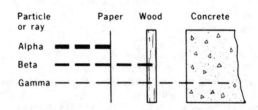

Figure 7.1.   Relative penetration of alpha, beta and gamma radiation. (US Atomic Energy Commission.)

Nursing Alert: During the period of greatest radioactivity (24–72 hours), limit amount of time spent with the patient to that required for essential care. Require patient to remain in his bed or room during course of treatment.

Vital Nursing Measures in Caring for the Patient with Internal Radiation

1   Be acquainted with the nomenclature describing dissipation of radioisotopes.
    a. *Physical half-life*—a constant rate in which one-half of radioactivity is dissipated in a given time.
    b. *Biologic half-life*—the time it takes for a radioisotope to disappear from the body via normal metabolic processes.
    c. *Effective half-life*—a combination of physical half-life and biologic half-life.
2   Recognize that an isotope that is completely dispersed throughout the body (or a major portion of it) is less hazardous to an organ or tissue than an isotope concentrated by the body into a limited area.
3   Recognize that an isotope that is excreted rapidly is less hazardous than radium, which may be kept in the body for long periods.
4   Take appropriate measures associated with *sealed sources of radiation* implanted within a patient (sealed internal radiation).
    a. Do not remain within 1 m (3 ft) of the patient any longer than required to give essential care.
    b. Know that the casing material absorbs all alpha radiation and most beta radiation, but that a hazard concerning gamma radiation may exist.
    c. Do not linger longer than necessary in giving patient care, even though all precautions are followed.
    d. Be alert for implants that may have become loosened (those inserted in cavities that have access to the exterior), e.g., check the kidney dish following mouth care for a patient with an oral implant.
    e. Notify the radiologist of any implant that has moved out of position.
    f. Utilize long-handled forceps or tongs and hold at arm's length when picking up any accidentally dislodged radium needle, seeds, tubes, etc., that may appear on dressings, bed, or floor. *Never pick up a radioactive source with your hands.*
    g. Do not discard any dressings or linens unless sure that no radioactive source is present.
    h. Wash hands with soap and water after caring for a patient who is being treated with a radioisotope. When wearing gloves, wash them with soap and water before removing them.

NOTE: This is not necessary for sealed sources.

    i. Encourage patients who are ambulatory to remain in their own rooms.
    j. Upon discharge of a patient, it is a good policy for the radiologist to check the room with a Geiger counter to be certain that all radioactive materials have been removed.
    k. Continue radiation precautions, when a patient has a permanent implant, until the radiologist declares precautions unnecessary. (See p. 291 for nursing care of the patient receiving radiation therapy.)
5   Take appropriate measures associated with *unsealed sources*; radioactivity may be (1) widely spread in the body, (2) localized or (3) present in any body tissue or fluid.

Examples:
a. *Radioactive iodine.*
  (1) Circulates in bloodstream, excreted by kidneys—urine and blood contain radioactive material.
  (2) Can be secreted by sweat glands.
  (3) May be found in vomit of patient who recently took oral dose.
b. *Radioactive colloidal gold.*
  (1) May be noted in wound seepage as pink, red or purple stain following intracavitary injection
  (2) May be noted in small amounts in urine.
c. *Radioactive phosphorus solution.*
  Be alert for contamination from excreta (urine and faeces) and vomitus.

IMMUNOTHERAPY

The *immune system* of the body has the ability to recognize and to defend itself against infection and invasion by foreign cells such as those of cancer. The immune system may be weakened or overwhelmed by the invasion of foreign cells so that it cannot function effectively.

Immunotherapy employs the immune mechanism of the body to combat cancer and overcome it. The immunotherapeutic approach to cancer is based on the fact that most tumours provoke an immune response (such as antitumour activity, production of tumour antigens) in the patient (host).

Although it is still considered investigational, significant research in immunotherapy is going on and progress is being made.

Objective of Immunotherapy

1 To successfully treat the cancer patient.
2 To challenge and to induce mobilization of the patient's immune defences by utilizing a chemical or microbial agent to which the patient has previously been sensitized.
  a. This produces a delayed hypersensitivity response that can be employed against the cancer.
  b. Once developed in this way, immunocompetence (either alone or in combination with radiation, chemotherapy or surgery) can fight the cancer.

Various Approaches of Immunotherapy

Active Specific Immunotherapy

1 Utilization of the patient's own immune mechanisms to reject or control his own malignant cells.
2 To date, active immunization, used alone, appears incapable of boosting the immune mechanism in the patient with advanced disseminated cancer.

Active Nonspecific Immunotherapy

1 Primarily activates macrophages and enhances delayed hypersensitivity of cellular immunity.

2   Utilization of bacteria or bacterial products as an immunologic adjuvant to enhance the immune response.
   a. *BCG* is a live attenuated strain of tubercle bacillus.
   b. *C. parvum* is a killed anaerobe.
3   These agents are easy to distribute widely, and the responses achieved in patients with melanoma and several other solid tumours, as well as acute leukaemia, make them attractive for a large number of therapy protocols.

Passive-Adoptive Immunotherapy

1   Utilization of the immunity of a competent donor.
2   The use of hyperimmune serum for rubella (passive) or for immunodeficiency diseases (adoptive) appears possible.
      Example: Immune RNA and lymphocyte transfer factor (LTF).
3   Again, further study is needed.

Adjunctive Immunotherapy

Because the above immunotherapeutic approaches appear inadequate, immunotherapy may be best utilized as an adjunct to other modalities (and even following curative methods, to eliminate the few remaining malignant cells).

1   *Immunotherapy and surgery.*
   a. Following surgical removal of the bulk of a tumour, immunotherapy may be effective in attacking small foci of cancer cells.
   b. Whereas surgery is directed towards larger primary tumours, immunotherapy can control small foci of metastatic disease at distant sites.
2   *Immunochemotherapy.*
   a. Timing is critical in successfully combining immunotherapy with chemotherapy.
   b. Cancer chemotherapeutic drugs are often immunosuppressive, but certain chemotherapeutic agents actually stimulate the immune response to some antigens.
3   *Immunoradiotherapy.*
   a. A problem associated with chemotherapy and radiation therapy is that they attack normal cells as well as cancer cells; because of the selectivity of immunotherapy, it could logically be combined with these other modalities.
   b. If the patient is given tumour-specific antibodies that are attached to isotopes, large doses of radiation could be directed to tumour cells; this would combine the destructive effects of radiation with the specificity of immunotherapy.

CARE OF THE PATIENT WITH ADVANCED CARCINOMA

Objectives of Nursing Management

To Halt the Spread of the Malignant Growth

1   Prepare the patient for the prescribed modality of treatment: surgery, chemotherapy or radiation.
2   Assist with diagnostic evaluation in an attempt to determine precise location(s) of involvement or spread.

3   Control local and generalized infections.
4   Promote optimum nutritional, fluid and electrolyte levels by correcting deficiencies.
5   Provide the patient with psychosociological support.
   a. Listen to his concerns.
   b. Observe and support his reactions where appropriate.
   c. Explain the aspect of treatment that is pertinent at that time.
   d. Empathize with him and offer reassurance where appropriate.
6   Assist with the prescribed form of therapy.

To Encourage the Patient to Pursue Purposeful or Diversional Activities as Long as Possible

1   Invite him to participate socially, visit with other individuals, take walks, etc.
2   Provide opportunities for communication and mind-occupying activities.
       Accept him as an individual with natural defence mechanisms; encourage him to talk about himself, his concerns, his understanding, his future—even the possibility of dying.
3   Support the patient as he taps his spiritual resources.
4   Understand his behavioural deviations, even when socially unacceptable; when the episode passes, assist in restoring his self-esteem.
5   Empathize with him in an effort to show concern and understanding.
6   Include the patient's family in planning with him meaningful day-to-day activities.

To Promote Comfort of the Patient and Relieve his Pain

1   Assist the patient in bathing and with personal hygiene; personal cleanliness is a comfort measure.
2   Provide warmth when required; in cool seasons the debilitated patient is more sensitive to chilling.
3   Assist him as required in moving, turning, getting out of bed, walking, etc., in an effort to promote maximum activity and minimum amount of pain.
4   Evaluate objectively the nature of his pain (location, duration, quality) and manner in which the patient tolerates or accepts it.
5   Convey the impression that his pain is understood and that relief is forthcoming.
6   Ascertain pain source—is it carcinoma-related? Is there some other physical source? Is it psychological?
7   Administer medications as specifically required:
   a. Sedative and hypnotics—to induce and promote sleep.
   b. Local anaesthetics—for localized pain.
   c. Specific medications—for nausea and vomiting.
   d. Muscle relaxant and antispasmodic drugs—to relieve tenseness.
   e. Tranquillizers—to promote a sense of well-being.
   f. Analgesics—for discomfort or pain.
   g. Narcotics—for more intense pain.

Nursing Alert: Recognize that elderly debilitated patients have increased sensitivity: Avoid this cycle: a narcotic → drowsiness → less food and fluid → dehydration → nausea and vomiting → increased pain → more narcotic (and a resumption of the cycle).

8 Prepare the patient for surgical pain-relieving interventions.
  a. Alcohol injections to block nerve pathways.
  b. Localized radiotherapy.
  c. Presacral neurectomy for visceral pain.
  d. Cordotomy for intractable pain.
  e. Neurosurgical nerve interruption.

To Cope with the Annoying and Discomforting Side Effects of Radiation Therapy

1 Radiation sickness.
  a. Administer sedatives, antiemetics and antihistamines as prescribed.
  b. Encourage adequate fluid intake.
  c. Tempt patient with small, frequent, high calorie, high protein feedings.
  d. Record his reactions.
2 Skin reactions.
  a. Observe skin for dryness, tautness, erythema, desquamation.
  b. Apply bland cream or oil to radiation site as directed.
  c. Cleanse skin gently with bland soaps (Neutrogena) and lukewarm water.
  d. Protect skin from sunlight, heat, trauma, constricting clothing.
  e. Note changes such as telangiectasis (small network of dilated arterioles).
  f. Offer medicated mouthwashes to soothe oral mucosa.
3 Diarrhoea.
  a. Give antidiarrhoea medications as prescribed.
  b. Avoid serving foods that aggravate the problem, such as stewed prunes.
  c. Diet restricted to low residue or bland foods.
4 Blood cell depression.
  a. Protect the patient from injury and infection.
  b. Observe for evidences of bleeding or infection and take measures to correct.

To Assist in Overcoming Bladder and Bowel Disturbances

1 Bladder frequency or incontinence.
  a. Keep an accurate input and output record.
  b. Establish a bladder control programme.
  c. Maintain perineal cleanliness.
  d. Insert an indwelling catheter if other measures fail.
2 Constipation.
  a. Maintain an adequate fluid level.
  b. Omit constipating foods from diet—ensure adequate fruits and vegetables.
  c. Administer glycerin suppository or mild laxative as prescribed.

Nursing Alert: Avoid giving enemas when patient has leucopenia or is taking drugs that irritate the intestinal tract (e.g., 5-fluorouracil).

To Maintain an Intact Skin and Prevent Tissue Breakdown

1 Offer regular gentle back and body massages; these can stimulate poor circulation and promote relaxation as well. Avoid brisk rubbing which may damage vulnerable tissue.
2 Ensure wrinkle-free, dry bedding—helps prevent skin breakdown in debilitated patients. Special mattress pads can be used.

3   Control skin breakdown following radiation treatment as indicated on p. 291.
4   Maintain an exercise programme utilizing range of motion activities.
5   Control oedema of extremities by elevating the part as well as supporting it.
6   Initiate measures to prevent pressure sores.

To Control Odours Which Tend to Emanate From the Affected Tissues

1   Promote an aesthetically comfortable environment.
2   Encourage good personal hygiene.
3   Irrigate external wounds with saline and use mechanical cleansers as prescribed (half-strength hydrogen peroxide, diluted antiseptic detergents, etc.).
4   Remove soiled dressings promptly and change all soiled linens frequently—wrap dressings in paper and place in covered container immediately.
5   Provide fresh circulating air—use aerosol deodorants when necessary.
6   Change packing or pads frequently, irrigate thoroughly any affected body cavities and shave where hair presents a problem—mouth, nasal area, vagina, rectum.
7   Avoid dressing changes at inopportune times—visiting hours, meal times, etc.
8   Consider use of antiodour dressings containing charcoal.

To Anticipate and Control Haemorrhage

1   Monitor vital signs to detect increase in pulse rate and respiration and decrease in blood pressure.
2   Apply pressure, if active bleeding occurs, at convenient pressure points between site and heart.
3   Employ emergency haemorrhage-control measures.
4   Note and record amount and nature of bleeding; notify doctor.
5   Reassure and comfort patient.
6   Use packing if bleeding involves accessible cavity, e.g., rectum, vagina.
7   Administer platelet or whole-blood transfusion as prescribed.
8   Prepare patient for cauterization and ligation if necessary.

To Assist Patient as He Strives for Peace of Mind in Preparing for Death

To Keep the Patient at the Optimum Physical and Psychological Level of Which He is Capable.

1   Provide a high calorie and high vitamin diet; cater to his personal food likes.
2   Offer between-meal feedings and milky drinks.
3   Change patient's environment if possible by encouraging him to walk and go outdoors.
4   Promote physical activities as much as possible; encourage rest periods.
5   Allow him to verbalize his feelings, thoughts; provide unhurried time for listening.
6   Maintain an optimistic atmosphere; limit the time plans to hour by hour or day by day (not week by week, month by month, or year by year).

PSYCHOSOCIAL SUPPORT OF THE DYING PATIENT

Reactions of the Patient to Dying*

Stage of Denial

1 Period of denial allows patient to mobilize his defences.
2 Patient will exhibit withdrawal and avoidance of subject of death.
3 Usually a temporary defence to be replaced in time by partial acceptance.
4 Patient may talk of death and then change topic abruptly.
5 Patient may be in a temporary state of shock.

Stage of Anger

1 Denial may be replaced by anger, rage, envy and resentment.
2 Anger may be displaced and projected into environment.
   a. Anger frequently directed at hospital staff. (Avoid reacting personally to this anger.)
   b. Try to tolerate rational and irrational anger. Patient may experience considerable relief in expressing anger.

Stage of Bargaining

Bargaining is an attempt to postpone the inevitable and to extend life.

Stage of Depression

1 This is a stage in which the patient is preparing himself to accept the loss of everything and everyone he loves.
2 Patient may be undergoing anticipatory grief to prepare himself for the final separation; may mourn the loss of meaningful people in his life.
   a. Allow the patient to express his sorrow—helps make the final acceptance easier.
   b. Sit with the patient.

Stage of Acceptance

1 Patient is neither depressed nor angry about his impending death; he bows to the sentence.
2 May contemplate his demise with quiet acceptance and expectation—detachment may make death easier.
3 During this stage patient may be almost devoid of feelings—his circle of interest diminishes.
4 Patient will sleep and rest more—does not desire news or visitors from outside world.
5 Patient may just wish someone to hold his hand—reassures him that he is not forgotten.
6 Patient may reach the point where death comes as a relief.
7 Family may require more support during this stage.

* Adapted from Kübler-Ross, E (1970) On Death and Dying, New York, Macmillan.

Supportive Attitudes and Actions to the Patient, Family and Health Team

Objectives

To allow the patient to live as fully as possible.
To relieve his discomfort and distress.
To be attuned to the special needs of the dying.
To help the patient achieve death with dignity.

Physical Support of the Dying Patient

See p. 298.

Emotional Support of the Dying Patient

1   Make sure the patient has continuing, personal and caring contacts—gives comfort and reassurance.
   a. Avoid changing personnel.
   b. Be willing to become involved with the patient—personal involvement is necessary if human interaction is to be supportive.
   c. Make sure the nursing approach reflects the mutuality of human interaction.
   d. Take *time* with the patient—gives him the feeling that he is being cared for.
   e. Do not withdraw from the presence of death.
2   Give the patient an opportunity to talk about himself, his illness and his dying.
   a. Accept the patient as he is now.
   b. Be able to accept the patient's anger—whether overt anger or that expressed as depression.
   c. Encourage him to talk about changes made by his illness.
   d. Demonstrate interest in patient's total life style.
      (1) Learn what supports his ego and self-esteem.
      (2) Be accessible.
3   Allow the patient to act out his feelings without judgement.
   a. Understand that the patient is increasingly overwhelmed by feelings of rage, anger, fear, guilt, futility, despondency and pain.
      (1) Understand the patient rather than judge him.
      (2) Demonstrate patience, tolerance and support.
   b. Allow the patient to keep his hold on *hope*—hope is therapeutic and will help maintain the patient through his suffering.
      (1) Maintain hope with the patient.
      (2) Avoid reinforcing hope after the patient has given up (stage of acceptance).
   c. Understand the patient's dread of being deserted.
4   Be alert for behavioural changes—patient may be trying to communicate something.
      Anticipate that the patient's behaviour will be altered by his deteriorating physical condition.
      (1) Withdrawal from customary interests.
      (2) Impairment of self-esteem.
5   Encourage the patient to retain confidence in his health team.
   a. Emphasize to the patient that he and the health team are in the battle together—patient will not be as fearful of loneliness, rejection, deceit.

b. Reassure him that everything possible will be done for him.

c. Let the patient know that he is respected and understood; treat him as a fellow human being.

d. Seek the opinions of the patient—bolsters his self-esteem.

e. Encourage the patient to take some initiative in his care.

f. Keep the room neat and confusion at a minimum.

6   Help the patient who must undergo the 'business' of dying.

a. Settling of affairs, settling problems in human relationships, planning future for children, parent, spouse.

b. Utilize services of chaplain, legal counsellor, social worker, etc.

7   Pay attention to the patient's day-to-day complaints.

a. Recognize the wide variety of symptoms accompanying anxiety—palpitation, nausea, insomnia, diarrhoea, irritability.

b. Be aware of the symptoms of depression—fatigue, lethargy, disturbances of sleep and appetite, inability to concentrate, psychomotor retardation.

c. Try to alleviate each symptom.

d. Reassure the patient that his pain will be relieved—helps the patient to cope with his discomfort.

e. Give appropriate drugs to help the dying patient face death, cope with his anxiety and depression, and alter his sensitivity to pain (see pp. 304–305).

f. Help make each day as good a day as possible.

Support of the Family of the Dying Patient

Anticipatory grief—mourning that occurs over an extended period of time before actual death:

Bereavement starts when one realizes that loss is inevitable.

Family experiences awareness of loss and depression.

Family may begin to adapt, physically and psychologically, to the consequences of death.

1   Understand that the family may be undergoing anticipatory mourning and reacting to anticipated loss.

a. Recognize that various family members behave differently while working out their anticipatory grief.

(1) Avoid showing disapproval of the behaviour of others—may produce feelings of shame, guilt and inadequacy.

(2) Understand that family members may feel guilty when they are unable to demonstrate grief—there may be little or no feeling at actual time of death because family members have worked through their grief during the anticipatory period.

(3) Family may withdraw emotional investment from the patient as they perceive he has no future.

b. Be alert for untoward reactions to death—family member may need supportive therapy and counselling.

2   Accept the feelings and attitudes of the family—helps avoid mutual hostility and recriminations.

Feelings include:

(1) Fear and anxiety.

    (2) Sorrow and grief.
    (3) Overt or suppressed hostility interwoven with guilt feelings; self-blame.
    (4) Ambivalent feelings toward dying member.
    (5) Overprotective attitude.
    (6) Depersonalization.
    (7) Projection of guilt to medical personnel.
    (8) Submission or excessive courtesy—may mask hostility.
3 Realize the problems faced by the family—anticipated separation of loved one, financial problems, disruption of family life, problems of communication.
4 Demonstrate concern for the family.
    a. Inform them of practical help—financial assistance, social worker, other supporting services of local helping agencies.
    b. Reassure family that they will not be left alone.
    c. Provide opportunity for family member to ventilate his conflicts—anger, depression, victimization by illness.

Support of the Health Team

1 Examine one's own attitudes and ability to face terminal illness and death.
    a. Look at possessions and relationships in context of inevitability of death.
    b. Plan for disaster and death.
2 Monitor one's own feelings.
    a. Accept the ideas of denial, fear and guilt.
    b. Assess and correct one's own biases and fears.
    c. Watch emotional responses to challenges of incurable disease and 'difficult' families.
3 Do not withdraw from the presence of death.
    a. Face the reality of the dying patient.
    b. Become skilled and sensitive in the art of human interaction.

Psychotherapeutic Agents* for the Support of the Seriously Ill Patient

The use of drugs is indicated when: (1) there is decreasing ability to function (eat, sleep, care for hygienic needs, etc.) and (2) duration of symptoms is abnormally long.

Objective

To assist the patient to maintain his daily activities.

Drug	Nursing Implications
Antianxiety Agents	
Sedatives	
Pentobarbitone sodium (Nembutal) Quinalbarbitone sodium (Seconal) Gluthethimide (Doriden)	1 Sedatives act as central nervous system depressants; given to relieve anxiety and induce sleep. 2 Dosage varies with physiologic and psychologic state of patient. 3 Evaluate patient for drowsiness, impaired judgement and performance, dizziness, drug habituation.

* Reader is referred to a pharmacology textbook for a more complete listing.

Drug	Nursing Implications
Tranquillizers Chlorpromazine (Largactil) Chlordiazepoxide hydrochloride (Librium) Diazepam (Valium)	1 Tranquillizers act in all parts of the brain; principally on the subcortical areas to produce mental relaxation and emotional calm. 2 Tranquillizers act at different subcortical levels, have different pharmacological properties and varying degrees of clinical usefulness. 3 Synthetic tranquillizers cause dry mouth, visual problems, constipation and tachycardia. 4 Watch for postural hypotension and syncope, drowsiness and delayed reflexes.
Antidepressant Agents Imipramine (Tofranil) Amitriptyline (Tryptizol)	1 Drug is started at a low dose and increased gradually until a maximum daily dose is reached (according to efficacy and side effects). 2 Treatment may be continued for several months; then the drug is gradually withdrawn. 3 Evaluate for weakness, drowsiness or deepening of depression; patient may also demonstrate agitation, tremulousness, visual hallucinations and agitation. 4 *Assess for postural hypotension*; dry mouth and constipation also occur.
Combinations Antianxiety agents and antidepressants may be used in combination—to treat combination of symptoms (anxiety and depression).	

FURTHER READING

Bouchard, P and Owens, N (1972) Nursing Care of the Cancer Patient, C V Mosby
Burkhalter, P and Donley, D (1978) Dynamics of Oncology Nursing, McGraw-Hill
Capra, L G (1972) The Care of the Cancer Patient, Heinemann Medical
Donovan, M I and Price, S G (1976) Cancer Care Nursing, Appleton Century Crofts

Downie, P A (1978) Cancer Rehabilitation: An Introduction for Physiotherapists and Allied Professions, Faber & Faber
Peterson, B H and Kellogg, C J (1976) Current Practice in Oncological Nursing, C V Mosby
Tiffany, R (1978) Oncology for Nurses and Health Care Professionals, Volumes I and 2, George Allen & Unwin
Tiffany, R (1978) Cancer Nursing—Medical, Faber & Faber
Tiffany, R (1979) Cancer Nursing—Radiotherapy, Faber & Faber
Tiffany, R (1980) Cancer Nursing—Surgical, Faber & Faber
TNM (1974) Classification of Malignant Tumours, UICC
Walter, J (1977) Cancer and Radiotherapy, Churchill Livingstone
Walter, J Millar, H and Conford, C K (1979) A Short Textbook of Radiotherapy, 4th edition, Churchill Livingstone

Terminal Care

Hannington-Kiff, J C (1974) Pain Relief, Heinemann Medical
Hinton, J (1963) Dying, Penguin
Kübler-Ross, E (1973) On Death and Dying, Tavistock Institute
Lamerton, R (1973) Bereavement, Pelican
McCaffery, M (1979) Nursing Management of the Patient with Pain, 2nd edition, J B Lippincott
Melzack, R (1973) The Puzzle of Pain, Penguin Educational
Saunders, C (1976) Care of the Dying, 2nd edition, Macmillan/Nursing Times
Saunders, C (1978) The Management of Terminal Disease, Edward Arnold

Chapter 8

SKIN DISORDERS

Dermatology

Burns

Dermatology

NURSING RESPONSIBILITIES IN DERMATOLOGY

Psychological Insights

1 Patients with dermatological problems can see and feel their problems and are more disturbed by their complaints than many patients with other conditions.
2 Skin eruptions evoke feelings of shame, disgust, avoidance, withdrawal and anger that compound the problems of management of patients with skin conditions.
3 Irritation is frequently a feature of skin disease and produces loss of sleep, anxiety and depression, which in turn reinforce discomfort and fatigue.
4 Cosmetic needs constitute the underlying motive that brings the patient to treatment.
5 Nursing support requires understanding, unending patience and continuing encouragement for these patients.

Nursing Assessment

Be aware that many systemic conditions may be accompanied by dermatological manifestations.

1   Obtain a dermatological history.
    a. How long has the patient had the skin condition?
    b. Has it occurred previously?
    c. Were there any other symptoms besides the rash?
    d. What site was first affected?
    e. What did the rash/lesion look like when it first appeared?
    f. How did it spread?
    g. What is the distribution of the lesion—symmetrical, linear, circular?
    h. Are there itching, burning, tingling or crawling sensations? Loss of sensation?
    i. Is it worse at a particular time?
    j. Does the patient have any idea how it started?
    k. Is there a history of hay fever, asthma, urticaria? (These problems are associated with eczema.)
    l. Was the appearance of the eruption related to the intake of food?
    m. Was there a relationship between a specific event and the outbreak of the rash/lesion?
    n. What medications is the patient taking?
    o. What is the patient's occupation?
    p. What is in his immediate environment (plants, animals) that might be precipitating the problem?
2   Describe the dermatosis (abnormal condition of the skin) clearly and in detail.
    a. What is (are) the colour(s) of the lesion?
    b. Is there redness, heat, pain or swelling?
    c. How large an area is involved; where is it?
    d. Is the eruption macular, papular, scaling, oozing, discrete, confluent?

Description of Skin Lesions

Primary Lesions (initial lesions)

1   Macule—flat discoloration of the skin; of various sizes, shapes and colours.
2   Papule—a solid, raised lesion.
3   Nodule—a raised lesion that is larger and deeper than a papule.
4   Vesicle—a small collection of fluid in or under the epidermis.
5   Bulla—a large vesicle or blister.
6   Pustule—an elevation of the skin that contains pus; may form as a result of purulent changes in a vesicle.
7   Wheal—transient elevation of the skin caused by oedema of the dermis and surrounding capillary dilatation.
8   Plaque—a patch on the skin or mucous membrane.

Secondary Lesions (changes that take place in primary lesions and possibly modify them)

1   Scales—heaped-up horny layer of dead epidermis; may develop as a result of inflammatory changes.
2   Crusts—a covering formed by the drying of serum, blood or pus on the skin.
3   Excoriations—linear scratch marks or traumatized area of skin. May be self-produced.
4   Fissure—a crack in the skin, usually from marked drying and long-standing inflammation.

5 Erosion—lesion formed by loss of epidermis from mucous membranes or skin.
6 Ulcer—lesion formed by local destruction of the epidermis and part or all of the underlying dermis.

SKIN TREATMENTS

Open Wet Dressings

Purposes

1 To cleanse skin of exudates, crusts, scales—thus making a cleaner and drier surface.
2 To reduce inflammation by producing vasoconstriction—thus decreasing vaso-dilatation and the local blood flow present in inflammation.
3 To maintain drainage of infected areas.

Clinical Uses

1 Vesicular, bullous, pustular and ulcerative disorders.
2 Acute inflammatory conditions.
3 Erosions.
4 Exudative, crusted surfaces.

Solution and Material	Desired Effect	Nursing Action
Solution Cool tapwater Normal saline Burrow's Solution (aluminium acetate solution) Magnesium sulphate Potassium permanganate	Effective in treating oozing dermatosis or swollen, infected dermatitis (furunculitis, cellulitis)	Keep dressing cool or at room temperature Moisten compress to the point of slight dripping Compresses may be remoistened with asepto syringe
Material Soft towelling Napkins Soft cotton sheeting	Relieves inflammation, burning and itching Has cooling effect Useful for removing crusts Cleansing and soothing	Add ice cubes to solution if coolness is desired Apply for 15 min every 2–3 hours unless otherwise indicated Keep patient warm if extensive areas are to be compressed Do not treat more than a third of the body at one time Discard dressing material daily *Caution*: Avoid burns

Baths

Baths are useful for applying medications to large areas of the skin, removing crusts, scales and old medications, and relieving inflammation and itching.

Bath Solution and Medication	Desired Effect	Nursing Action
Water Saline Colloidal–Oatmeal or Aveeno	Same effects as wet dressings Used for widely disseminated lesions Antipruritic and drying	Fill the tub half full—120 l (25 gal) Keep the water at a comfortable temperature (approximately 36°C (96–98°F))
Sodium bicarbonate	Cooling	Do not allow the water to cool excessively
Starch		Use a bath mat—*medications may cause tub to be slippery*
Medicated tars (follow package directions) Polytar emollient, psoriderm bath emulsion, liquor picis carbonis Bath oils Oilatum emollient, emulsifying ointment	Tar baths are used for psoriasis and chronic eczematous conditions Bath oils are used for antipruritic and emollient actions Used for acute and subacute eczematous eruptions	Apply a lubricating agent to wet skin after bath if emollient action is desired —increases hydration Dry by blotting with a towel Keep room warm to minimize temperature fluctuations Encourage patient to wear light, loose clothing after the bath
Antiseptics Potassium permanganate, hexachlorophane Antifungal Sterzac	Used for infected lesions and when mild antiseptic action is required	

Topical Medications

Type of Medication	Desired Effect	Nursing Action
Lotions Liquid vehicles for carrying medication; act by evaporation	Lubricate Cool through water evaporation May be protective, antiparasitic, antifungal, antipruritic; may act as sunscreen	May be applied with cotton gauze or soft paintbrush

(continued)

Type of Medication	Desired Effect	Nursing Action
Ointments and Creams Have greasy, nongreasy, or penetrating base depending on nature of lesion and drug applied	Lubricate Protect the skin Serve as vehicle for medications Retard water loss Used in chronic or localized skin conditions Cause vasoconstriction; reduce blood flow to skin	Apply ointments with a wooden tongue depressor Creams are rubbed into the skin by hand Teach patient to apply his own ointment or cream Ointments may have to be covered with a dressing to prevent soiling of clothing
Topical Adrenocorticosteriod Agents (many preparations available	Have anti-inflammatory action	Apply to localized area requiring medication Use only a small amount and rub in thoroughly Use with occlusive dressing as directed—enhances penetration Nurse should wear gloves when applying steroids to prevent absorption through her skin
Powders (usually with a talc, zinc oxide, bentonite or cornstarch base)	Act as hygroscopic agents (take up moisture) Increase evaporation; absorb perspiration Reduce friction	Dispense with shaker top Avoid accumulating powder in intertriginous areas
Pastes Suspension of powder in a greasy base, usually soft paraffin	Serve as a vehicle for medication, e.g., Dithranol in Lassar's paste	Apply thickly with a spatula Apply Dithranol only to affected areas Dust with powder Cover with tubular gauze Remove old paste with liquid paraffin
Intralesional Therapy Injection with a tuberculin syringe of sterile suspension of medication (usually suspension of corticosteroid) into or just below a lesion	Has anti-inflammatory action	Be aware that local atrophy may result Check patient for anaphylactoid reaction which may occur
Systemic Medications Adrenocorticosteroids Antibiotics Antihistamines Sedatives and tranquillizers Analgesics Antineoplastics		

Dressings for Skin Conditions

Occlusive Dressing

An airtight plastic film is applied to cover medicated skin (usually corticosteroid) (Fig. 8.1).

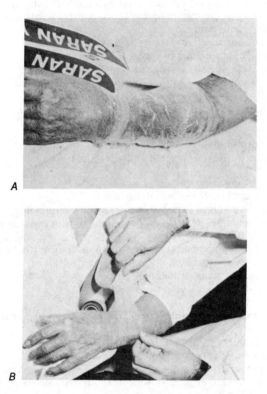

A

B

Figure 8.1.   a. Occlusion of treatment area with plastic film greatly enhances the effectiveness of topical corticosteroid. Sealing the ends with tape adds airtightness and humidity. b. Plastic surgical tape containing corticosteroid in the adhesive layer can be cut to size and applied to individual plaques. (From Weinstein, G D (1972) Postgraduate Medicine, 52 (5): 193.

1   Enhances absorption of topically applied medication.
2   Increases penetration of corticosteroids into the skin, thus enhancing anti-inflammatory effect.
3   Produces moisture retention; prevents medication from evaporating.

Nursing Alert: Prolonged use of occlusive dressings may cause skin atrophy, striae, telangiectasia, folliculitis, nonhealing ulceration, erythema or systemic absorption of corticosteroids. Dressings should be removed for 8 out of 24 hours, to prevent some of these complications.

Other Dressings

1 Fingers and toes—tubular gauze or, when required, bigger gauze or cotton dressings held in place with tubular gauze (Tubinette, Tubegauze).
2 Hands—disposable polyethylene gloves, sealed at wrists; cotton gloves.
3 Feet—cotton socks or disposable plastic bags; tubular gauze socks.
4 Extremities (arms and legs)—cotton cloth covered with tubular material.
5 Groin, perineum—disposable nappies; cotton cloth folded in nappy fashion; napkin, tubular gauze pants.
6 Axillae—cotton cloth taped in place or held by cotton bandage or tubular gauze.
7 Trunk—cotton or light flannel pyjamas or tubular gauze suit.
8 Scalp—turban or plastic shower cap or tubular gauze cap.
9 Whole body—a suit is made of the various sizes of tubular gauze.

THE PATIENT WITH AN ABNORMAL SKIN CONDITION (DERMATOSIS)

Objectives of Treatment and Nursing Management

To Control Itching and Relieve Pain

1 Examine area of involvement.
  a. Attempt to discover the cause of discomfort.
  b. Record observations in detail, using descriptive terminology.
2 Encourage rest and immobility to reduce stimuli of pain and itching and to raise the threshold of discomfort.
3 Advise patient to employ measures that produce vasoconstriction.
  a. Maintain cool environment.
  b. Reduce excess clothing or bedding.
  c. Provide tepid, cooling baths.
  d. Apply cool wet dressings.
4 Treat dryness (xerosis) with lubricating creams or lotions applied after bathing and before drying to enhance hydration.
5 Apply prescribed lotions or ointments.
6 Supply analgesic and antipruritic medications as prescribed.
7 Administer tranquillizing agents or sedative drugs, as necessary.
8 Instruct patient to refrain from self-medication with salves or lotions that are commercially advertised.
9 Assist the anxious patient to improve his insight and to identify and cope with his problems.

To Treat an Inflammatory Lesion

1 Apply continuous or intermittent wet dressings to reduce intensity of inflammation.
2 Remove crusts and scales before applying topical medications.
3 Use topical applications containing corticosteroid drugs, as prescribed.
  a. Rub topical medicaments well into skin to enhance penetration.
  b. Observe lesion periodically for changes in response to therapy.

To Control Oozing and Prevent Crust Formation

1 Provide tub baths and wet dressings to loosen exudates and scales.

2 Remove medications with mineral oil before re-applying.
3 Use mildly astringent solutions to precipitate proteins and decrease oozing.
4 Supply a high protein diet if oozing is voluminous and serum loss substantial.
5 Administer antibiotics by topical application or by mouth, as prescribed.

To Avoid Damage to Skin

1 To protect healthy skin from maceration when applying wet dressings.
2 Remove moisture from skin by blotting gently and avoiding friction.
3 Guard carefully against risk of thermal trauma from excessively hot wet dressings.
4 Advise patient to use sun-screening agents to prevent actinic damage (chemical changes from ultraviolet light).

To Ensure Efficacy of Topical Applications

1 Use occlusive dressings, as prescribed, to retain medication in constant contact with affected skin.
2 Elicit the patient's co-operation by having him perform his own skin treatments.
3 Instruct patient clearly and in detail to ensure that treatments are carried out as prescribed.

SEBORRHOEIC DERMATOSES

Dermatoses refers to abnormal skin conditions.
  Seborrhoea is excessive production of sebum (secretion of sebaceous glands) in those areas where glands are normally found in large numbers (face, scalp, scrotum).
  Seborrhoeic dermatitis is a chronic inflammatory disease of the skin with a predilection for areas that are well supplied with sebaceous glands or that lie between folds of skin where the bacterial count is high.

Clinical Features

1 Characteristic lesion (remarkably varied).
  a. Dry, moist or greasy scales.
  b. Crusted pinkish-yellow or yellowish patches of varying shapes and sizes.
  c. Possible erythema (redness), fissuring (cracking) and secondary infection.
  d. Dry, flaky desquamation on scalp with profuse amount of fine, powdery scales (dandruff).
2 Sites:
     Scalp (dandruff), eyebrows, eyelids, nasolabial crease, lips, ears, axillae, under breast, groin, gluteal crease.
3 Seborrhoeic dermatitis is associated with genetic predisposition; hormones, nutrition, infection and emotional stress influence its course.
4 There is a tendency to lifelong recurrences lasting for weeks, months or years.

Treatment

Objective

To control the disorder (no known cure at this time) and allow the skin to repair itself.

1   Advise patient to remove external irritants and avoid excess heat and perspiration—rubbing and scratching will prolong the disorder.
2   Suggest local remedies.
   a. *For scalp*—to control dandruff.
     (1) Give the hair an initial cleansing shampoo to remove accumulated scale.
     (2) Use shampoo with zinc pyrithione suspension (Head and Shoulders or ZP11); leave shampoo on scalp 10 min; rinse thoroughly.
     (3) Shampoos containing tar are also effective, especially in controlling itching.
     (4) Shampoo daily or once or twice weekly, depending on condition of the scalp.

     CAUTION: Observe precautions on container.

   b. Seborrhoeic dermatitis of the body and face.
     (1) May respond to a topically applied corticosteroid cream.
     (2) Use with extreme caution on the eyelids, since it can induce glaucoma in predisposed individuals.
     (3) Prolonged use of fluorinated steroids on face can produce an acne-like eruption. Prolonged use in intertriginous areas can produce striae and atrophy. Therefore, plain hydrocortisone is used.
3   Systemic steroids are given on rare occasions for severe and acute seborrhoeic dermatitis.
4   Use antibacterial measures if exudation and crusting occur.
   a. Systemic antibiotic may be required to prevent infection spreading.
   b. Topical antibiotics (cream or lotion) may be applied.
5   Watch for occurrence of secondary moniliasis (yeast infection) that may occur in body creases or folds.
   a. Advise patient to cleanse intertriginous areas carefully; ensure maximum aeration of skin.
   b. Patient with coincidental moniliasis should be investigated for diabetes mellitus.

Health Teaching

1   Encourage patient to eat a well-balanced diet; reduce carbohydrate and fat intake.
2   Advise patient to avoid systemic aggravating factors—overwork, lack of sleep, infection, emotional stress.

ACNE VULGARIS

Acne vulgaris is a chronic disorder of the sebaceous (oil) glands, characterized by the presence of comedones (blackheads), whiteheads, papules, pustules, nodules and cysts. It usually begins at puberty (or earlier) and usually clears by 30 years of age.

Predisposing Factors

1   Genetic predisposition—strong genetic overtones.

2 Hormonal changes of adolescence—sebaceous glands start to enlarge under the influence of adrenal hormones; there is increased seborrhoea.
3 In adults—can occur postpartum or related to use of oral contraceptive drugs.
4 Can be aggravated by anxiety, stress, emotional tension.

Altered Physiology

Increase in amount and thickness of oil secretion → colonization by bacteria producing irritating, oily products → obstruction of sebaceous glands by blackheads (comedones) → disruption of the follicular epithelium, allowing discharge of the follicular contents in the dermis → inflammatory reaction → papules → pustules → nodules → cysts.

Treatment

Objectives

To reduce colonization by *Corynebacterium acnes* bacteria.
To prevent follicular obstruction.
To reduce inflammation and combat secondary infection.
To minimize scarring.
To eliminate factors that may predispose to acne.

The therapeutic regimen is tailored to the individual patient's needs.

Prevent Obstruction of the Oil Glands

1 Wash face gently three times daily with mild soap and water—to remove surface oil.
   Mild abrasive soaps and drying preparations may be used for mild involvement (mainly comedones).
2 Shampoo scalp nightly or twice weekly with medicated shampoo.
3 Use bath brush if back is involved.

Topical Agents for More Severe Involvement

Objective

To clear keratin plugs from follicular ducts.

1 Topical vitamin A acid, tretinoin (Retin-A)—speeds up the cellular turnover, which forces out the comedones; produces a clinical improvement in patients with comedonal acne. Instructions to patient:
   a. Avoid washing the face for at least 2 hours before applying the cream and several hours afterwards.
   b. Apply Retin-A as tolerated (available as gel, cream, liquid). Some individuals tolerate applications daily; others only every 2–3 days.
   c. Warn the patient that the symptoms may worsen during the early weeks of treatment due to action of medication on previously unseen comedones; there is possibility of some erythema and peeling. Improvement may take 4–8 weeks.
   d. Be cautious during first few weeks about exposure to sun (including sun-lamps)—antikeratinizing effect of treninoin makes patient more sensitive to sunburn.

    e. Avoid other irritants, such as strong soaps.

    f. Read the product information brochure.

2 Topical benzoyl peroxide, in gel base (PanOxyl)—exerts an antibacterial effect and is useful for inflammatory acne.

    a. Apply sparingly once daily and adjust to needs of patient thereafter.

    b. May dry the skin and produce some peeling.

3 Topical antibiotic—recent developments have shown some success with the use of Clindamycin 50% in IMS.

    a. Apply sparingly once or twice daily after washing.

    b. Apply to the acne/affected areas as one would an astringent or aftershave lotion.

Systemic Antibiotics

Appear to reduce fatty acids on skin surface; thought to suppress anaerobic lipase-producing bacteria (*C. acnes*) in the skin with reduction of the inflammation-inciting free fatty acids of sebum; useful when patient does not respond to topical therapy.

1 Tetracycline or erythromycin is given and adjusted according to therapeutic response (250–500 mg daily).

2 Long-term, low-dose antibiotic may be given (usually at least 3–6 months).

3 May take several weeks for effect of antibiotics to show.

4 Instruct the patient to take tetracycline at least 1 hour before or 2 hours after mealtime; avoid taking any dairy products (milk, ice cream) within 2 hours before or after taking medication—tetracycline is poorly absorbed with food.

5 Side effects of tetracycline include photosensitivity, nausea, diarrhoea, super-infection and moniliasis. (Vaginitis in women; cutaneous infection in either sex, but more often in men.) Should not be taken during pregnancy.

Hormones

Usually in form of oral contraceptive that combines an oestrogenic and a progestational agent.

1 Oestrogens may be given to antagonize androgens—counteracts production of sebum.

2 Usually reserved for young women with severe cystic acne.

Acne Surgery

1 Comedo extraction (see below).

2 Incision and drainage of cysts—may be required in large, fluctuant, nodular-cystic lesions.

3 Intralesional injection of corticosteroids (triamcinolone acetonide)

    Diluted steroid suspension is injected using a small syringe with a needle to distend the cyst—leads to rapid resolution.

4 Cryosurgery (freezing with liquid nitrogen)—for indurated lesions and cysts.

5 Dermabrasion—surgical planing of the skin.

    NOTE: Carries risk of causing hyperpigmentation.

Health Teaching

1   Keep hands away from face.
2   Do not squeeze pimples or blackheads—squeezing the skin makes acne worse. The majority of blackheads are pushed down into the skin by squeezing. This may cause the follicle to be ruptured.
3   Acne is not caused by dirt and cannot be washed away; it is a chemical imbalance that causes the oil in the skin to form blackheads.
4   Acne is *not* related to sexual activity.
5   Eat a healthful diet; eliminate any food that you feel worsens your acne.
6   Keep hair off the face; wash hair daily if necessary.
7   Avoid friction and trauma.
    a. Do not prop your hands against your face.
    b. Avoid overzealous washing of face, rubbing the face, pressure from tight collars/helmets.
8   Avoid cosmetics (including cleansing creams)—contain chemicals that can aggravate acne.
9   Avoid perspiration around the face.
10 Be able to talk over your problems with an understanding person—acne may become a source of power struggle between teenager and parent.
11 Continue treatment even though your skin clears.

GUIDELINES: Comedo Extraction*

A *comedo* (blackhead) is a mass composed of lipids and keratin that forms a solid plug in a dilated follicular opening (pore).

Underlying Considerations

1   Blackheads are approximately 4 mm deep and cannot be washed away.
2   Comedones are considered end-stage lesions and their removal is only of temporary benefit. However, their removal is necessary in some patients.

Equipment

Light   Alcohol and sponges
Magnifying loupe   Comedo extractor

Procedure

Action	Reason
1 Apply warm compresses to face for a few minutes.	1 Facilitates emptying of the lesions.
2 Wipe off the site with an alcohol sponge.	2 For antisepsis.

---

* This procedure must be performed with skill by a prepared person.

Action	Reason
3 Gently express the contents of the lesion through the hole of the comedo extractor.	3 Overly vigorous attempts to express comedones may result in an increased inflammatory response.
4 Wipe off the site with a fresh alcohol sponge.	

BACTERIAL INFECTIONS

Furuncles

A *furuncle*, or boil, is an acute inflammation arising deep within one or more hair follicles. *Furunculosis* refers to multiple or recurrent lesions. A *stye* is a furuncle that forms on eyelid margin.

Clinical Features

1 Initial occurrence—usually begins around a hair follicle.
2 Sites of predilection—back of neck, axillae, buttocks.
3 Causative factors—irritation, pressure, friction, excessive perspiration, shaving of axillae (in persons with lowered resistance).
4 Symptoms—tenderness, pain and surrounding cellulitis; after furuncle localizes, the centre becomes boggy and fluctuant and a soft yellow or white head appears on the surface.

Nursing Alert: Every person with boils should be checked for diabetes mellitus.

Treatment

1 Protect area from irritation, squeezing and trauma.
2 Apply hot wet compresses—to increase vascularization and hasten resolution.
3 Cleanse surrounding skin with antibacterial soap.
4 Apply antibacterial ointment as prescribed to surrounding skin—to prevent spillage and seeding of the bacteria when furuncle ruptures or is incised.
5 Prepare for surgical drainage when furuncle has become localized and shows fluctuation (wave-like motion upon palpation); furuncle may rupture spontaneously.
6 Systemic antibiotic therapy is given (selected by sensitivity study) if spreading still occurs or if area of involvement poses a risk of complications.

Nursing Alert: Take special precautions with boil on face, since the skin area drains directly into the cranial venous sinuses. There is danger of cavernous sinus thrombosis.

1 Place patient with boils on nose, lip, groin, perineal or perianal region on bed rest.
2 Course of systemic antibiotic therapy is given—to control spread of infection.

Health Teaching

Instruct the patient as follows:

1 Keep draining lesion covered with a dressing.

2 Wash hands thoroughly after caring for lesion.
3 Wrap soiled dressings in paper and burn.
4 Discard razor blades after each use; keep razor in alcohol between shaves.
5 Bathe with bacteriostatic soap.

Carbuncles

A *carbuncle* is an abscess of the skin and subcutaneous tissues—an extension of a furuncle invading multiple follicles; usually caused by staphylococcal infection.

Clinical Features

1 Seen most frequently within the thick, fibrous, inelastic skin of the back of the neck and upper back.
2 More apt to occur in older and debilitated persons; especially frequent in diabetics.

Nursing Alert: Every patient with a carbuncle should be suspected of diabetes until it is disproved.

3 Symptoms:
   a. Fever, leucocytosis, extreme pain and prostration.
   b. Bacteraemia is common because the extensive inflammation makes it difficult to completely wall off the infection, so that absorption of toxins takes place; extension of infection to bloodstream may take place.

Treatment

1 Administer antibiotic (based on sensitivity studies)—antibiotic is continued until infective process is controlled.
2 Determine whether there is an underlying disease condition (diabetes, haematologic disease, etc.).
3 Prepare for surgical incision and drainage when definite fluctuance occurs. (Local surgical incision is usually necessary.)
4 Symptomatic treatments (infusions, tepid sponges, etc.) are used for the toxic patient.

Impetigo

Impetigo (impetigo contagiosa) is a superficial infection of the skin caused by streptococci, staphylococci or multiple bacteria.
   Bullous impetigo is a superficial infection of the skin caused by *Staphylococcus aureus* characterized by the formation of bullae from the original vesicles.

Clinical Features

1 Lesion appears as discrete, thin-walled vesicle that ruptures and becomes covered with a loosely adherent, honey-yellow crust.
2 Crusts are easily removed and reveal smooth, red, moist surface on which new crusts soon develop.

3   Areas affected—exposed parts of body (face, hands, neck and extremities).
4   Impetigo is a contagious disease. It is seen in all ages, but is particularly common among undernourished children living in poor hygienic conditions.
5   Sources of infection—children's pets, dirty fingernails, other children, adults, barber shops, beauty parlours, swimming pools.
6   May be secondary to pediculosis capitis, scabies, herpes simplex, insect bites, poison ivy, eczema.

Treatment

1   Give a prescribed systemic antibiotic (benzathine penicillin, erythromycin, oral penicillin). Glomerulonephritis is a complication of impetigo, depending on strain of streptococcus found. However, this therapy has not been proved to prevent nephritis.
2   Give penicillinase-resistant penicillin for staphylococci that may be penicillin-resistant.
3   Wash lesions with bacterial soap or treat with warm, moist compresses to remove the loci of bacterial growth and to give topical medication an opportunity to reach the infected site.
4   Apply a prescribed topical antibiotic cream (neomycin, bacitracin, polymyxin B) after crust removal.
5   Wear gloves while treating patient.

Health Teaching

1   The patient and family should bathe at least once daily with bacteriostatic soap as recommended.
2   The child with impetigo should be observed for at least 7 weeks for signs of acute glomerulonephritis.
3   Keep infected child away from other children.
4   Dispose of tissues and materials that come in contact with lesions.
5   Encourage good hygienic practices to prevent spread of disease from one skin area to another and from one person to another.

FUNGAL INFECTIONS

Fungi are plantlike organisms that feed on organic matter; they are responsible for a variety of common skin infections.

Tinea Pedis (Athlete's Foot) or Ringworm of the Feet

Tinea pedis (athlete's foot) is a superficial fungal infection which may manifest itself as an acute, inflammatory, vesicular process or as a chronic rash involving the soles of the feet and the interdigital web spaces.

Clinical Features

1   Tinea pedis is the most common fungal infection.

2 Causes intense itching and burning.
3 Lymphangitis and cellulitis may occur when bacterial superinfection is present.

Diagnosis

1 Direct examination of scrapings (skin, nails, hair).
2 Isolation of the organism in culture.

Treatment

1 Use soaks (potassium permanganate, Burow's solution, saline) to remove scales, crusts, debris and residual medications; also for mild antiseptic effect.
2 Apply fungistatic creams or lotions as prescribed such as tolnaftate (Tinactin), miconazole (Daktarin) or clotrimazole (Canesten) to involved skin.
3 Continue with topical therapy for several weeks—there is a high rate of recurrence.
4 Systemic antifungal agent (griseofulvin) (500 mg daily) is given if indicated.

Preventive Measures and Health Teaching

Instruct the patient to keep feet dry—moisture encourages the growth of fungi.

1 Dry carefully between the toes.
2 Alternate shoes—to permit adequate drying of shoes between wearings.
3 Change socks frequently.
4 Wear light cotton socks or stockings with cotton feet—synthetic material does not absorb perspiration as well as cotton.
5 Wear perforated shoes if feet perspire excessively—to permit aeration of feet.
6 Foot powder can be applied twice daily—to keep feet dry.
7 Use clogs in community pools, showers, etc.
8 Use small pieces of cotton between toes at night—to absorb moisture.

Tinea Capitis (Ringworm of the Scalp)

Tinea capitis (ringworm of the scalp) is a fungal disease of the scalp.

Clinical Features

1 Lesions appear as round, grey, scaly bald patches on the scalp.
2 Sometimes boggy swelling (kerion) occurs in an area of involvement; this may be followed by scarring.
3 Tinea capitis is contagious; usually occurs in prepubertal children.

Treatment and Health Teaching

1 Griseofulvin, a fungistatic and fungicidal antibiotic, is given.
   Take medication with or just after a meal. The presence of fat aids in absorption of the drug.
2 Instruct the patient as follows:
   a. Shampoo scalp two or three times weekly.

b. Apply topical antifungal preparation as directed—to reduce dissemination of organisms.

c. Each person should have his own comb and brush. Avoid exchanging headgear.

d. All infected members of family and all household pets should be treated.

Tinea Corporis or Tinea Circinata

Tinea corporis or tinea circinata is ringworm of the body.

Clinical Features

1 Appearance—rings of vesicles with central clearing; appear in clusters.
2 Lesions usually appear on exposed areas of body; may extend to scalp, hair or nails.
3 An infected pet is a common source of infection.
4 Ringworm of the body causes intense itching.

Treatment

1 Apply topical antifungal medication as prescribed to small areas (Tinaderm, Daktarin, Canesten).
2 Griseofulvin may be used in very extensive cases. Side effects include photosensitivity, skin rashes, headache, nausea, etc.

Health Teaching

Instruct the patient as follows:

1 Wear clean cotton clothing next to the skin.
2 Use a clean towel daily; dry thoroughly all areas and skin folds that retain moisture.

PARASITIC SKIN DISEASES

Three varieties of lice infest man; their itching bites are the cause of many skin problems. Lice bite the skin to obtain blood, which they feed on. They leave their eggs and excrement on the skin and are passed from person to person.

Pediculosis Capitis

Pediculosis capitis is an infestation of the scalp by the head louse, *Pediculus humanus* var. *capitis* (Fig. 8.2a).

Clinical Features

1 Appearance—minute white nits (eggs) (Fig. 8.2b) attached to hair shaft in series: usually on scalp and hair at back of head and behind ears.
2 Most often found in children and persons wearing long hair.

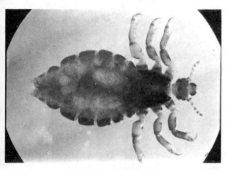

A. Head louse

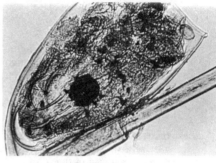

B. Nit

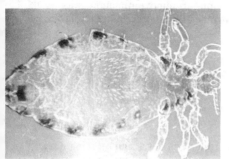

C. Body louse

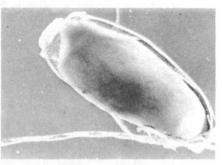

D. Body louse ova

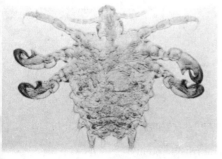

E. Crab louse, male

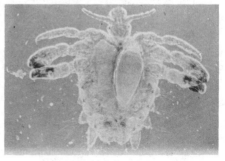

F. Crab louse, female

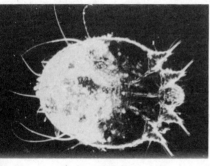

G. Scabies

Figure 8.2. Parasites causing skin diseases. (Courtesy Reed and Carnrick Research Institute.) a. Head louse. b. Nit. c. Body louse. d. Body louse ova. e. Crab louse, male. f. Crab louse, female. g. Scabies.

3 The bite of the insect causes intense itching, and the resulting scratching may lead to complications such as impetigo, furuncles and enlarged cervical lymph nodes.
4 May be transmitted by direct physical contact or contact with infested combs, brushes, wigs, hats and bedding.

Treatment

1 Instruct the patient as follows:
   a. Use a shampoo containing gamma benzene hexachloride (Lorexane, Quellada) or malathion 0.5% lotion (Prioderm).
   b. Shampoo the scalp at least 4 min with this preparation; rinse thoroughly.
   c. Comb hair with a fine-tooth metal comb—to remove remaining nits.
   d. Disinfect comb and brushes with Lorexane or Prioderm shampoo; sterilize all washable fomites.
   e. Repeat in 24 hours if necessary.
2 Treat all family members and close contacts.
3 Treat complications—severe pruritus, pyoderma (pus-forming infection of the skin), and dermatitis—with antipruritics, systemic antibiotics and topical corticosteroids.

Health Teaching

1 Head lice infestation may happen to anyone; it is not a sign of being dirty.
2 Treatment should be started immediately, since the condition spreads rapidly.
3 Control of school epidemics may be helped by having all of the students shampoo their hair on the same night.

Pediculosis Corporis

Pediculosis corporis is an infestation of the body by the body louse, *P. humanus* var. *corporis* (Fig. 8.2c).

Clinical Features

1 The body louse lives chiefly in the seams of undergarments and other clothing, to which it clings.
2 Its bite causes characteristic minute haemorrhagic points.
   a. Widespread excoriations may appear on the back and shoulders.
   b. May produce secondary lesions—hyperaemia, parallel linear scratches and hyperpigmentation in persistent cases.
3 Areas of skin involved are those that come in closest contact with the undergarments (neck, trunk, thighs).
4 The lice may be seen in the seams of clothing. They move to the skin for blood feedings and then return to the clothing.

Treatment

1 Instruct the patient as follows:
   a. Bathe with soap and water.

b. Apply gamma benzene hexachloride (Lorexane, Quellada) cream or lotion to trunk and extremities—leave medication on skin 24 hours.
c. Eliminate parasites and nits from clothing, bedding and sleeping bags. Launder, dry clean, press with hot iron.
2 Examine and treat all family members and contacts.
3 Treat pruritus, secondary bacterial infections and dermatitis.

Nursing Alert: Body lice are vectors for rickettsial disease, epidemic typhus, relapsing fever, trench fever. The causative organism may be in the gastrointestinal tract of the insect and excreted on the skin surface.

Pediculosis Pubis

Pediculosis pubis is an infestation by *Phthirus pubis* (crab louse) (Fig. 8.2e and f); it is chiefly transmitted by sexual contact and is generally localized to the genital region.

Clinical Manifestations

1 Chief symptom is itching.
2 Reddish brown 'dust' (formed from the excretion of the insects) may be found on the underclothing.
3 Lice may infest hairs of chest, axillary hair, beard and eyelashes.
4 Grey-blue macules (1–3 cm in diameter) may be seen on the trunk, thighs and axillae as a result of the action of the insects' saliva on bilirubin—converts it to biliverdin.

Treatment

1 Instruct the patient as follows:
   a. Bathe with soap and water.
   b. Apply gamma benzene hexachloride (Lorexane, Quellada) cream or lotion or malathion 0.5% (Prioderm) to areas of involvement.
      (1) Leave on for 24 hours.
      (2) Treat again in 4–7 days for heavy infestations.
      (3) Do not apply Lorexane or Quellada to eyebrows.
         (a) Remove nits manually from eyebrows or eyelashes with cotton-tipped applicator or toothpick.
         (b) Apply yellow oxide of mercury or physostigmine ophthalmic ointment before removing nits.
   c. Machine wash all clothing and bedding in a hot wash.
2 Treat all sexual contacts and family members.
3 Screen patient for coexisting venereal disease.
4 Treat secondary bacterial infection, itching and dermatitis.

Scabies

Scabies is an infestation of the skin by *Sarcoptes scabiei* (itch mite) (Fig. 8.2g). Scabies is transmitted by close personal contact.

Clinical Features

1   *Primary lesion.*
   a. Adult female burrows into superficial layer of skin after fertilization has occurred on skin surface; burrows are short, wavy, brownish or blackish thread-like lesions.
   b. She extends the burrow, laying 2–3 eggs daily for up to 2 months, and then dies; larvae hatch in 2–3 days and migrate to skin surface where they reach maturity in 2–3 weeks.
   c. Male mites die shortly after mating.
2   Ask patient where itch is most severe at the time you are examining him; look for burrows with a magnifying glass (may or may not see them).
3   Sites—between fingers, on flexor surfaces of wrists and palms, around nipples, in axillary folds, under pendulous breasts, in or near groin or gluteal fold, penis, scrotum.
4   Secondary lesions include vesicles, papules, pustules, excoriations and crusts; bacterial superinfection or eczematization may complicate the picture.
5   Symptoms—intense itching, more pronounced at night; usually occurs 1 month after initial infection.
6   The disease may be found in poor persons living under substandard hygienic conditions, but is also found in very clean individuals.
   a. Promoted by close physical contact.
   b. However, infestations are not dependent on sexual activity, since the mites frequently involve the fingers—hand contact may produce infection.
   c. Infestations with mites may also result from contact with dogs, cats and small animals.

Treatment and Health Teaching.

Instruct patient as follows:

1   Take a hot, soapy bath or shower—to remove scaling debris from the crusts.
2   Apply a scabicide such as gamma benzene hexachloride (Quellada lotion) or crotamiton (Eurax cream and lotion) at bedtime.
   a. Apply emulsion all over the body including between fingers and toes and the soles of the feet. Leave out no part except the head and face.
   b. Allow time for the emulsion to dry and repeat the application at once. When this has dried, go to bed.
   c. Next morning repeat the application—the whole body except the face and head. No bath.
   d. In the evening take a bath to remove the emulsion.
   e. Put on freshly laundered or dry cleaned clothes and change all bed linen, underclothes and night clothes.
   f. A bland ointment may be applied to the skin after completion of treatment.
   g. Treatment should only be repeated on doctor's instructions and not within 3 weeks.
   h. Benzylbenzoate, malathion (Prioderm) and carbaryl are also used.
3   All family members and close contacts should be treated simultaneously whether they are infected or not to eliminate the mites.

4   All used linen must be washed. The cuffs of all coats worn during the previous 3 weeks must be ironed. Gloves must be washed or laid aside for 3 weeks. Blankets and other bed linen need not be treated provided that sheets are used.
5   Advise patient that he may be uncomfortable for some weeks—the treatment solution is irritating to the skin and pruritus may remain for a time. Calamine cream will help to relieve itching.

Bedbug Infestation

Two species of bedbugs, *Cimex lectularius* and *C. hemipterus* invade human habitations. These are nocturnal blood-sucking insects.

Clinical Features

1   Appearance—bites tend to be grouped in a straight line and consist of haemorrhagic spots associated with papular or wheal-like lesions; there may be a tiny red point marking the original site of the bite.
2   Sites—buttocks, back and extremities are most frequently bitten—patient experiences itching and burning; urticaria (hives) may accompany the lesions.
3   Secondary infection and pyoderma may occur.

Health Teaching

1   Direct patient to apply lotions containing menthol and phenol to local areas of bites. Antihistamines may be prescribed for intense itching (e.g. Piriton).
2   Advise patient to eliminate insect by vacuum cleaning and then spraying in crevices of furniture, walls, floors, mattresses and beds.

HERPES ZOSTER

Herpes zoster (shingles) is an inflammatory condition in which the virus produces a painful vesicular eruption along the distribution of the nerves from one or more posterior ganglia.

Aetiology

Virus appears to be identical with the causative agent of varicella (chickenpox); herpes zoster may be a reactivation of the latent varicella virus and reflects a lowered immunity.

Clinical Manifestations

1   Malaise and gastrointestinal disturbances may precede the eruption.
2   Vesicles appear within 12–24 hours.
   a. Characteristic patches of grouped vesicles on erythematous and oedematous skin.
   b. Early vesicles contain serum—they appear purulent and rupture, forming crusts.
   c. Some vesicles dry up without scarring.

3   Eruption appears posteriorly and progresses to the anterior and peripheral distribution of the nerves from one or more posterior ganglia.
4   Eruption usually accompanied or preceded by itching, tenderness and pain, which may radiate over entire region supplied by the nerves.
     Inflammation is usually unilateral, involving the thoracic, cervical or cranial nerves in a band-like configuration.
5   Clinical course varies from 1–3 weeks; healing time varies between 7–26 days.
6   The disease is considered infectious only for the first 2–3 days and only to persons with immunosuppression or to those who have not previously had varicella.
7   There is a greater tendency towards complications and sequelae in the older patient.

Treatment

Objectives

To make the patient comfortable.
To reduce or avoid complications (infection, paralysis, scarring, postherpetic neuralgia).

1   Control the pain—controlling the pain may reduce incidence of postherpetic neuralgia.
    a. Give analgesics— aspirin, codeine, dextropropoxyphene, propoxyphene hydrochloride (Distalgesic)—to control pain and promote rest.
    b. Give sedatives—to control nervousness associated with neuralgia and itching.
    c. Give antihistamines—to control itching.
2   The following treatment regimen may be given.
    a. Apply local treatment to skin lesions.
       (1) Apply cool wet dressings to pruritic lesions.
       (2) Apply topical idoxuridine (5%) in dimethyl sulphoxide (Herpid) to individual lesions.
    b. Treat secondary bacterial infection of skin lesions—culture and sensitivity studies will indicate appropriate antibiotic.
    c. Systemic corticosteroids may be given to the elderly to prevent postherpetic neuralgia—usually initial high dose gradually tailed off over 2–5 weeks.
    d. Support the patient undergoing diagnostic studies to investigate the possibility of underlying disease.

Nursing Alert: Herpes zoster may indicate the presence of serious internal disease, especially in persons past middle age (Hodgkin's disease, leukaemia, malignancy).

3   Watch for complications.
    a. Persistent pain (neuralgia) of affected nerve following healing, especially in the elderly.
    b. Ophthalmic herpes zoster—pain in the orbit radiating up over the forehead; constant, boring pain.
       (1) Pain particularly severe in elderly following ophthalmic herpes zoster.
       (2) Patients with ophthalmic herpes zoster should be examined by ophthalmologist to avoid serious ocular complications.
    c. Facial nerve paralysis.
    d. Encephalitis.

4   Treatment of severe postherpetic pain.
    Procaine or alcohol injection to nerve ganglia.

CONTACT DERMATITIS

Contact dermatitis (dermatitis venenata) is a common inflammatory, often eczema-tous, condition caused by a skin reaction due to contact with a variety of irritating or allergenic materials. There is damage to the epidermis by repeated physical and chemical insults.

1   *Primary irritant contact dermatitis* is a nonallergic reaction caused by exposure to an irritating substance.
2   *Allergic contact dermatitis* results from exposure of sensitized individuals to contact allergens.

Causes

1   Plants.
2   Cosmetics.
3   Soaps, detergents and scouring compounds.
4   Industrial chemicals.
5   Hair dye, nickel, rubber, chemicals.

Predisposing Factors

1   Extremes of heat and cold.
2   Frequent immersion in soap and water.
3   Pre-existing skin disease.

Clinical Manifestations

1   Skin eruptions begin at point of contact with causative agent.
2   Itching, burning, erythema, vesiculation and eczema.
3   Weeping, crusting, drying, fissuring and peeling.
4   Thickening of skin and pigmentation changes, if repeated reactions occur or if there is continual scratching by patient.
5   Secondary bacterial invasion may occur—prevention of normal sweating pro-duces vesicles, itching and inflammation.

Treatment

Objective

To protect and rest the involved skin.

1   Inspect the entire body for a distribution pattern—helps differentiate between allergic contact dermatitis and the irritant type.
2   Obtain a detailed history.
3   Instruct the patient as follows:
    a. Identify and remove the offending irritant.
        (1) Avoid the use of soap until healing occurs.

    (2) Avoid exposing skin to the causative agent after recovery.

    (3) Wear lined rubber gloves while working, if hands are involved.

b. *Topical treatment.*

    (1) Use bland, unmedicated lotion for small patches of erythema.

    (2) Use cool, wet dressings for small areas of acute, vesicular dermatitis—for soothing and to help stop oozing.

    (3) Cleanse away softened crusts and other debris.

    (4) Apply a thin layer of cream or ointment containing one of the steroids, as directed—usually not as beneficial when blisters are present, although some authorities feel it is helpful in these instances if used more frequently; i.e., at least five times daily.

    (5) Use medicated baths at room temperature (p. 311) for larger areas of dermatosis.

4   Give sedatives and antihistamines if necessary to relieve itching and burning.

5   Give systemic antibiotics if secondary bacterial infection is present—purulent exudate and systemic symptoms (fever, lymphadenopathy, etc.).

6   Administer short course of systemic steroids if a more widespread and disabling condition is involved—can shorten the course of a severe disease; allays inflammation.

7   See also the patient with a dermatosis, p. 314.

Health Teaching

Instruct the patient as follows:

1   Avoid heat, soap, rubbing—all these are external irritants.

2   Avoid topical medications except when specifically prescribed.

3   Wash thoroughly immediately after exposure to antigens.

4   Do not touch uninvolved body areas with involved areas.

Patch Testing

Patch Testing is the method used for diagnosis of allergic contact dermatitis.

Equipment

Patch testing strips, A1-Test or Finn chambers
Adhesive tape if A1-Test is used
Substances to be applied (usually a standard battery as well as substances indicated by patient's history)
Felt-tip marker

Method

1   Strips are prepared with substances to be tested.

2   Patient is informed of procedure.

3   The prepared strips are fixed to normal skin—usually on the back.

4   Patches are marked with a felt-tip marker to indicate position and order of test substances.

5   Patches are removed after 48 hours and results of any reaction recorded.

6 Felt-tip marks are renewed.
7 Reactions are recorded again after a further 48 hours.
8 Patients who have positive reactions are advised on how to avoid future contact with the substances responsible.

NONINFECTIOUS INFLAMMATORY DERMATOSES

Eczema

Eczema is one of the most common abnormal skin conditions. (The terms eczema and dermatitis are often used synonomously.)

Clinical Features

1 Characteristics:
   a. Epidermis becomes erythematous and thickened followed by a vesicular eruption.
   b. When the vesicles rupture, the serous exudate dries and forms a crust.
   c. Skin becomes scaly and may be thickened in patches of varying shapes and sizes.
   d. Itching can be severe, causing the patient to scratch and lichenification can develop.
2 Types:
   a. Atopic eczema.
      (1) Chronic fluctuating disease.
      (2) May occur at any age.
      (3) Genetically determined disorder; there may be a family history of eczema, asthma or hay fever.
      (4) Distribution of the lesions may vary considerably.
      (5) Common symptom is itching.
   Forms:
      (1) Infantile eczema.
      (2) Atopic eczema of childhood.
      (3) Adolescent and adult atopic eczema.
         (a) May follow childhood eczema or may occur as the first manifestation of atopic eczema.
         (b) Affects the limbs, flexures, face and may spread to the neck and trunk.
         (c) The total skin surface may be affected in severe cases.
   b. Nummular eczema.
      (1) Appears as well-defined round or oval coin-like patches of eczema.
      (2) Common sites are the calves, shins, forearms, backs of fingers and hands.
      (3) Itching is usually severe, as in atopic eczema.
   c. Pompholyx (eczema of thick skin, e.g., of the hands and feet).
      (1) Occurs on the sides and palms of the fingers and hands and the sides and soles of the toes and feet.
      (2) The thick horny layer at these sites inhibits rupture of vesicles—thus the vesicles may remain for days looking like whitish grains in the skin.
      (3) Seborrhoeic eczema (seborrhoeic dermatitis) (see p. 315).
      (4) Contact dermatitis (see p. 331).

Treatment

1 Advise patient to remove any known irritants. Patch test any suspect patient to confirm any contact dermatitis.
2 Topical therapy to be used regularly.
   a. Apply moisturizing cream (e.g., Boots E45) liberally and frequently during day and after washing to all dry or inflammed areas.
   b. Use oilatum emollient in bath.
   c. Emulsifying ointment should be used instead of soap.
   d. Moisturizer and emulsifying ointment should be used even after eczema has cleared to help prevent skin becoming dry and a recurrence of the eczema.
3 *Steroid therapy*
   a. Topical corticosteroids (Hydrocortisone, Betnovate, Dermovate, Haelan, Synalar) should be used only when prescribed and only on the affected areas. Nurse must wear gloves to apply topical steroids.
   b. More potent preparations (Betnovate, Dermovate) should never be used on the face.
   c. Systemic corticosteroid therapy (Prednisone) may be used in acute exacerbations.
4 *Antibiotic therapy* is given for secondary infection.
   a. Systemic antibiotics are given as prescribed.
   b. Topical antibiotics may be prescribed.
5 *Baths* (see p. 311).
   a. Antiseptic baths are given for infected eczema.
   b. Bath oils are used for emollient and antipruritic effect.
6 *Open wet dressings* are applied as prescribed (see p. 310).
7 *Systemic therapy*.
   a. Antihistamines (Piriton) are given as prescribed to relieve itching.
   b. Sedatives may be prescribed to help patient sleep and prevent scratching.

Health Teaching

1 Advise patient on importance of continuing moisturizing therapy.
2 Advise patient to avoid aggravating factors.
3 Help patients with chronic condition in planning their own management.
4 Reassure and support patient and family in coping with long-term problems.
5 Advise patient of the existence of the National Eczema Society, Tavistock House North, Tavistock Square, London WC1.

Psoriasis

Psoriasis is a chronic, proliferative, inflammatory dermatosis of unknown aetiology appearing as an eruption of dry, red patches of all sizes, sharply defined against the normal skin and covered with heavy, dry, silvery scales (Fig. 8.3). In time the patches can coalesce, forming extensive irregularly shaped patches.

Clinical Features

1 In psoriasis, the rate of production of the epidermis of the skin is about nine times

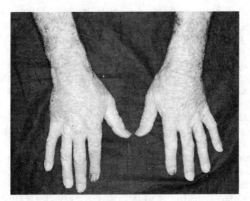

Figure 8.3.   Psoriasis of the hands. (Courtesy of Armed Forces Institute of Pathology.)

faster than normal; this abnormal process does not allow for formation of normal protective layers of skin.

2 There appears to be a hereditary biochemical defect that causes an overproduction of keratin; there is also thought to be a hormonal influence.

3 Onset is usually before the age of 20, but all age groups are affected.

4 Psoriasis may be coupled with polyarthritis and cause crippling disability.

5 *Sites* (bilateral symmetry):

  a. Bony prominences (knees, elbows, sacrum), scalp, external ears, genitalia, perianal area, nails and dorsa of hands.

  b. Psoriasis of the ears—scaling and dryness.

  c. Psoriasis of palms and soles—vesicular and pustular pruritic lesions.

  d. Psoriasis of nails—thickening, discoloration, crumbling beneath free edges; pitting of nails.

  e. Psoriasis between skin folds—smooth, shiny red lesions, easily fissured.

6 The disease may range from a benign cosmetic source of annoyance to a physically disabling and disfiguring affliction.

Treatment and Nursing Management

Objective

To reduce scaling and itching; the goal is control since no cure is known.

1 Instruct patient to take daily tub bath—to help soak off scales.

  a. Gently remove excess scales with a soft brush while bathing.

  b. Apply prescribed ointment after removal of scales.

2 Topical therapy (includes corticosteroids, coal tar, dithranol, salicylic acid, etc.).

  a. Corticosteroids.

    (1) Apply wet dressings to irritated areas of psoriasis.

    (2) Apply corticosteroid preparations—betamethasone (Betnovate) to skin.

    (3) Hold dressings in place with occlusive film (traps heat and moisture, softens scaly plaques and enhances transepidermal penetration).

      (a) Occlusive dressings over the entire body may be held in place with polythene pyjama suit or a large plastic bag with holes cut out for the head and arms; another bag may be used for the legs; extremities (arms) may be wrapped in plastic film. Total body occlusion is rarely used and should only be done under strict medical supervision.

Caution the patient not to smoke while wrapped in these dressings.

(b) In patients being treated at home, hands can be wrapped in gloves, the feet in plastic bags and the hair covered by a shower cap.

b. Dithranol preparations (a distillate of crude coal tar).

(1) Useful for especially thick and resistant psoriatic plaques.

(2) Instruct patient to apply dithranol medication to affected areas only; do not apply to normal skin, face or flexures.

(3) Dithranol should always be applied with a spatula—*never* with the hands. Wash hands thoroughly after application—medication can produce a chemical conjunctivitis.

c. Coal tar preparations (ointments/baths)—retard and inhibit the rapid growth of psoriatic tissue.

(1) Coal tar is applied for a period of time; may then be removed; this treatment can be followed by carefully graded doses of ultraviolet radiation, after performing ultraviolet test.

(2) Begin ultraviolet radiation with low dose (10 s) and build up dosage time gradually.

(3) Ultraviolet may produce mild redness and slight desquamation.

3   Systemic medications

a. Methotrexate—folic acid antagonist may be used in patients with extensive psoriasis that is resistant to all other forms of treatment. It is taken in a small weekly dose.

(1) Liver biopsy may be done before initiation of treatment.

(2) Patient should avoid alcohol intake while on methotrexate—increases possibility of liver damage.

(3) Laboratory studies should be conducted to ensure adequate function of hepatic, haematopoietic and renal systems; these parameters should be monitored before the course of drug treatment is started.

(4) Methotrexate is a potent abortive or teratogenic agent and is used with extreme caution in women of childbearing age.

b. Hydroxyurea—inhibits cell replication by affecting DNA synthesis.

4   Photochemotherapy (PUVA).

a. Involves interaction of light and drug.

b. Oral psoralens (8-methoxypsoralen) is followed by long wave ultraviolet light (UVA) exposure.

c. The drug binds the DNA and appears to halt its replication in the presence of ultraviolet radiation therapy.

d. Following PUVA, patient must wear dark glasses for 10–12 hours, as PUVA produces photosensitization.

Health Teaching

1   The patient must be taught to live with psoriasis; it is a chronic disease often requiring continuous therapy.

2   Advise the patient that treatment is time-consuming and expensive.

3   If possible, the patient should try to schedule exposure to sunlight on a regular basis. Avoid sunburn, since it can cause a generalized inflammation.
4   Advise patient of the Psoriasis Association, 7 Milton Street, Northampton NN2 7JG

Exfoliative Dermatitis (Generalized Erythroderma)

Exfoliative dermatitis is a serious condition characterized by progressive inflammation in which erythema and scaling often occur in a more or less generalized distribution. It may be associated with chills, fever, prostration, severe toxicity and an itchy scaling of the skin.

Clinical Features

Systemic Effects

Exfoliative dermatitis has a marked effect on the entire body.

1   There is a profound loss of stratum corneum (outermost layer of the skin)—causes capillary leakage, hypoproteinaemia and negative nitrogen balance.
2   Iron loss from the skin produces anaemia.

Appearance

1   Starts acutely as either a patchy or generalized erythematous eruption (Fig. 8.4) accompanied by fever, malaise and occasionally gastrointestinal symptoms.
2   The skin colour changes from pink to dark red; then after a week the characteristic exfoliation (scaling) begins, usually in the form of thin flakes which leave the underlying skin smooth and red, new scales forming as the older ones exfoliate (cast off).
3   Hair loss and nail shedding may accompany the disorder.

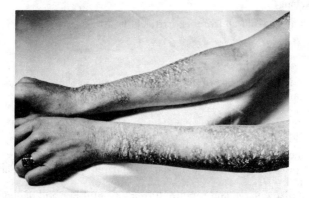

Figure 8.4.   Exfoliative dermatitis of arms. (Courtesy of Armed Forces Institute of Pathology.)

Multiplicity of Causes

1   May arise as a primary condition.
2   May follow a previous skin condition (eczema, psoriasis) that had become generalized.
3   May appear as a part of the lymphoma group of diseases and may precede the appearance of lymphoma or leukaemia.
4   Also appears as a severe reaction to a wide number of drugs, including penicillin, phenylbutazone and phenytoin (Epanutin).

Treatment and Nursing Management

Objectives

To maintain fluid and electrolyte balance.
To prevent intercurrent or cutaneous infection.

1   Hospitalize the patient and place him on bed rest.
    Maintain comfortable room temperature—patient does not have normal thermoregulatory control owing to temperature fluctuations from vasodilation and evaporative water loss.
2   Maintain fluid and electrolyte balance—considerable water and protein loss from skin surface.
3   Give systemic corticosteroids as prescribed—for anti-inflammatory action; may be a life-saving procedure.
4   Apply compresses and soothing baths—to treat acute extensive dermatitis.
5   Maintain nursing surveillance for intercurrent or cutaneous infection; the erythematous, moist skin is receptive to infection and becomes colonized with pathogenic organisms which produce more inflammation.
    Antibiotics are given if infection is present; selected by culture and sensitivity.
6   Watch for symptoms of heart failure—hyperaemia and increased cutaneous blood flow can produce a cardiac failure of high-output origin.

Health Teaching

Advise patient to avoid all irritants, particularly drugs.

Pemphigus

Pemphigus is a serious disease of the skin characterized by the appearance of blisters (bullae) of various sizes on apparently normal skin and mucous membranes (Fig. 8.5).

Clinical Features

1   Appearance:
    a. Asymptomatic large bullae appear on apparently normal skin and mucous membranes.
    b. The bullae enlarge and rupture, forming painful raw and denuded areas.
    c. Bullae and erosions occur on the skin, mouth and vagina; large areas of skin may be denuded.

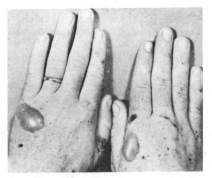

Figure 8.5. Pemphigus; bullous dermatitis of hand (vesicles). (Courtesy of Armed Forces Institute of Pathology.)

d. Bacterial superinfection is common.

2 Available evidence indicates that pemphigus is an autoimmune disease.

Treatment and Nursing Management

Objectives

To bring the disease under control as rapidly as possible.
To prevent loss of serum and development of secondary infection.
To promote re-epithelialization of skin.

1 Administer corticosteroids (prednisone) in large doses, as prescribed—to control the disease.
   a. High dosage level is maintained until remission is apparent.
   b. Dosage is reduced to minimum daily maintenance dose as soon as possible.
   c. Give medication with or immediately after a meal; may be accompanied by an antacid as prophylaxis against gastric complications.
2 Take fluid measurements of body weight, blood pressure; test urine for glucose. Record fluid balance (input and output).
3 Give immunosuppressive agents (methotrexate; cyclophosphamide) as prescribed—may be given to help control the disease and reduce the maintenance dose of corticosteroids.
4 Assess patient for evidence of local and systemic infection—bullae are susceptible to infection, and septicaemia may follow.
5 Evaluate for fluid and electrolyte imbalance—extensive denudation of the skin leads to fluid and electrolyte imbalance.
   a. Give soft, high-protein, high-calorie diet—patients with painful oral involvement have difficulty maintaining nutrition.
   b. Administer saline infusions as directed—significant loss of tissue fluids and therefore of sodium chloride occur through the skin.
   c. Encourage patient to maintain adequate fluid intake.
6 Give blood or component therapy (packed red cells, plasma, etc.) as necessary—large amount of protein and blood lost through denuded skin; nursing management is similar to that of patient with an extensive burn. (See p. 362.)

7 Administer cool wet dressings and/or baths—patients with large areas of blistering have a characteristic odour that is lessened when secondary infection is under control.
8 Give meticulous oral hygiene—lesions and painful erosions in the mouth are common.
9 Usually associated with serious underlying medical condition, e.g., systemic lupus erythematosus. Some authorities suggest the cancer may be associated with pemphigus.

ULCERS AND TUMOURS OF THE SKIN

Ulcers of the Skin

Ulceration is a superficial loss of surface tissue due to death of cells.

Causes

Ulcers of the skin usually arise from (1) infection or (2) an interference with the blood supply.

1 Infection as cause of skin ulcers.
   a. Usually develop from an infection with anaerobic streptococci or from combination of infections (haemolytic streptococci and staphylococci).
   b. Tend to progress peripherally—characterized by an overhanging edge.
2 Deficient circulation as cause of skin ulcers.

Tumours of the Skin

Cysts

Epidermal cysts are common, slow-growing, firm, elevated tumours consisting of a mass of eipidermal cells; frequently found on the back.

Sebaceous cysts are rounded tumours of variable size caused by retention of the excretion in the sebaceous follicles; also referred to as *wens*.

Benign Tumours

Verrucae (Warts)

Common, benign skin tumours caused by a virus.

1 Many times warts do not need treatment, since they tend to disappear spontaneously.
2 Treatment:
   a. Freezing with liquid nitrogen—liquid nitrogen has a somewhat destructive action, although it tends to spare the epidermis (Fig. 8.6).
   b. Area may be treated locally with salicylic acid plasters, or paint, formalin 3% or podophyllin. In some cases currettage and electrocautery may be used.

Angiomas (Birthmarks)

Benign vascular tumours involving the skin and subcutaneous tissues.

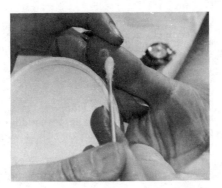

Figure 8.6. Liquid nitrogen is delivered to a wart by a cotton applicator. It should be repeatedly applied until the freezing part extends to 1–2 mm around the tissue. (From Kumar, A A (1975) Liquid nitrogen cryotherapy in the treatment of benign skin lesions, J Fam Pract, 2(3): 222. Courtesy of Adarsh A Kumar, MD.)

1 May occur as flat, violet-red patches (port-wine angiomas) or as raised, bright-red nodular lesions (strawberry angiomas). Strawberry angiomas may involute spontaneously.
2 Port-wine angiomas usually persist indefinitely.

Pigmented Naevi (Moles)

Common skin tumours of various sizes and shapes ranging from yellowish to brown to black.

1 May be flat macular lesions or elevated papules or nodules that occasionally contain hair.
2 Majority of pigmented naevi are harmless; however, in rare cases malignant changes supervene and a melanoma develops at the site of the naevus.
3 Treatment:
  a. Naevi at sites subject to repeated irritation from clothing, etc., should be removed—for comfort.
  b. Naevi that show change in size or colour, or which bleed, should be removed—to determine if malignancy has occurred.
  c. Excised naevi should be examined histologically.

Keloids

Benign overgrowths of fibrous tissue at site of scar or trauma.

1 More prevalent among black race.
2 Usually asymptomatic—may cause disfigurement and cosmetic concern.
3 Treatment—topical corticosteroids (Haelan), intralesional injection with corticosteriods, or radiotherapy.

Cancer of the Skin

Clinical Features

1   Skin cancer has a greater incidence than cancer of any other organ.
2   There is a 95% cure rate due to early diagnosis, the slow progression of most skin cancers and the effective methods of treatment available.

Causes

1   Exposure to sun over a period of time (outdoor workers).
2   Texture of skin and its pigment content—persons with ruddy or light complexions seem to develop skin cancer more frequently than those with coarser or darker skin.
3   Exposure to irradiation (history of x-ray treatment for benign skin lesions).
4   Exposure to certain chemical agents (arsenic, nitrates, tar and pitch, oils and paraffins).
5   Cancer of skin may develop on scars of severe burns 20–40 years later.

Nursing Assessment

Look for:

1   Chronic sunburn.
2   Actinic damage—pigment change, splotches, wrinkling, leathery complexion.

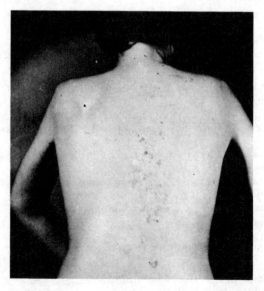

Figure 8.7.   Basal cell carcinoma on skin of back. (Courtesy of Armed Forces Institute of Pathology.)

3   Precancerous lesions (keratosis; leucoplakia).
4   Change in a skin lesion.

Nursing Alert: Any skin lesion that changes in size or colour, bleeds, ulcerates or becomes infected may be skin cancer.

Diagnosis

1   Biopsy.
2   Histological evaluation.

Types of Skin Cancer

Basal Cell Carcinoma or Rodent Ulcer

1   Most common skin cancer; higher incidence in regions where population is subjected to intense and extensive exposure to sun.
2   Lesions are small nodules with a rolled, pearly, translucent border with telangiectasia (dilation of end blood vessels), crusting and occasionally ulceration (Fig. 8.7).
3   These tumours may be pigmented, multiple, superficial or cystic.
    a. Basal cell carcinoma is chiefly caused by prolonged skin exposure to irritants.
    b. Characterized by invasion and erosion of continuous tissues—rarely metastasizes.
    c. Lesions appear most frequently on face, between hairline and upper lip.

Squamous Cell Carcinoma

1   A malignancy that arises on sun-exposed areas of skin and mucous membrane and is considered a truly invasive carcinoma.
2   Appears as an infiltrated, plaque-like or nodular, rapid-growing tumour.
3   May be preceded by leucoplakia (premalignant lesion of mucous membrane), actinic keratoses, scarred or ulcerated lesions.
4   Seen most commonly on lower lip, tongue, head, neck and dorsa of hands.
5   Requires more aggressive approach (wider margin of normal skin included in excision)—greater chance of metastases from squamous cell carcinoma and significantly lower cure rate.

Treatment

1   Method of treatment depends on tumour location; cell type (location and depth); history of previous treatment; and whether or not it is invasive and if metastatic nodes are present.
    Usual modes of treatment are (1) curettage and electrocautery, (2) surgical excision and (3) radiotherapy.
2   *Curettage followed by electrocautery*—usually done on small tumours (less than 1–2 cm).
    a. Curettage—excision of skin tumour by scraping with a curette; electrocautery is used to achieve haemostasis and to destroy any viable malignant cells in margins or in base of wound.
    b. This form of treatment takes advantage of the fact that the tumour in each

instance is softer than the surrounding skin and can be outlined by curette, which 'feels' the extent of the tumour.

   c. Tumour is removed and the base cauterized; process repeated a number of times.

3 *Surgical excision*

   a. Wide surgical excision—adequacy of excision verified by microscopic study of sections of the specimen.

   b. Histological study of excised tissue allows determination of whether or not margins are free of tumour.

   c. Skin grafting may be necessary.

4 *Radiotherapy*—usually done for cancer of eyelid, tip of nose, in or near vital structures (facial nerve) where tissue sparing is difficult with other forms of treatment; used for extensive malignancies when goal is palliation or when other medical conditions contraindicate other forms of therapy.

   a. Explain to patient that he may experience skin reddening and swelling about the time of the third treatment; may progress to blistering.

   b. Stress importance of follow-up care—there is always the possibility of recurrence or a new primary lesion.

   c. Caution the patient against exposure to the sun.

5 *Cryosurgery*—deep freezing to selectively destroy tumour tissue.

   a. Liquid nitrogen is applied by cryospray or cryoprobe technique.

   b. Site thaws naturally and then becomes gelatinous and heals spontaneously.

6 Mohs' chemo-surgery—combined use of topically applied chemicals and serial surgical excisions to remove tissue; immediate microscopic examination is made for tumour extensions.

   Useful for recurrent skin cancers, since surgical excision is guided by microscopic study.

7 *Topical chemotherapy*—application of topical antitumour agent (fluorouracil) to destroy cancer cells.

Health Teaching

Most skin cancer can be prevented by avoidance of and protection from excessive direct exposure to sun. Susceptible patients should show any suspect lesions to their doctor.

   Instruct the patient as follows:

1 Avoid unnecessary exposure to the sun, especially during times when ultraviolet radiation is most intense (10 a.m. to 2 p.m.).

2 Wear appropriate protective clothing (e.g., broad-brimmed hat, long-sleeved garments).

3 Use shading devices (e.g., umbrella).

4 Apply a protective sunscreen cream or lotion if an activity requires long periods of exposure.

5 Watch for indications of potential malignancy in moles (e.g., change in colour, increase in size, ulceration, bleeding or serous exudation).

6 Follow-up after treatment of squamous cell cancer and malignant melanoma should be carried out for the patient's lifetime and should include palpation of adjacent lymph nodes.

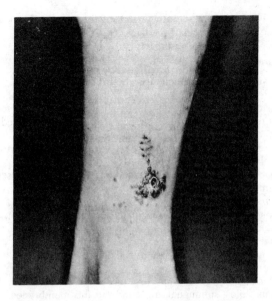

Figure 8.8. Melanoma. (Courtesy of Armed Forces Institute of Pathology.)

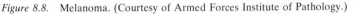

Malignant Melanoma

Malignant melanoma is a malignant tumour of the skin (Fig. 8.8) which occurs in three forms: lentigo-maligna melanoma, superficial spreading melanoma and nodular melanoma. It has higher mortality rate than other forms of skin cancer.

Classification

Lentigo-maligna Melanoma

1   Slowly evolving pigment lesions; occur on exposed skin surfaces of elderly.
2   First appears as tan, flat lesion—in time undergoes change in size and colour.

Superficial Spreading Melanoma

1   Occurs anywhere on body; usually affects persons of middle age.
2   Tends to be circular with portion of its outline irregular (either protruding or indenting).
3   Has combination of colours—hues of tan, brown and black admixed with grey, bluish-black or white.
4   May be dull pink-rose colour in a small area within the lesion.

Nodular Melanoma

1   Spherical blueberry-like nodule with relatively smooth surface and relatively uniform blue-black colour.

2   May be polypoidal, with smooth surface of rose-grey or black colour; may be present as elevated, irregular plaque.

Clinical Features

1   Signs that suggest malignant change:
  a. *Variegated colour*
    (1) Colours that may indicate malignancy in a brown or black lesion are shades of red, white and blue; shades of blue are considered ominous.
    (2) White areas within a pigmented lesion are suspicious.
    (3) Some malignant melanomas are not variegated but are uniformly coloured (bluish-black, bluish-grey, bluish-red).
  b. *Irregular border*—look for angular indentation or notch present in the border of a malignant melanoma.
  c. *Irregular surface.*
    (1) Look for uneven elevations of the surface; irregular topography may be palpable or visible.
    (2) Some nodular melanomas have a smooth surface.
2   Common sites of melanoma—skin of back, legs, between toes, and on feet, face, scalp, fingernails, back of hands.
3   In the black race, melanomas are most apt to occur on less pigmented sites—palms, soles, subungual areas and mucous membranes.

Diagnosis

1   Any change or alteration in size or colour; symptoms such as itching, oozing, bleeding.
2   Biopsy—excision of suspicious mole from both raised and invasive areas and from flat, noninvasive area.
3   Prognosis—survival is related to depth of dermal invasion of malignant melanocytes in the primary lesion; melanoma is curable only when confined to primary site.

Treatment

The therapeutic approach depends on the depth of the lesion.

1   Radical surgery—wide excision with possible regional node dissection, usually followed by plastic repair or skin grafting.
2   Regional isolation perfusion; specific area is isolated by mechanically controlling its arterial inflow and venous outflow. This allows high concentration of cytotoxic drugs to be delivered to cancer-bearing sites.
3   Chemotherapy.
4   Grenz ray therapy for lentigo-maligna melanoma.

Health Teaching

1   Educate people to observe their moles and to report moles that *change* colours, enlarge or become raised or thicker.
2   Treatment should be initiated immediately.

SYSTEMIC DISEASES WITH SKIN MANIFESTATIONS

Lupus Erythematosus

Systemic lupus erythematosus (SLE) is an inflammatory disease of unknown origin involving the vascular and connective tissues of many organs (primarily skin, joints, kidneys and serous membranes) with resultant multiple local and systemic symptoms.

Discoid lupus erythematosus is a chronic eruption of the skin which, although often disfiguring, does not pose a threat to life.

Clinical Features

1 Aetiology is not understood—evidence indicates that it is an autoimmune disease.
2 Appears to be familial in nature.
3 Most frequently found in young women with signs and symptoms referable to the joints and skin.
4 May be drug-induced (procainamide; hydralazine).
5 Is characterized by remissions and exacerbations.

Clinical Manifestations

1 Vary greatly, since they can affect every organ system; mimic many other diseases.
2 Weakness, malaise, weight loss.
3 *Skin manifestations.*
   a. Malar rash, alopecia, dermal vasculitis, Raynaud's phenomenon, purpura.
   b. Possible skin rash with butterfly distribution over bridge of nose and malar bone prominences (butterfly distribution).
   c. Similar lesions over neck, chest, upper and lower extremities—may become pruritic and scaly.
   d. Broken-off hair ('lupus hair').
4 Generalized lymphadenopathy.
5 Long-continued low grade fever.
6 Arthritis and arthralgia.
7 Cardiac involvement (pericarditis, myocarditis, pleural effusion).
8 Renal involvement (proteinuria, haematuria, renal insufficiency and failure).
9 Central nervous system involvement (convulsive disorders, abnormalities in mental function and cranial nerves, depression, emotional lability, neurosis).

Diagnosis

Many laboratory abnormalities may be found.

1 Positive LE cell test.
2 Immunologic abnormalities present in most persons with SLE.
   a. ANA (antinuclear antibody test) positive—high titres of antibody to nuclear antigens.

b. Serum complement fixation test—decreased complement titres in patients with renal disease.

c. Increased gamma globulins.

3 Urine—may reveal proteinuria and cellular casts.

4 Cerebrospinal fluid examination—may have elevated protein concentration and mononuclear cells.

5 Blood evaluation—shows evidence of anaemia, leucopenia, thrombocytopenia.

6 Abnormal renal function tests.

Treatment

No known cure at this time.

Objective

To control the disease by suppressing inflammation and relieving symptoms.

1 Treat intercurrent illness—exacerbations of SLE may follow infection, drug administration, emotional stress, surgical procedures.

2 Other forms of treatment—selection depends on nature and severity of disease.
   a. Corticosteroids (prednisone)—used for suppressing inflammation and thus relieving symptoms.
   (1) Observe patient carefully—may be difficult to distinguish between drug effects and those of SLE.
   (2) See Volume 2, Chapter 5 for Side Effects of Steroids.
   b. Salicylates—for musculoskeletal pain; will also lower temperature.
   Patient should take salicylates on a regular schedule so that adequate blood levels are maintained.
   c. Antimalarials (chloroquine)—to control the skin and joint manifestations.
   Patient should be examined by ophthalmologist at least twice yearly—retinal degeneration resulting in visual impairment may be a problem.
   d. Immunosuppressive agents (cyclophosphamide; azathioprine)—to suppress manifestations of SLE.
   (1) Still considered experimental in treatment of SLE.
   (2) Usually reserved for patients who are unresponsive to steroids or who develop unacceptable side effects from steroids.

3 Treat the patient as each problem arises (depending on the organ system involved and its physiological consequences)—nephritis, renal failure, congestive heart failure, central nervous system lupus, etc.

4 Give continuing emotional support. Psychiatric treatment may be indicated for debilitating depression, etc.

5 Be aware that some patients do not react favourably to immunization procedures.

6 Watch for development of complications—uraemia, central nervous system disorders, malignancies, infection (namely 'opportunist' bacterial pathogens), acute abdominal catastrophes.

Health Teaching

Instruct the patient as follows:

1 Avoid whatever you know may aggravate the condition.

2 Avoid undue exposure to sunlight—can produce exacerbations and worsen dermal lesions.
3 Use a sunscreening agent when exposure to sun is necessary.
4 Avoid sensitizing drugs (penicillin; sulphonamides) and avoid using hair sprays and hair colouring agents.
5 Avoid taking contraceptive pills—anovulatory drugs may precipitate lupus syndrome in susceptible person.
6 Try to avoid (and cope with) stress—emotional turmoil may precipitate a flare-up.
7 Obtain more rest.
8 Eat a well-balanced diet.
9 The makeup 'Cover-Mark' or Keromask may conceal facial lesions and scarring (of discoid LE).
10 Report to the doctor immediately any worsening of symptoms—fever, cough, skin rash, increasing joint pain, etc.

Periarteritis Nodosa (Polyarteritis)

Periarteritis nodosa (polyarteritis) is a disease of unknown cause characterized by inflammation and necrosis of medium-sized and small vessels, especially arteries, which results in altered function of the organ system in which the arterial supply has been impaired.

Clinical Features

1 The walls of the vessels are involved; spotty inflammation causes changes in circulation and tissue damage.
2 Clinical manifestations vary according to organ(s) involved and amount of necrosis produced by obstructing vascular lesion.
   a. Prolonged fever; myalgia and arthralgia; renal involvement; gastrointestinal manifestations (abdominal pain, nausea, vomiting, diarrhoea); cardiovascular manifestations (coronary insufficiency, myocardial infarction); palpable nodules along the arterial trunks—may occur.
   b. Ocular manifestations (retinal exudates and haemorrhages) are fairly common.
   c. Skin lesions are usually in the form of painful nodules that may ulcerate.
      (1) Subcutaneous nodules vary in size and may be located in any part of the body.
      (2) Overlying skin may be reddened or ulcerated.
      (3) Purpuric papules may be present.
3 Periarteritis is apt to run a course of a few years' duration; recovery is unpredictable—death may ensue from renal decompensation, congestive cardiac failure, etc.

Treatment

Treatment is similar to that of systemic lupus erythematosus.

Objective

To give the patient symptomatic and supportive care.

1 A search is made for any offending drug that may precipitate the disease.
2 Corticosteroids (prednisone)—given to control symptoms and to prevent progression of disease.
   a. Large doses may be given initially; patient is observed for evidence of disease regression.
   b. See Management of Patient Having Steroid Therapy (Chap. 5, Vol. 2).
3 Immunosuppressive drugs (cyclophosphamide; azathioprine) may be given in combination with corticosteroids.
4 Watch for and treat intercurrent infections.
5 Advise patient to avoid drugs that may exacerbate symptoms.

Scleroderma (Progressive Systemic Sclerosis)

Scleroderma (progressive systemic sclerosis) is a disease of unknown aetiology in which there is chronic hardening or shrinking of the connective tissue throughout the body. It is characterized by vascular abnormalities (sclerosis of the blood vessels), fibrosis of the skin, atrophy of smooth muscle and loss of visceral function.

Clinical Features

1 The disease starts insidiously on face and hands; skin acquires a tense, wrinkle-free, bound-down appearance (cannot be picked up from adjacent structures).
   a. Wrinkles and lines are obliterated.
   b. Skin is dry—sweat secretion over involved area is suppressed.
   c. Face appears mask-like, immobile and expressionless; mouth becomes rigid.
   d. Condition spreads slowly; extremities become stiff and immobile; the fingers semiflexed, immobile and useless; the hands claw-like.
2 Detectable clinical changes may occur in the internal organs.
   a. Heart becomes fibrotic—causing dyspnoea and other symptoms.
   b. Oesophagus is hardened, with disruption of normal oesophageal peristalsis—gastro-oesophageal reflux, with heartburn and dysphagia.
   c. Lungs are scarred—impeding respiration.
   d. Intestines become hardened—digestive disturbances.
   e. Progressive renal failure may occur.
   f. Variety of other disturbances develop, including Raynaud's phenomenon and arthritis.

Treatment

Methods of treatment may include:

1 Steroid therapy for anti-inflammatory effect.
2 Salicylate therapy—to relieve joint stiffness.
3 Physical therapy—helpful in preventing joint contractures and in maintaining joint mobility.
4 Surgical procedures (as in surgery for arthritis)—for hand deformities.
5 Vasoactive drugs, anti-inflammatory and antifibrotic agents—may be helpful for Raynaud's phenomenon.

6 Operative control of gastro-oesophageal reflux (reconstruction of oesophago-gastric junction) may be considered for reflux oesophagitis.
7 Cardiac, pulmonary and renal involvement are treated symptomatically.
8 The skin is kept lubricated with a bland cream (e.g., E45 cream).

Health Teaching

Instruct the patient as follows:

1 Keep warm; take warm hand baths/paraffin dips for hand involvement.
2 For gastrointestinal disturbances:
   a. Chew well and eat slowly to allow oesophagus time to empty by gravity, since there is disruption of normal oesophageal peristalsis.
   b. Elevate head of bed on blocks.
   c. Take antacids between meals and before bedtime.

SURGERY TO THE SKIN

Plastic Reconstructive Surgery

Reconstructive surgery (plastic surgery) is performed to repair extravisceral defects and malformations, both congenital and acquired, and to restore function as well as prevent further loss of function.

Cosmetic surgery involves reconstruction of the cutaneous tissues around the neck and face; done to restore function, correct defects and remove the marks of time. (See Table 8.1).

Definitions

1 *Skin graft* (free graft)—a section of skin tissue which is separated from its blood supply and transferred as a free section of tissue to the recipient site.
2 *Skin flap* (pedicle graft)—a section of skin tissue used to cover or fill a defect; it is lifted from its bed but still has partial attachment by a pedicle from which it receives its blood supply until healing takes place in its new location.
   Flaps are used to cover defects in which there is poor vascularity; for reconstruction of eyelids, ears, nose and cheeks.
3 *Autograft*—transfers or transplants from same person.
4 *Allograft*—transfer or transplants between two individuals of same species.
5 *Isografts*—grafts between identical twins.
6 *Xenografts*—grafts between two animals of different species, e.g., rabbit to mouse, baboon to man.
7 *Split-thickness graft* (Thiersch's graft)—graft of approximately one-half the thickness of skin which is removed by a knife or dermatome; deeper layers of dermis are left behind. (Used for coverage and closure of skin defects.)
8 *Full-thickness skin graft*—contains the epidermis and all of the dermis.
   a. Used frequently for reconstruction of facial defects, for it neither contracts nor develops unsightly pigmentation.
   b. Grafts may be further subdivided into thin and thick:
   (1) Thin (0.010–0.015 in thick)—used to resurface contaminated granulations or recipient sites in which blood supply is jeopardized.

Table 8.1.   Common Cosmetic Plastic Operations

Operation	Purpose	Surgery	Postoperative Expectations
Rhinoplasty (nose)	To improve the shape of the nose in relation to the rest of the face	1–1½ hours. Excess bone or cartilage is removed; nose is reshaped	Nasal splint; soft intranasal packing; foam rubber dressings
Mentoplasty (chin)	To improve the profile, as is necessary with a receding chin	Incision approach is within the mouth. Silicone or plastic implant is positioned	Healing complete in a week
Rhytidoplasty (face lift)	To remove excess skin due to elastosis and to tighten remaining skin	Incision is anterior to ear and extended down to nasolabial fold to the mental foramen near the chin and to the midline in the upper neck; the stretched subcutaneous tissues and fascia of the face are folded to provide a basic firmness	Improvement lasts up to 10 years
Glabellar rhytidoplasty	To remove two vertical furrows between eyebrows	Dermabrasion and excision; skin graft may be required	
Otoplasty (ear)	To correct deformed, flattened or protruding ears	1–1½ hours. Silicone or plastic implant may be used	Ear bandaged for a week; protection during sleep required for 3 weeks
Blepharoplasty (eyelid)	To remove wrinkles and bulges caused by herniation of fat, ageing or inheritance	1–1½ hours. Two incisions; one on upper lid and one on lower lid	Neosporin ointment applied around eyes and lids. Individual eye dressings are applied. Swelling and discoloration subside in about 10 days

(2) Thick (0·015–0·010 in thick)—used where durability is the important factor.

9 *Pinch graft*—a small piece of skin graft obtained by elevating the skin with a needle or forceps and cutting it off with scissors or knife.

10 *Take*—refers to the appearance of the graft between the third and fifth day after transfer, signifying that the vascular connections have developed between the recipient bed and the transplant.

Causes of Graft Failure

1 Fluid beneath the graft.
2 Haematoma—avoid by early inspection and removal of clots.
3 Infection.

Nursing Management (for Grafting Procedures)

Preoperative Care

Objective

To bring the patient to his optimal physical and emotional level.

1 Assess for nutritional status.
 a. Give vitamins and increase protein intake as directed—to facilitate healing.
 b. Note haemoglobin level and clotting time—these levels can affect healing process.
2 Prepare donor and recipient sites for surgical excision. (See p. 354.)
3 Inform the patient about what to expect postoperatively.
 a. Appearance of the wound—redness, distortion, swelling and unattractive suture lines are characteristics that will change with time.
 b. Pressure dressings, immobilization devices, etc.
4 Prepare the patient psychologically.
 a. Attempt to establish the reasons why the patient seeks surgery.
 (1) Patient's attitudes towards his disfigurement, his motivations for seeking surgery and his assessment of how his disfigurement has influenced his life and his psychosocial relationships are taken into consideration before surgery is considered.
 (2) Desirable to have unimpaired body image and realistic acceptance of surgical limitations.
 (3) Poor candidate for cosmetic surgery is one who has delusions concerning his deformity, unhealthy psychological responses and unrealistic expectations of results.
 b. Explain the limitations of the contemplated procedure, the possibility of complications and the unpredictability of the result (responsibility of the surgeon).

Postoperative Care

1 Inspect graft under dressing daily, using a good light—to be sure that oedema, blistering or haematoma has not formed and is not jeopardizing successful graft.
 a. Surgeon carefully teases dressing away from wound—changing dressing may cause avulsion (tearing away) of recent graft around margin of wound.

      b. Surgeon will nick graft to evacuate blood clots.

      (1) Fluid may be rolled out of graft with cotton-tipped applicator or by aspirating with needle and syringe.

      (2) Seromas or haematomas may impede healing.

2 Apply mittens to patient if he is inadvertently scratching the graft during sleep—to protect graft and donor site from subconscious scratching.

3 Apply wet dressings to infected graft as directed.

4 Use prophylactic antibiotic therapy for patient with infected graft as prescribed. Utilize sensitivity testing to identify organism.

5 Elevate grafted extremity for 7–10 days.

      a. Immobilize part—movement of body areas beneath graft may predispose to loss of graft.

      b. Apply cast or immobilizing bandages to restrict all regional movements of the extremity.

      c. Begin ambulation activities very gradually.

6 Inform the patient of the changing hues of the graft—to help him accept his situation.

      a. Free graft is at first pale, then pink and red—it then fades and appears similar to neighbouring skin.

      b. Full-thickness grafts may remain deeply red for months.

      c. Anticipate skin scaling in full-thickness grafts.

      d. Teach the patient that the graft is vulnerable to sun; avoid overexposure to the sun.

7 Instruct the patient to apply mineral oil or lanolin on wound after second or third week—to remove superficial crusts, moisten the graft and stimulate circulation to the wound area.

Care of the Donor Site

1 The donor site is usually covered with lightly lubricated paraffin or antibiotic-impregnated gauze and held in place with a gauze dressing to absorb blood and serum from the wound.

      a. The outer dressing may be removed in 24 hours.

      b. Area may be left exposed after first or second postoperative day.

      c. Paraffin gauze may be left in place until it loosens as epithelialization becomes complete—prevents heavy crusting.

2 Prevent area from coming in contact with clothing or bedding—to provide adequate circulation of air to the donor site.

3 Apply wet dressing (as directed) if donor site becomes infected.

4 Lubricate donor site with lanolin after healing—to keep it soft and pliable.

5 Donor sites heal by re-epithelialization; healing should be complete in 2 weeks' time.

Nursing Management of Patient Undergoing Maxillofacial Surgery

Preoperative Care

See p. 75 for nursing support.

Postoperative Care

1 Maintain an adequate airway.
2 Observe dressings for impairment of circulation and for oedema—pressure dressings are frequently used.
   a. Control oral haemorrhage by inserting gauze pad in the mouth and exerting pressure at bleeding point.
   b. Wipe blood from wound—blood under suture line may cause haematoma and infection and spoil the cosmetic result.
3 Watch colour of skin flaps—may appear blue and congested due to partial obstruction of the venous circulation.
   a. Surgeon may make small incisions in the flap to relieve the blood congestion and avoid gangrene of the flap.
   b. Moisten flap dressing with warm sterile solution as directed.
4 Relieve pain—expect more pain on operations involving jaw and facial bones.
   a. Apply heat or cold according to direction.
   b. Give analgesics as ordered.
5 Keep the patient well hydrated and nourished.
   a. Offer cracked ice and water as soon as nausea subsides.
   b. Give soft diet as tolerated
      (1) Provide an adequate quantity and caloric quality to patient on prolonged liquid diet (following jaw surgery, etc.).
      (2) Give frequent feedings in order to obtain caloric equivalent of a full diet.
6 Offer appropriate psychological support—numerous operations may be required.

Dermabrasion

Dermabrasion is surgical planing of the superficial portion of the skin.

Clinical Indications

1 Done on selected patients with facial disfigurements from scars due to acne, trauma, naevi, freckles, chickenpox or smallpox.
2 Removal of precancerous lesions (keratosis).

Surgical Procedure

The epidermis and some superficial dermis are removed, but enough of the dermis is preserved to allow re-epithelialization of the dermabraded areas.

1 The patient is anaesthetized.
2 The skin is sprayed with a topical anaesthetic to stabilize and stiffen the skin.
3 The superficial layer of skin is removed by an abrasive machine (Dermabrader) or by sandpapering.
4 Copious saline irrigations are carried out during and after the planing procedure.
5 Paraffin gauze or plastic-faced (Op-site) dressings are applied immediately after the procedure.

Nursing Management

Postoperative

1 Apply saline compresses over paraffin gauze dressings—to absorb oozing and clotting, which are subject to infection.
   a. Mild oozing may be expected for 24 hours.
   b. Crusts then form; are shed in 7–10 days.
   c. Skin remains pink 6–12 weeks.
2 Discontinue saline compresses after 12–24 hours, or as directed.
3 Assist with removal of dressing in 48 hours—patient will experience a 'recent sunburn' sensation.
4 Apply lanolin, hypoallergenic cream, etc., as directed—to relieve sensation of tightness when crusts form.
5 Warn the patient to avoid exposure to direct sunlight for 3–4 months—planed area may become darker or lighter than surrounding skin due to sunlight.

Burns

CARE OF THE BURN PATIENT

Burns are wounds caused by excessive exposure to four categories of agents: thermal, electrical, chemical and radioactive.

Incidence

1 Over 150 000 burn injuries occur annually in England and Wales.
2 Approximately 14 000 burn victims require hospitalization each year in this country.
3 Nearly 1000 persons die from burns each year in England and Wales.
4 Most burn accidents occur in the home and are caused primarily by carelessness or ignorance.
5 Authorities estimate that at least 75% of all burns could be prevented.
6 The nurse is in a strategic position for teaching burn prevention and for promoting legislation for safety practices.
7 One-third of burn victims are children.

Surgical Prediction

1 Best survival expectancy occurs in young-adult groups, aged 15–45 years.
2 A burn affecting over 20% of the body endangers life.
3 Prognosis depends on age of patient, depth and extent of burn, condition of patient and imminence of complications, as well as on dedication of the treating team.
   a. Sudden drop in haemoglobin concentration may be diagnostic.
   b. Sudden drop in white blood cells and platelets is seen in terminal sepsis—largest killer in burns.

4   Prognosis is largely affected by whether or not a respiratory injury is incurred—respiratory injury (usually reported as pneumonia) is the second most frequent cause of death (after infection) in burn victims.

Toxic Fume Hazard

1   Toxic fumes from burning plastic are more dangerous than smoke.
2   Resulting gases, particularly hydrogen chloride, rapidly increase level of carbon monoxide in a fire.
3   Survival time to get out of a fire is cut in half.
4   What can be done?
   a. Reduce amount of plastic items in a home (or building).
   b. During a fire, move quickly and stay close to the floor where oxygen availability is greatest.
   c. Wear masks even after a fire has been brought under control.
   d. If exposed to burning plastic, notify your doctor.

Assessment of Patient's Burn Injury

NOTE: This can be done most accurately when wounds are cleaned—otherwise estimate is often erroneous due to presence of soot and debris.

Assess Extent of Body Surface Burned

1   Anatomical location—greater morbidity and mortality for burns affecting hands, feet, face and perineum.
2   Determination is based on the use of tables for this purpose, such as the 'Rule of Nine' Chart (Fig. 8.9) and the Burn Evaluation Chart (Fig. 8.10). For children, use paediatric evaluation chart. These tables or charts serve as a guide for fluid therapy.

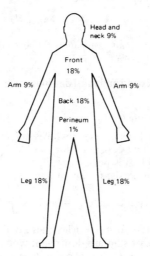

Figure 8.9.   'Rule of Nine' chart.

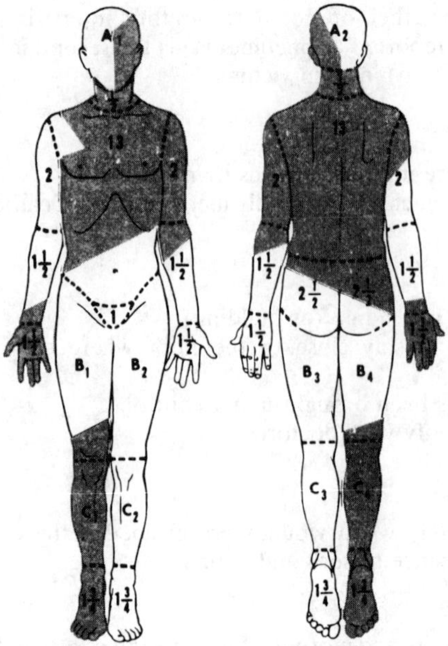

	ANTERIOR	POSTERIOR
HEAD	A_1 1.5	A_2 1.0
NECK	.5	.5
RT. ARM		1.0
RT. FOREARM	.5	.25
RT. HAND	1.5	1.5
LT. ARM	2.0	2.0
LT. FOREARM	.5	.5
LT. HAND		
TRUNK	10.0	13.0
BUTTOCK	(L) .5	(R) 1.0
PERINEUM		
RT. THIGH	B_1 1.0	B_4 .75
RT. LEG	C_1 3.5	C_4 3.5
RT. FOOT	1.75	1.75
LT. THIGH	B_2	B_3
LT. LEG	C_2	C_3
LT. FOOT		

% PARTIAL THICKNESS ____
Mixed
% FULL THICKNESS ____
TOTAL   50%

PERCENT OF AREAS AFFECTED BY GROWTH:

	0	1	5	10	15	ADULT
A = ½ HEAD	9½	8½	6½	5½	4½	3½
B = ½ ONE THIGH	2¾	3¼	4	4¼	4½	4¾
C = ½ ONE LEG	2½	2½	2¾	3	3¼	3½

Figure 8.10. Burn Evaluation Chart—estimation per cent body burns. (Courtesy Crozer-Chester Medical Centre.)

3 Repeat assessment on second and third day inasmuch as demarcation may not be visible until then.

Assess Depth of Burn: Classification

1 *First-degree burn* (partial thickness)—involves epidermis only.
   a. Redness, pain and slight oedema—this subsides quickly.
   b. In about 5 days, epidermis peels.
   c. Itching and pink skin persist for about a week.
   d. No scarring.
2 *Second-degree burn* (partial thickness)—involves epidermis and part of dermis.
   a. Superficial
      (1) Pink or red; blisters form (vesicles); also oedema.
      (2) Superficial layers of skin are destroyed; wound moist and painful.
      (3) Heals within 10 days to 2 weeks if it does not become infected.

    b. Deep dermal.
      (1) Mottled white and red; reddened areas blanch on pressure.
      (2) Blisters form—may or may not be sensitive to touch.
      (3) Hair does not pull out easily.
      (4) Takes several weeks to heal.
3 *Third-degree burn* (full thickness).
    a. Destruction of epithelial cells—entire epidermis and dermis destroyed.
    b. Reddened areas do not blanch on touch.
    c. Because of surface dehydration, eschar (leathery cover) may form.
    d. For most full thickness burns grafting is required.
    e. Not painful; coloration varies from waxy white to brown.
    f. Severe full thickness burn can include destruction of epithelium, fat, muscles and bone.
    g. Area appears black and depressed.

NOTE: Major burns—Second-degree burns of over 30% of body.
                Third-degree burns of over 10% of body.

RAPID ASSESSMENT: Use hair test—if hair can be pulled out easily, there is likelihood of full-thickness injury.

Assess Unique Contributing Factors

1 Causative agent (boiling water, chemical, etc.).
2 Duration of exposure.
3 Thickness of skin.
4 Patient's age.
5 Pre-existing medical complicating factors.
6 Prior psychological status of the patient.
7 Circumstances where burn was sustained, e.g., in a closed area—this may cause respiratory damage.
8 Chemical, electrical and radiation burns can cause more damage than appears obvious.
9 Concomitant injuries, e.g., patient may have fallen or been thrown in an explosion.

Assess the Possibility of Postburn Pulmonary Damage.

1 Look for burns around the mouth or neck.
2 Look for singeing of nasal hairs.
3 Inspect mouth for burns of the oral or pharyngeal mucous membranes.
4 Observe for voice changes or coughing up soot.
5 Determine whether victim sustained burn in a restricted or confined area (forced to inhale hot smoke, etc.).
6 Respiratory status may appear satisfactory initially, but intrinsic and extrinsic oedema may cause airway obstruction at any time during first 48 hours postburn. When in doubt, intubate patient to ensure an adequate airway until oedema subsides several days postburn.

Obtain a Brief History

1 Previous state of health.

2   Allergies.
3   Tetanus immunization status.
4   Height and weight of patient (pre- and postburn).
5   Vital signs.

Emergency First-aid Measures

1   Immediately stop the burning process.
2   When clothes catch fire, have victim fall to floor or ground and roll him in a carpet or blanket—if available within 1 or 2 m (5 or 6 ft); otherwise drop, roll and beat out flames with anything (including hands as last resort).
   a. Running would fan flames.
   b. Standing would force him to breathe flames and smoke, cause his hair to be ignited, or cause facial disfigurement.
   c. After fire is extinguished, soak hot clothing with cold water.
3   Apply cold to the burn—immerse in cold water for 10 min, intermittently (if pain present, repeat up to three time) or apply towels soacked in cold water—this relieves pain and reduces tissue oedema and damage.
4   Cover burn as quickly as possible with sterile dressings or any clean cloth—to prevent further wound contamination.
   a. Bacterial contamination is minimized.
   b. Pain is decreased by preventing air from contacting injured surface.

Nursing Alert: Grease, ointment or antiseptic solutions should *not* be applied to any large burn as an emergency measure.

5   Irrigate chemical burns immediately—continue irrigating for 10–15 min.
   a. Flush eyes, if affected, with clean, cool water.
   b. Consult doctor.
6   Allow victim to lie down while awaiting transportation to medical facility.
   a. Do not remove clothing unless it is hot or burning.
   b. Cover victim with a blanket to prevent loss of body heat.
   c. Place ice bottles or ice strategically to reduce pain. (Do not do this if burn is large—patient may become hypothermic and go into shock.)
7   Determine best disposition of the patient depending upon severity of burns.
   a. Critically burned person should be moved to a well-equipped burn unit that has a medical and nursing staff experienced in burn care. This includes victims with:
      (1) Respiratory tract burns.
      (2) Partial-thickness burns—more than 30% of body surface.
      (3) Full-thickness burns—more than 10% of body surface.
      (4) Burns of face, hands, feet, genitalia.
      (5) Burns complicated by fractures, major soft tissue injury, electrical injury.
      (6) Patients at extremes of age (under 2 or over 60) or with chronic disease (COAD, cardiac, diabetic).
   b. Moderately burned person may be taken to a community hospital. This includes victims with:
      (1) Partial-thickness burns—15–30% of body surface.
      (2) Full-thickness—less than 10% of body surface.

c. Minimally burned person may be treated in a doctor's office or hospital outpatient department. This includes victims with:
  (1) Partial-thickness burns—less than 10%.
  (2) Full-thickness—less than 2%.

Systemic Changes in Major Burn

Fluid Shifts

1 In addition to changes in the local burned area, there are alterations and disruptions in the vascular and other systems of the body.
2 The water-vapour barrier for the body is the outermost layer of epidermis. When it is rendered nonfunctioning, severe systemic reactions from fluid losses can occur (Table 8.2).
3 Blanching of the skin following burn injury is caused by contraction of skin capillaries; redness occurs when arterioles and capillaries dilate.
4 Fluid volume deficit is directly proportional to extent and depth of burn injury.
5 Capillary permeability increases, permitting fluid and protein to move from vascular to interstitial spaces (oedema results). Protein-rich fluid is lost in blebs of the burned tissues as well as by weeping of second-degree wounds.
   With reduced vascular volume, the patient will go into shock in untreated.
6 Vascular fluid loss occurs in first 24–48 hours.
7 Capillary permeability returns to normal in about 48 hours—but protein lost in interstitial spaces remains there for 5 days to 2 weeks before returning to the vascular system.
   a. When fluid mobilizes (moves from interstitial spaces back to vascular compartment) patients with good cardiac and renal function will diurese.
   b. Observe carefully for fluid overload and pulmonary oedema; patient requires decreased fluid intake, frequent observation of vital signs, central venous pressure and urine output.
8 Red cell mass is also diminished, due to thrombosis and sludging; as fluid escapes from capillary walls, blood concentrates and the flow is sluggish—haematocrit rises.
9 Capillary stasis may cause ischaemia and even necrosis.
10 The body attempts to compensate for losses of plasma volume.
   a. Constriction of vessels.
   b. Withdrawal of fluid from undamaged extracellular space.
   c. Patient is thirsty. (Oral fluids not given until bowel sounds are heard.)

Table 8.2.   Fluid Loss

Adult	Amount per Hour per Square Metre of Body Surface
Normal unburned individual	15–20 ml
Average adult with a flame burn of 40% of his body	100 ml

Haemodynamics

1   Lessened circulating blood volume results in decreased cardiac output and increased pulse rate.
2   There is a decreased stroke volume as well as a marked rise in peripheral resistance (due to constriction of arterioles and increased haemo-viscosity).
3   This results in inadequate tissue perfusion, which may in turn cause acidosis, renal failure and irreversible burn shock.
4   A burn injury often upsets the acid-base balance; therefore, careful monitoring of arterial blood gases, serum electrolytes and urine volume is needed for proper fluid therapy; this will allow one to replace fluid loss and prevent dilatation and paralytic ileus.

Calorie and Nitrogen Losses

1   Immediately following an extensive burn, there is a breakdown of cells (catabolism) resulting in a marked outpouring of potassium and nitrogen.
2   When adequately treated, an extensively burned patient will probably increase his weight the first 3–4 days, due to collection of fluid in the interstitial spaces; thereafter, weight loss will be progressive, at the rate of about 1 lb a day in a young adult, for about a month. *Adequate nutritional therapy* can reduce this loss to no more than 5–10% of preburn body weight before weight stabilizes.
3   In spite of all nutritional support it is almost impossible to counteract a negative nitrogen balance; the sooner a burn wound is closed, the more rapidly a positive nitrogen balance is reached.
4   The postburn adult requires 6000–8000 calories a day; high calories, high protein may be given orally and in some instances by intravenous feeding or by nasogastric feeding along with normal meals and snacks.

Objectives of Medical and Nursing Management

Objectives

To prevent burns by initiating and promoting safety practices.
To employ lifesaving measures in the care of the severely burned person.
To provide early specialized and individualized treatment of the burn victim in order to promote tissue repair and to prevent disability and disfigurement.
To recognize that the burn patient is a person with feelings, thoughts and concerns.
To include the burn patient and his family in the plan of treatment and rehabilitation.

To Remove Burning Agent, Alleviate Pain and Initiate Plan of Treatment

1   Observe for any breathing impairment; prepare for insertion of endotracheal tube if necessary.
2   Remove burned clothing and assess extent of burned area. (This may have to be done in hydrotherapy).
3   Make patient as comfortable as possible (morphine intravenously for pain, etc.) while history and physical examination progress; immediately covering burn sites aids in eliminating pain.

To Prevent and Treat for Burn Shock

1 Prepare for fluid replacement immediately—electrolytes, colloid (plasma or serum protein albumin) and fluid.
   a. Weigh patient on admission if possible (baseline weight) and 4 hourly thereafter for 48 hours then daily at the same time each day.
   b. Measure circumference of burned extremities; this may be useful later in determining oedema formation (believed unnecessary by some authorities), and photograph.
   c. Insert an indwelling catheter; measure hourly output and describe. Maintain urine output in range of 30–50 ml/hour. Check pH, specific gravity, sugar and acetone.
   d. Prepare for continuous intravenous therapy.
       Patient may require very large amounts of fluid:
   Roehampton Burns Unit Formula:

   120 ml dextran for 1% body surface area burned.

   This gives the total quantity of intravenous fluid in 48 hours and is divided: one-half in first 48 hours, one-quarter in next 16 hours and one-quarter in final 24 hours (Note: maximum of 6 l); with deep burns, up to one-third of total quantity may be given as whole blood.
   e. Record intake and output conscientiously.
   f. Observe for signs of dehydration or overhydration by use of haematocrit, central venous pressure and urinary output; notify doctor if signs occur.
   g. Note any untoward signs indicative of a transfusion reaction; if apparent, terminate transfusion and notify doctor.
   h. Elevate all burned extremities; check radial and pedal pulses hourly.
       Be alert to decreased circulation in fingers and toes due to circumferential burns (can cause oedema to form a tourniquet). Report to doctor immediately and prepare for escharotomy (an incision through dead eschar to relax constriction).
   i. Change patient's position 2 hourly and treat pressure areas.
2 Administer oxygen; it may have to be administered under pressure because of reduced blood volume, in order to saturate plasma.
3 Observe depth and rate of respirations. Circumferential chest burns may constrict chest movement and decrease tidal volume, causing a drop in Po_2 and an increase in Pco_2. Escharotomy may be required to allow adequate chest expansion.

To Prepare Burn Area for Assessment and Treatment

1 Excise blisters and remove loose necrotic material. Cleanse wound gently with 1–200 Savlon solution, then saline and dry. Hydrotherapy (p. 364) is more common in the USA.

To Assess the Physical and Psychological Reaction of the Patient to His Condition

1 Take and record vital signs hourly, including central venous pressure; blood pressure may be taken using a 'Doppler' to hear pressure if it is inaudible otherwise due to oedema. Arterial pressure monitors are available.

Hydrotherapy consists of immersing the burn patient in warm water to which electrolytic solutions are added to approximate tissue fluids and nonirritating agents are added to facilitate cleansing the patient.

Purpose:

1   To cleanse and loosen slough, exudate, eschar, topically applied medications.
2   To assist the debriding process.
3   To facilitate the patient's performance of range of motion exercises.

Patient protection:

1   The temperature is usually 37.8°C (100°F); the patient is closely supervised to prevent chilling.
2   Allow patient to assist in removing dressings; it keeps him occupied and is less painful when he does it himself.
3   The nurse and attendants wear long plastic gloves and plastic aprons in addition to caps and masks.
4   The tub may be lined with plastic to prevent cross-contamination and facilitate cleaning.
5   Repeat cleaning process two or three times rather than cleanse vigorously the first time.
6   Shave all areas within 5 cm (2 in) of the burn wound to prevent hair from causing bacterial growth.
7   Assess vital signs immediately before and after hydrotherapy. Be alert for septic episode after wound manipulation in hydrotherapy.

2   Note whether blood specimens are taken by the laboratory technician as requested.
3   Obtain 24-hour urine specimen if ordered. Measure urine output hourly while patient is critical.
4   Talk to patient to determine his concerns; include him in his therapy plan.
5   Observe patient for his reaction to his condition; set goals for him and be consistent in the therapeutic plan.

To Provide Physical Comfort and Emotional Support of the Patient

1   Administer sedatives and analgesics as prescribed for pain (intravenously, while patient is critical).
2   Elevate the burned extremities for comfort and to lessen oedema.
3   Place patient in physiologically comfortable position, keeping in mind the need to prevent contractures.
4   Provide diversional therapy; allay fear and anxiety.

To Meet Nutritional Needs and Control Gastrointestinal Disturbances

1   Initially, patient is usually fed by nasogastric tube; an antacid such as mist magnesium trisilcate, is given every 2 hours.
2   When bowel sounds return, administer oral fluids *slowly*, so that patient's tolerance can be observed. If no problem, advance diet to regular, as tolerated.

3 If serum potassium levels drop, give fruit juices that contain potassium.
4 After several days, supplement the diet with high protein drinks and vitamins.
5 Offer more solid food towards the end of the first week as tolerance for food improves.
   a. Build up daily caloric intake to match daily caloric expenditure.
   b. Provide: 3 g protein/kg body weight; 20% of needed calories in form of fats; remainder in carbohydrates.
6 Imagination and ingenuity may be required to stimulate a sluggish appetite.
7 Encourage patient to feed himself; adapt utensils to his individual needs.
8 If patient does not maintain an adequate intake voluntarily, it may be necessary to pass a nasogastric tube for administration of high protein formula.
9 Keep record of patient's weight and caloric intake—let him participate in meeting caloric goal by selecting foods he desires.
10 Be alert for evidence of Curling's ulcer—the incidence is in proportion to the extent of the burn.

To Prevent Complications

1 *Infection.*

> *Burn Wound Sepsis*—the proliferation and/or active invasion of the burn wound by micro-organisms numbering 100 000 or more per gramme of tissue (10^5 per gramme of tissue)
> Clinical manifestation: elevated temperature, abdominal distension, ileus, disorientation.
> Most common organism—*Pseudomonas*.

a. Assist in the cleansing and debridement of tissues.
b. Practise rigid asepsis when wound is exposed.
c. Wear mask, cap and gown in addition to sterile gloves during change of dressings.
d. Obtain wound culture when requested; often, burn-wound biopsy cultures are required every other day until eschar has begun to separate.
e. Keep environment as clean as possible; laminar airflow is used in many burn units.
   (1) Employ good housekeeping practices; do not permit wet mops and dry dust cloths, but utilize wet and dry vacuuming and damp-dusting with a disinfectant.
   (2) Keep temperature just below the level that would cause patient's uninvolved skin to perspire; keep humidity low.
   (3) Maintain isolation precautions.
   (4) Restrict visitors.
f. Change dressings, usually twice daily, in hydrotherapy; the tank is filled with warm tap water, 37.8°C (100°F), to which are added prescribed amounts of sodium chloride, potassium chloride, calcium hypochlorite, and perhaps a mild soap powder for cleansing purposes.
g. Administer antibiotics as prescribed (usually after first day, since blocked

capillaries at burn site will prevent medications from reaching the area); subeschar antibiotic therapy may be initiated for concentration at site of colonization.

h. Recognize changes in vital signs that may indicate infection.

i. Apply topical bacteriostatic substance as directed (silver nitrate, sulfamylon, etc.).

j. Promote the best personal hygiene for the patient.

(1) Cleanse unburned areas of the body with antibacterial soap or detergent-germicide; maintain clean nails—hydrotherapy is most effective for this.

(2) Shave hairs from burned areas and adjacent areas; shampoo hair daily.

(3) Provide meticulous mouth care.

(4) Keep all orifices especially clean; give special attention to indwelling catheter and meatus.

k. On admission administer tetanus toxoid (if immunized previously) or administer tetanus immune globulin (if toxoid not given previously).

l. Continue to monitor action of topical agent by wound cultures; if such an agent is not controlling infection, subeschar antibiotic therapy may have to be instituted.

2   *Contractures and deformities.*

a. Maintain proper body alignment, using supports and splints as necessary.

b. Initiate passive, then active exercises where possible, with doctor's permission, on first postburn day.

c. Turn frequently, encourage deep breathing, and initiate early ambulation as soon as feasible.

d. Perform range of motion activities in hydrotherapy and at bedside three times daily.

e. Use a footboard to prevent footdrop.

f. Splint hands at night and even during day when not being used for feeding or other activity.

g. Have patient feed himself with burned (second-degree) hands as early as first or second postburn day.

h. Use overhead frame for trapeze and slings to assist with positioning and exercise.

3   *Respiratory difficulty.*

a. assess respiratory rate, chest movement and any respiratory stress.

b. Determine whether patient inhaled smoke, fumes or flame—whether he has singed nasal hair, red pharynx, hoarse voice, cough, stridor, etc.

c. Have endotracheal tube and oxygen equipment easily accessible.

d. Keep airway free of secretion by frequent oral and nasotracheal suctioning, preferably under sterile conditions.

e. Monitor for signs of pulmonary oedema—increased tracheobronchial secretions, râles over both lung fields, blood-tinged expectorations, shortness of breath.

f. Initiate turning, coughing and deep-breathing regime.

4   *Hazards of immobility.*

a. Prevent pressure sores—use Stryker bed to turn if circumferential burns are present.

(1) Teach patient to change position slightly himself.

(2) Turn patient and observe possible pressure points every 2 hours.

b. Prevent pneumonia—provide excellent respiratory hygiene.

To Recognize and Treat an Inhalation Burn Injury

1 Be familiar with the patient's history—note whether he was 'overcome with smoke' or in a closed space when injured.

2 Early symptoms are significant and require immediate concern and treatment:

a. Does he exhibit irrational behaviour, have a cough, progressive hoarseness, dyspnoea, haemoptysis?

b. Look for burns in area of head, neck and chest (circumoral and nasal).

c. Is there constricting oedema of the neck or chest? May require escharotomy.

d. Are the nasal vibrissae (hairs) singed? (Check with a torch.)

e. Auscultate chest for wheezes, râles and rhonchi—any sign of airway obstruction?

f. Examine nasal and oral mucosa for soot stains; check expectorations for carbon particles.

3 Perform laboratory tests—Serial chest x-rays (first may be normal, but oedema and atelectasis may be detected later); serial blood gases (PO_2 and pH decrease, PCO_2 increases); carboxyhaemoglobin levels.

4 Attempt to determine other related significant factors such as whether patient took alcohol or other drugs, has other medical problems.

5 Initiate treatment:

a. Maintain adequate airway.

(1) Insert soft endotracheal tube for 2–3 days while oedema persists.

(2) Employ tracheotomy if patient cannot tolerate intubation, or beyond the 3-day period. (This may be delayed longer—up to 7 days if cuffed endotracheal tube is used.)

b. Reduce thick and dry secretions:

(1) Administer humidified oxygen therapy.

(2) Encourage the patient to cough; utilize postural drainage and chest percussion if feasible.

(3) Administer bronchodilators such as aminophyllin.

(4) Promote liquefying of secretions by using such broncholytic agents as parenteral sodium iodide or supersaturated potassium iodide.

c. Insert nasogastric tube.

This will aid in preventing gastric dilatation, vomiting, aspiration.

d. Prevent hypoxaemia and maintain acceptable arterial PO_2 levels.

(1) Administer supplemental oxygen by using a face tent, venti-mask, croup tent, etc.

Nursing Alert: Nasal cannulae are usually not recommended because air swallowing is likely (would promote gastric dilatation).

Nasal oxygen administration promotes undesirable mucus and drying of bronchi. Nasal oxygen should be humidified.

(2) Monitor blood gases and pH every 6 hours.

(3) Use mechanical ventilator if justified following blood gas determinations.

   e. Prevent pulmonary oedema.
     (1) Observe central venous pressure readings.
     (2) Utilize pulmonary capillary wedge pressure readings for accurate observation of left ventricle function.
     (3) Utilize digitalis carefully.
        Monitor serum potassium and diuretics.
   f. Restore blood and fluid volume when appropriate.
   g. Attempt to prevent (or initiate treatment of) pneumonia.
     (1) Obtain sputum and tracheal aspiration for culture daily.
     (2) Many authorities recommend broad-spectrum systemic antibiotic therapy.
     (3) After specific organisms are identified, treat with specific antibiotics.

METHODS OF TREATING BURNS

Open Air or Exposure Method

(This is the method of choice at Roehampton for the treatment of burns.) Exposing the burn to the drying effect of air allows the exudate to dry; a hard crust forms in 3 days and then acts as a protection to the wound.

Advantages and Mode of Action

1 Effective during disaster, when large numbers of persons must be cared for.
2 Most frequently used to treat burns of face, neck and perineum, and extensive burns of the trunk.
3 There are no painful dressing changes; therefore, less equipment is used and there is less discomfort for the patient.
4 Infection can be detected earlier.
5 Second-degree burns, beneath crust—regeneration of skin in 2–3 weeks.
6 Third-degree burns, beneath eschar—usually requires grafting.
7 Eschar loosens and must be debrided.

Imperative—Keep Immediate Environment Free of Organisms.

1 Everything that comes in contact with patient must be clean.
   a. Clean, freshly laundered linens on bed. (If sterile, sterility lost rather quickly.)
   b. Masks, sterile gowns and gloves for persons in contact with patient.
   c. Gowns and masks for visitors—instruct not to touch patient or hand him anything.
   d. 'Burn pack' desirable since it contains all linens for patient and gown and mask for attendant.
2 Room must be kept clean.
   a. Screens on windows.
   b. Dusting and mopping to be done with damp cloth or mop—not dry.
3 Humidity and temperature should be regulated—humidity 40–50%; temperature preferably 24.4°C (76°F).
   a. If too warm, patient may lose needed body fluids.
   b. Warmth encourages bacterial growth.

c. Bed or partial cradle with cover (or a heat shield overhead) can be used to prevent chilling.
d. Electric dehumidifier can be used if necessary.

Nursing Management

1 Prevent burn area from sticking to the sheet—use nonadherent disposable sheeting or burn pads to absorb excess exudate.
2 Avoid unnecessary trauma when changing linens by wetting those parts of tissue adhering to linen with sterile saline.
3 Have patient turn frequently to prevent cardiopulmonary complications and contractures.
4 Have patient feed himself if hand burns are not chiefly third degree.
5 Walk patient if complicating fractures are not present.
6 Patient may be nursed on:
    a. Standard hospital bed covered with sterile linen.
    b. Nylon mesh exposure bed covered wtih sheets of sterilized polyurethane foam. The foam sheets are sprayed with a silicone spray (Rikospray) to reduce adherence to the burn surface. (These sheets are easier to change than conventional bed linen.)
    c. An air bed, i.e. treatment by levitation making use of the inverted hovercraft principle.

Occlusive (Pressure) Dressings

Advantages

1 Less pain in first 48 hours postburn.
2 Takes less nursing time.
3 Useful for outpatients who may not have a clean environment or who cannot be relied upon to change dressing with good technique.

Disadvantages

1 High incidence of burn wound sepsis.
2 Discomfort and pain when changed.
3 If not put in proper position—may encourage development of contractures.

Nursing Management

1 Observe for signs of infection—temperature elevation, increased pulse, increased pain, perhaps an odour.
2 Change dressings if exudate stain is noted; this may indicate the presence of moisture which may lead to bacterial growth.
3 Elevate extremity to prevent oedema.

Topical Antibiotics

1 Topical medications are used to cover burn areas and to reduce the number of organisms.
2 They are applied directly to the burn area as ointments, creams or solutions, or they may be incorporated in single-layer dressings.

3 Usually these dressings are held in place by a single layer of stretch bandage or by net tube dressings.
4 When the patient is lying, fluffy absorbent dressings or pads are placed on the bed where the burn area will make contact.
5 Desired characteristics in a topical antibiotic:
   a. Ability to diffuse through the wound.
   b. Nontoxic and noninjurious to body tissue.
   c. Inexpensive, pleasant to use, odourless, or has pleasant odour.
   d. Will not cause resistant strains of pathogenic organisms to develop.
6 To date there is no 'ideal' topical antibiotic.

Sulfamylon Acetate (p-aminomethylbenzene–sulphonamide acetate)

Advantages and Mode of Action

1 Burn area is treated with this antibiotic agent because it will penetrate the eschar (slough) to reduce the number of infecting organisms.
2 In cream form, mafenide acetate diffuses rapidly through the burned skin and is relatively nontoxic.

Disadvantages

1 Causes a burning pain within $\frac{1}{2}$ hour following application.
2 Has a tendency to cake; tub bathing permits easy removal.
3 Inhibits carbonic anhydrase activity in the renal tubules and may cause metabolic acidosis.
4 Usually not recommended for patients with pulmonary disease since they cannot use respiratory mechanism sufficiently to maintain acid-base balance in most instances.
5 Some patients are allergic to sulfa drugs.

GUIDELINES: Application of Sulfamylon Ointment

Equipment

Sulfamylon Acetate cream
Sterile gloves
Sterile scissors
Sterile forceps

Nonadherent absorbent pads
Fine mesh gauze strips
Stretch gauze bandage.

Procedure

Nursing Action	Reason
1 Administer analgesic as prescribed.	1 To relieve burning pain which occurs during first few minutes following application of Sulfamylon cream.
2 Cleanse burn areas by most feasible method: a. Hubbard tub.	2 To facilitate removal of necrotic tissue and at the same time provide relaxation for the patient.

Nursing Action	Reason
b. Bathtub.	
c. Shower.	
d. Local bathing in bed with non-irritating cleansing solutions.	
3 Place nonadherent absorbent pad under patient's burned area.	3 To absorb exudate and provide a means of holding cream in contact with burn area.
4 Remove loose or necrotic tissue from wound using a sterile forceps and scissors; may be done during tub bathing.	4 To permit Sulfamylon cream to contact viable tissue and to eliminate pressure areas where dried and dead tissue accumulate.
5 Apply a layer of Sulfamylon cream (2–4 mm) to the burned area, using a sterile gloved hand.	5 To provide adequate contact via diffusion through avascular burn tissue.
6 Cover creamed areas with a single layer of fine mesh gauze; fasten with single-layer stretch gauze bandage. (Varies with clinics; some do not use this.)	6 To maintain contact with tissue—cream often rolls or slides off burned areas because of exudate.
7 Reapply Sulfamylon cream when absorbed; for first 2 to 3 days this may be required every 4–5 hours.	7 To maintain constant action of ointment on burn area.
8 Assess for any unusual reaction such as increased redness, increase in pulse or respiration.	8 To detect allergic manifestations.
9 Place patient in Hubbard bath once or twice every 24 hours (or as suggested by doctor).	9 To remove dressings and loosen tissue. To permit motion of joints. To provide comfort and relaxation for the patient.
10 Reapply Sulfamylon.	
11 Check electrolytes.	11 To rule out metabolic acidosis or respiratory alkalosis.

Silver Sulfadiazine 1% (Flamazine)

In an ointment base.

Advantages and Mode of Action

1 Chlorides of the body are not readily precipitated, as with silver nitrate. Therefore no electrolyte abnormality occurs and no acidosis develops.
2 Applied as a cream with a spatula or in impregnated gauze.
3 Little pain experienced with application of cream.
4 Viscous dressings are easily and painlessly removed.
5 Silver sulfadiazine is odourless.
6 Action occurs by oligodynamic action (active in minute quantities) of silver and is dependent upon chloride and other anions in the wound exudate.
7 It utulizes the special antibacterial action of sulphonamide; it is particularly

effective against infections due to gram-negative and gram-positive micro-organisms and to *Candida albicans*.

8　It can be bactericidal up to 48 hours; however, when wounds are not clean, dressings are changed 2–3 times daily.

Disadvantages

1　Some patients develop skin rash, probably due to sensitivity to sulphonamides.
2　When dressings are removed, they often have a grey-green appearance—this does not necessarily mean a gross infection.
3　Because sulfa drugs are known to increase possibility of kernicterus, silver sulfadiazine should not be used on infants through the first month of life or on pregnant women near term.
4　If topical proteolytic enzymes are used in debriding, silver sulfadiazine may inactivate them.

Mode of Application

1　Silver sulfadiazine can be applied directly to the burn wound, spread thinly, 2–4 mm, and left exposed; wound should be so covered that no part is visible.
2　Some surgeons prefer that after ointment or cream is applied, it should be covered with a single layer of mesh gauze.
3　Reapply as it rubs off; if occlusive dressings are used, change every 48 hours.

Silver Nitrate (0.5%) Solution

Being used less because of its disadvantages.

Advantages and Mode of Action

1　Silver nitrate is a bacteriostatic chemical and is effective in reducing colonization.
　a. Above 1% produces tissue necrosis.
　b. Below 0.5% solution is ineffective as an antiseptic.
2　Cap, gown and mask are not required.
3　An effective method for treating large numbers of burns, as during war; is relatively inexpensive.
4　Several layers of 4-ply gauze dressings *must be thoroughly wet every 2–4 hours with silver nitrate solution* to be effective. It is held close to the wound by stretch bandage or net tube dressings.
5　Silver nitrate can be used over grafted areas and donor sites as well as burn surfaces.

Disadvantages

1　Since silver nitrate solution only penetrates 1–2 mm of burn eschar, only surface contaminants can be controlled.
2　The wound must be completely free of oil or grease for silver nitrate solution to be effective.
3　Hyponatraemia (loss of sodium ions), hypokalaemia (loss of potassium ions) and hypochloraemia (loss of chlorine ions) may occur. (For this reason, should not be used for children.)
4　Frequent blood samples are required to determine sodium, potassium and calcium ion levels.

5 It is necessary to replace electrolytes that are lost.
6 Methaemoglobinaemia (a modified form of oxyhaemoglobin) may be caused due to the reduction of nitrates to nitrites, resulting in cyanosis.
7 Silver nitrate turns black in sunlight.
  a. Clothes, hands, floor, etc., are stained black.
  b. Gloves must be worn by the nurse and assistants.

Gentamicin Sulphate (Garamycin cream) 0.1%

Advantages and Mode of Action

1 Useful against a wide variety of gram-negative and gram-positive organisms. (Even effective against *Providenica stuartii.*)
2 Application and use are similar to Sulfamylon acetate (see p. 370).
3 Ointment spreads easily and tends to become invisible.
4 No pain is associated with this cream.

Disadvantages

1 Since this drug has a tendency to promote the emergence of gentamicin-resistant organisms that may spread to other patients in the burn unit, it is usually reserved for life-threatening situations.
2 Is nephrotoxic—monitor creatinine levels.

Povidone-iodine Ointment 10% and Betadine Solution

Advantages

1 This agent appears to be effective against a wide variety of gram-negative and gram-positive organisms as well as yeasts, fungi and viruses.
2 It can be applied as an ointment (similar to Sulfamylon), the solution can be sprayed on, or it can be incorporated into mesh gauze dressings.
3 Usually the dressings are changed every 6 hours, during tub bathing; however, it may be more convenient to merely remove outer dressings and rewet inner layer of dressings with Betadine solution.

Disadvantages

1 This agent tends to cause crusting—this may be a help in some situations, a hindrance in others.
2 Materials may be stained, but stain can be removed by laundering immediately.
3 Some stinging is noted by patients, but it soon disappears.
4 Some patients are allergic to iodine preparations.

SKIN GRAFTING OF BURN SITE

Removal of Eschar

This dead tissue is removed in preparation for skin grafting as soon as is feasible in the overall plan for grafting. Grafting is usually done after 14 days.

Effective Methods

1 Surgical excision.

2   Change dry dressings every 2 days; light anaesthesia may be necessary to remove loose tissue; scissors are used to cut strands that hold eschar.
3   Bathe daily in a Hubbard tank; use scissors and forceps to debride small areas daily.
4   Apply wet soaks every 4 hours (saline) using coarse mesh gauze; frequent removal of gauze also facilitates pulling away of dead tissue.
5   Proteolytic enzymes with saline to dissolve eschar.

Autografts

Autografts are skin grafts taken from an uninjured part of the patient's body and applied elsewhere on his body, as needed.

Types of Autografts (Fig. 8.11)

Split thickness (skin between 0.010–0.035 in thick—useful for burn areas)

Free—a segment of skin completely removed from one area and transferred to the desired grafting area, where it will be nourished by the capillary ingrowth from the granulating bed.

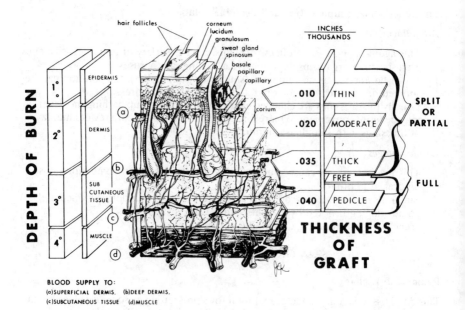

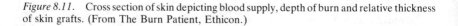

Figure 8.11.   Cross section of skin depicting blood supply, depth of burn and relative thickness of skin grafts. (From The Burn Patient, Ethicon.)

Full Thickness (greater than 0.035 in)

Pedicle graft—a graft of skin in which three sides are freed from the donor site but the fourth remains attached, so that blood supply is maintained.

Application of Autograft

1   Grafting may be done in two or more stages depending upon readiness of burn surface and condition of patient.
    a. Priority areas in skin coverage (in order):
       (1) Hands.
       (2) Face.
       (3) Neck.
       (4) Areas of motion: elbows, axillae, knees, lower leg.
    b. These areas should be grafted as soon as possible to lessen scarring and contracture formation.
2   Grafting is done in the operating room under aseptic conditions.

Meshing of Grafts (Use of Device such as Zimmer Mesher)

1   Slits can be cut in graft before application to allow skin to be 'stretched'—i.e., to cover an area larger than that from which it was taken.
2   This permits good drainage and prevents collection of fluid under graft.

Care of Postgraft Recipient Site

Methods of Initial Care

1   *Exposure method.*
    a. Note the progress of vascularization.
       Permits detection of haematomas and seromas—when such formations are present, graft will not take unless fluid is released and grafts are sutured.
    b. Roll out the graft using a sterile cotton applicator stick to flatten graft and permit fluid to escape.
    c. Apply saline compresses for short intervals every 2–3 hours—this can provide the high humidity required for a graft to take.
    d. Immobilize the grafted area for 2–3 days by use of sand bags, trochanter rolls, etc.
2   *Occlusive dressing method.*
    a. Effective for young children or older persons who are irrational or unco-operative.
    b. Compression is desirable to lessen the formation of fluid beneath the grafts.
    c. Pressure dressings of the preformed variety are most effective.
       (1) Single layer of commercially prepared nylon fabric.
       (2) Preformed gauze pads.
       (3) Fluffed gauze.
    d. These dressings are removed after 3–5 days in some clinics. In other clinics they are removed daily—using saline during careful removal and reapplication of saline-soaked gauze.

Use of Hubbard Tank

1   About fourth day in exposure method.
2   Removal of occlusive dressings is facilitated when patient is submerged.
    a. Stimulates circulation.
    b. Keeps graft area clean.

Care when Patient is Ambulatory

1   Have patient wear elastic rubberized bandages on lower extremities over graft sites for 3 months.
    a. Prevents epithelium breakdown.
    b. Eliminates burning sensation often felt when no supporting bandage is used.
2   Provide diversional, recreational or occupational therapy.
3   Healed graft sites may require use of elastic garments (Jobst) to prevent hypertrophic scarring.

Allografts (Homografts)

An *allograft* is a graft of skin taken from a person other than the burn victim and applied to a burn wound temporarily (a cadaver is most common source).

A *xenograft* or *heterograft* is a segment of skin taken from an animal such as a pig or dog. It is useful in preparing debrided area for grafting and is really a biological dressing.

Donor Criteria

1   Skin colour unimportant since it is only a temporary graft.
2   Donor should be an adult free of infection.

Purpose

1   Closes wound temporarily.
2   Prevents fluid and protein loss.
3   Reduces risk of infection.
4   Reduces pain.

Clinical Procedure

Graft is replaced about every 3 days; otherwise, there is too much trauma and bleeding when the homograft is pulled away.

Discharge Planning and Health Teaching

1   Often a patient who has been critically ill with burns has difficulty adjusting to the fact that he is improving; he may still believe he is going to die from his burns and that he actually is being discharged from the hospital to go home to die.
    a. To overcome this feeling, the nurse must stress the positive, healthy future of the patient. Be hopeful but realistic in helping patient accept a new self-image.
    b. Permit the patient to take brief trips out of the hospital before his discharge—car rides, etc.

c. Prepare family for his coming home—particularly those who haven't seen his changed appearance.

d. Assist the family in making a transition in their feelings about the patient; they may have expected and adjusted to the fact that the patient was going to die. Now he is coming home to live. They must encourage him to become more and more independent.

2 Develop a plan with the family for helping the patient to become active and interested in a vocation; to prepare to return to work; to make social adjustments. Be alert to need for psychological counselling.

3 Explore the possibility of overcoming scarring and contracture formation by using special formed splints and elastic supports where effective—e.g., for hand and fingers. (Available for whole body.)

4 Explain to the family the gamut of activities the patient can perform, and also inform them of activities for which he will need assistance.

5 Know community resources which will assist with his adjustment; community nursing service agencies may have a physiotherapist and medical social worker in the area where the patient lives.

6 Provide written instructions to the patient on skin care, wound care, exercises prescribed, use of elastic garments and splints; what to do for common problems such as blisters, discoloration, itching, flaking of skin.

NOTE: When patients go home, they most often report difficulty sleeping, dreaming about reliving the burn injury, fearing return to work or other activity that may have been involved with the burn injury. They often become very fire-safety conscious. There may be expressions of boredom (particularly in patients who cannot return to work for a while); difficulty resuming sexual activity; feeling out of control, i.e., living from one reconstructive procedure to the next, being unsure when they can resume control and direction of their own lives rather than allow the health professions to dictate this to them.

FURTHER READING

Books

Cason, J S (1981) The Treatment of Burns, Chapman & Hall

Cronin, E (1980) Contact Dermatitis, Churchill Livingstone

Fregart, S (1981) Manual of Contact Dermatitis, 2nd edition, Munksgaard

Macallan, E S and Jackson, I T (1971) Plastic Surgery and Burns Treatment, Heinemann Medical

Malten, K E, Nater, J P and Venketel, W G (1976) Patch-testing Guidelines, Dekker & van de Vegt

Murray, D (1981) The Anti-Acne Book, Arlington Pocket Books

Rook, A, Wilkinson, D S and Ebling, A (1979) A Textbook of Dermatology, 3rd edition, Blackwell Scientific

Sneddon, I B and Church, R E (1976) Practical Dermatology, 3rd edition, Edward Arnold

Wilkinson, D S (1977) Nursing and Management of Skin Diseases, 4th edition, Faber & Faber

Articles

Amann, L P (1981) The management of psoriasis, Nursing, 26: 1123–1125

Armstrong-Esher, C A (1981) Skin and hypersensitivity, Nursing, 26: 1152–1156

Chaplain, S (1981) Skin problems in the community, Nursing, 26: 1116–1118

Dencer, D (1980) Plastic surgery: result—a lip to be kissed with relish, Nursing Mirror, 151: 30–33

Evans, A J (1975) The modern treatment of burns, British Journal of Hospital Medicine, March, 287–298

Jeffcott, M (1981) Management of burns, Nursing, 26: 1126–1127

Lawrence, J C (1981) Burns: causes, management and consequences, Nursing, 26: 1123–1125

Martin, V (1981) Preventing hypertropic scarring: a burning issue, Nursing Mirror, 153: 32–33

Ryan, T J (1981) The handicap of skin diseases, Nursing, 26: 1144–1145

Stoughton, R D (1979) Topical antibiotics for acne vulgaris, Archives of Dermatology, 115: 486–489

Tring, F C (1981) Warts and their treatment, Nursing Times, 77: 1415–1417

Chapter 9

ALLERGY PROBLEMS

ALLERGIC REACTIONS

Definitions

1 *Antigen*—a substance that, when repeatedly in contact with the body, stimulates production of a counteracting substance, a globulin 'antibody'.

2 *Antibody*—a globulin produced by the lymphoid cells as a result of stimulation of these cells by an antigen; the antibody is capable of combining with the antigen in a very specific manner.

3 *Immunity*—a state of increased resistance to a particular substance.

  a. *Active immunization*—resistance brought about by the injection of an antigenic substance (e.g. tetanus toxoid).

  b. *Passive immunization*—resistance brought about by the transfer of antibody-containing serum from an immunized donor to a normal recipient (e.g. tetanus antitoxin).

4 *Allergic reactions*—a type of hypersensitivity resulting from the interaction between an antigen and an antibody.

Pharmacological Mediators of Immediate Hypersensitivity Reactions

1 *Histamine*—released from tissue mast cells by the interaction of an antigen and its corresponding antibody.
   a. Causes contraction of smooth muscle of bronchioles, uterus, intestines.
   b. Dilates and causes increased permeability of capillaries of skin and mucous membrane.
   c. Produces itching of skin and mucous membrane.
   d. Stimulates secretion of nasal, lacrimal, salivary and gastrointestinal glands.
   e. Lowers blood pressure.
2 *SRS-A*—slow reacting substance of anaphylaxis now referred to as a leucotriene. A lipidopeptide with powerful constricting action on bronchial smooth muscle. Probably a very important mediator in asthma.
3 *Bradykinin*—acts chiefly by increasing capillary permeability and contractility of smooth muscle.

There are many other mediators.

Hypersensitivity Reactions

Hypersensitivity is said to exist when the body reacts adversely against substances in the environment which elicit no response from most persons. This may, or may not, be due to antibody–antigen interaction.

Antibody–antigen interactions consist of (a) those that are protective and beneficial to the body ('immunity') and (b) those that are not always protective and beneficial to the body. They may cause tissue damage resulting in discomfort to the patient ('allergy').

Common Causes of Allergy

1 Inhaled allergens.
   a. Plant pollens—grasses, shrub and tree pollens.
   b. Moulds, fungi, spores, animal dander, house dust and the house dust mite.
2 Ingested allergens—cow's milk, egg white, fish, nuts, chocolate, certain fruits.
3 Contact allergens—contact dermatitis.

Delayed Hypersensitivity

1 Term for a reaction that reaches its peak 24–48 hours after an antigen is injected intradermally into a sensitized individual.
2 The reaction usually consists of erythema and induration.
3 Delayed hypersensitivity is mediated by sensitized 'T' (thymus-dependent) lymphocytes (not by immunoglobulins).
4 Example: tuberculin skin test.

Immunoglobulins

Antibodies that are formed by plasma cells (which are derived from lymphocytes) in response to an immunogenic stimulus comprise a group of serum proteins called *immunoglobulins*.

1 The abbreviation for immunoglobulin is Ig.
2 Antibodies combine with antigens in a 'lock and key style'.

3   There are five classes of immunoglobulins:
    a. IgM (gamma 'M')—a macromolecule; tends to stay in bloodstream and is primarily engaged in defence in intravascular compartment.
    b. IgG (gamma 'G')—most abundant. Readily diffuses into tissue spaces and crosses the placenta. Assists in combating infection.
    c. IgA (gamma 'A')—circulates in the blood, but its role here is uncertain; it is prominent in external secretions (saliva, tears) where it provides a primary defence mechanism.
    d. IgD—function has not yet been determined.
    e. IgE (gamma 'E')—responsible for most of the 'immediate types' of allergic reactions.

TESTS FOR ALLERGY AND IMMUNOTHERAPY (HYPOSENSITIZATION)

Immunotherapy is a procedure designed to increase a person's resistance to offending antigens by administration of small, gradually increasing amounts of a specific antigen over a period of time.

Skin Tests

1   Skin prick test—the skin is pricked with a needle through a drop of allergen containing solution.
2   Intracutaneous method—allergen is injected between the outermost layers of the skin.
3   Patch test—this is used in the diagnosis of allergy due to delayed type hypersensitivity.
4   Skin tests are also used as an aid in the diagnosis of active infection, e.g., the tuberculin test for tuberculosis, the Schick test for diphtheria.

Interpretation

1   A positive reaction—reddened, flushed area and a blanched weal at skin site appearing within minutes reaching maximal reaction between 15–20 min.
2   Systemic reactions may occur from a concentrated dose to a hypersensitized person *if the intracutaneous method is used.*
    a. Administer adrenaline and antihistamines.
    b. Give hydrocortisone, bronchodilators, if necessary.

Hyposensitization

1   This form of therapy consists of injections of dilute allergenic extracts of such substances as pollens, dusts, mould spores and insect venom.
2   It is thought that as amounts of injected substances are gradually increased, the body builds up a supply of blocking antibodies (mainly immunoglobulin G type—IgG). This is a theory which is yet to be proven.
3   When the patient comes into contact with allergens that previously caused allergic reactions, it may be that the blocking antibodies combine with the allergens in a way that reduces or prevents symptoms.

GUIDELINES: Skin Testing

Skin Testing consists of the introduction of an allergen into or on the skin surface to determine hypersensitivity.

Purpose

1   Assisting in the diagnosis of allergy.
2   Confirming the need for hyposensitization when the history is suggestive.

Methods and Equipment

1   Skin prick test—a drop of antigen is applied to the skin then a needle is used to prick the surface of the skin through the drop.
   Equipment: Sterile 25 gauge 16 mm needle—a separate needle for each test, biro or felt-tip pen to mark the sites, paper tissues.
   Advantage: Little risk of a general constitutional reaction.
   Disadvantage: Risk of misinterpretation if the allergens are not correctly standardized.
   Depends on normal skin response to histamine. For that reason a solution of histamine should be used as a positive control.
2   Intradermal—Injection of a small amount of antigen into the superficial layers of skin.
   Equipment: Tuberculin 1.0 ml syringes, felt-tip or biro pen to mark the sites, 25 gauge 16 mm needles, paper tissues. A separate syringe and needle is used for each antigen and its dilutions.
   Advantage: Slightly more accurate than prick test method.
   More dilute solutions of antigen are required.
   Disadvantage: There is a serous risk of systemic reactions.
3   Patch test—Application of test material either to skin or to skin immediately covered with a small gauze dressing (or gauze part of a Band-Aid).
   Advantage: Effective in cases involving contact hypersensitivity to topically applied substance, e.g., nickel, chromium, primula.
   Disadvantage: Not as accurate as other methods.

Interpretations of Skin Prick Testing and Intracutaneous Skin Testing Methods

1   Positive.
   a. Indicates IgE antibody response to previous contact with antigen.
   b. False positive reactions may occur with nonspecific histamine liberators sometimes present in certain allergen extracts, e.g., fish, shellfish.
2   Negative.
   a. Indicates antibodies have not been formed against the antigen.
   b. Patient is not reacting normally to histamine.
3   Suppressed reaction—may occur if the patient:
   a. Is on antihistamines.
   b. Feels faint or is cold.

Sites for Skin Prick Testing or Intracutaneous Testing

1 Volar or anterior surface of the upper third of the forearm approx. 10 cm (4 in) below the bend of the elbow.
2 The back, below top of the scapula, avoiding the spine. A useful site for children.

Procedure

1 Place tests approx. 5 cm (2 in) apart (to prevent results of one test from coalescing with those of another).
2 Avoid hairy area (will interfere with interpreting the results).
3 Avoid areas near bone or tendons or areas without adequate subcutaneous tissue.

Preparation of Patient

1 Explain to patient what is being done and why.
2 Provide adequate lighting.
3 Thoroughly cleanse testing area with alcohol or ether and allow the area to dry.

Patch Test

Technique

Apply test material directly to skin for purpose of producing a small area of allergic dermatitis, e.g., nickel, chromium, primula, plant oils, hair tonic, shaving cream. Either leave the area exposed or cover with a small lint dressing and adhesive or use a Band-Aid.

Reaction

1 Remove patch after 48 hours.
2 It is important to wait for 20–30 min to allow any unrelated reaction to subside. A true allergic reaction will persist for several days.
3 Observe reaction and describe:
     + Erythema.
    ++ Erythema, papules.
   +++ Erythema, papules, vesicles.
  ++++ Erythema, papules, vesicles and severe oedema.
4 Positive reactions often show an increase in severity in next 24 hours. It is important that the site is re-examined in 72 hours.
5 Record nature of sensitizing agents and reactions.

Skin Prick Testing

Technique

1 Mark each site where a skin test is to be performed using a biro or felt-tip pen. They should be spaced about 5 cm (2 in) apart (spacing is required to prevent the coalescing of one reaction with another).

2　Place a drop of glycerine-saline and at another site a drop of histamine solution on the skin (the glycerine-saline acts as a negative control, the histamine as a positive control).
3　Place a drop of each antigen to be tested at the other marked sites then with a separate needle for each test very gently prick the surface of the skin through each drop. (A separate needle is essential to eliminate the possibility of false positive recordings.)
4　When all the tests have been performed blot the whole area dry using absorbent paper tissues taking care not to smear the solutions.
5　Cover the arm, if possible, instructing the patient not to scratch the sites if they itch and wait 15–20 min before reading the results.
6　Record type of antigen used and the results in the following manner:
　　　－　No weal or flare.
　　　＋　Weal absent or slight. Erythema no more than 3 mm diameter.
　　＋＋　Weal not more than 3 mm diameter. Erythema not more than 5 mm.
　＋＋＋　Weal between 3 mm and 5 mm diameter, with erythema.
＋＋＋＋　Any larger reaction.

Intradermal Test

1　Limit number of intradermal tests to no more than 20.
2　Use sterile tuberculin syringe with graduations of one-hundredths of a millilitre.
3　Use a hypodermic needle, size 25 g × $^5/_8$ in, 16 mm.
4　Use a separate syringe and needle (preferably disposable) for each antigen.

Technique

1　Eject all air from syringe and needle. (Air injected will affect reading.)
2　Hold forearm with one hand and use thumb to stretch skin.
3　Hold syringe between thumb and forefinger and place plunger against heel of hand.
4　Position bevel upwards and place needle and syringe almost parallel along long axis of arm (with bevel upwards, needle can penetrate superficial layer of skin and antigen can be deposited directly under skin surface).
5　Depress needle into arm and advance until bevel just disappears into the epidermis.
6　Contract hand and advance plunger injecting amount necessary to raise a bleb of approx. 3 mm (0.01–0.05 ml).
7　Remove needle (transient bleeding is usually of no significance). Wait 15–20 min before reading results.
8　Record type of antigen used and the results as for skin prick testing.

ANAPHYLAXIS

Nursing Alert: With injection of allergenic extracts, the risk of systemic reaction is always present. Skin testing, particularly of the intradermal type, has resulted in systemic reactions.

Early Manifestations

1 Feeling of uneasiness or apprehension, weakness, perspiration, sneezing or nasal pruritus.
2 Generalized pruritus, urticaria, angioedema.
3 Dyspnoea, wheezing, dysphagia, vomiting, abdominal pain.
4 Pulse—may be rapid, weak, irregular or unobtainable.
5 Syncope or shock—may follow rapidly.
6 Possible urgency, faecal and urinary incontinence, convulsions and coma.

Treatment

Administer adrenalin—the pharmacologic antagonist of the action of chemical mediators on smooth muscle and other effector cells.

Immediate

Always have an emergency tray of drugs readily available.

1 Inject 0.3 ml of 1:1000 adrenaline subcutaneously into upper arm; gently massage site of injection.
2 Have hydrocortisone ready for injection.
3 Have antihistamine ready for injection.
4 Aminophylline ready when bronchospasm is a feature of the reaction.

If Reaction is not Reversed by Adrenaline

1 Vasopressors or volume expanders for hypotension.
2 Oxygen and tracheotomy pack for laryngeal obstruction.
3 Equipment necessary for performing cardio-pulmonary resuscitation.

Further Observations.

1 Evaluation of patient reaction and response to treatment.
2 Repeat adrenaline, if necessary.
3 Monitor blood pressure/pulse at regular intervals.
4 Assess pulmonary function.

RESPIRATORY HYPERSENSITIVITY

Allergic Rhinitis

Allergic rhinitis is induced by grass and tree pollens (hay fever), house dust, especially the house dust mite (*Dermatophagoides pteronyssinus*), animal danders, fungi and mould spores and other airborne allergens. The body reacts by releasing histamine and other pharmacological agents which produce the symptoms.

Classification of Seasonal Allergic Rhinitis

1 Spring—March to early May. Often caused by pollens of certain trees (birch, plane, oak).

2 Summer—May to September. Often caused by pollens of certain grasses (timothy) and sometimes by the mould *Alternaria*.
3 Autumn—September to November. Often caused by various moulds (e.g., *Cladosporium herbarum*) and fungi.

Clinical Manifestations

1 Rhinitis—leading to oedema, blocked nostrils.
2 Nasal mucous membranes—itch, burn and secrete thin, irritating discharge.
3 Sneezing—violent paroxysms.
4 Eyes—red, burning, lacrimating.

Sensitivity Tests

Skin tests confirm patient's hypersensitivity to causative allergen.

Treatment

1 Avoid causative allergen if possible.
2 Use antihistamines; this will not only control symptoms in four out of five patients but will also have an atropine-like drying effect.
3 Hyposensitization, when appropriate.
4 Local disodium cromoglycate (Lomusol, Rynacrom) or corticosteroids (beclomethasone diproprionate (Beconase)) when antihistamines are ineffective or cause too many side effects; these act by reducing responsiveness of mucous membranes to histamine.

Bronchial Asthma

Bronchial asthma manifests itself clinically by intermittent episodes of wheezing and dyspnoea; it is always associated with bronchial hyper-reactivity and allergies are often an important cause. Bronchial asthma differs from other causes of wheeze in that it is reversible either with time or as a result of treatment.

Incidence

Asthma affects approximately 3–4% of the population and represents about 25% of chronic diseases of childhood.

Pathophysiology

1 Antigen–antibody reaction.
   a. Susceptible individuals form abnormally large amounts of IgE when exposed to certain allergens.
   b. This immunoglobulin (IgE) fixes itself to the mast cells of the bronchial mucosa.
   c. When the individual is exposed to the appropriate allergen, it combines with cell-bound IgE molecules, causing the mast cell to degranulate and release chemical mediators.
   d. These chemical mediators, primarily histamine and leucotrienes (formerly

known as SRS-A, slow reacting substance of anaphylaxis) are thought to produce bronchospasm.
2 Infections, i.e., common cold, sinusitis.
3 Autonomic nerves probably stimulated by nonspecific triggers, e.g., exercise, cold, smoke, laughter, fumes, coughing.

Clinical manifestations.

1 Can be symptom-free periods between attacks (episodic asthma).
2 During an attack of asthma, the amount of airway obstruction determines the degree of severity of symptoms.
   a. During early or mild episodes—cough or mild chest tightness.
   b. As asthmatic episodes become more severe—wheezing, coughing, shortness of breath.
   c. Dyspnoea may become apparent, inspiratory wheezing and use of accessory respiratory muscles.
   d. As severity of attack increases, the patient becomes more anxious, restless and apprehensive.
   e. A fatigue state may follow—respirations are less laboured and there is less audible wheezing.
   f. This may lead to respiratory failure with hypercapnia, respiratory acidosis and hypoxaemia.

Diagnosis

1 Generalized rhonchi on auscultation.
2 Obstruction to airflow as shown by spirometry.
3 Reversal of obstruction after administration of a bronchodilator.
4 Sputum eosinophilia.

Classification

Extrinsic Bronchial Asthma

1 Cause.
   a. Hypersensitivity reaction to inhalant allergens.
   b. Mediated by immunoglobulin E (IgE-mediated).
2 Diagnosis
   a. Correlation with exposure to aeroallergens (and less commonly ingestants).
   b. Positive skin tests.
3 Major inhalant allergens, e.g., house dust mite, pollens, animal danders, mould spores.
4 Prognosis.
   Favourable, with avoidance of offending allergens; good response to bronchodilators and specific therapy.

Intrinsic Bronchial Asthma

1 Cause.
   a. Unknown.
   b. Infection.

    c. Skin tests of common inhalant antigens and foods are usually negative (non-IgE-mediated).
2 Occurrence.
    After age 35, most commonly in women.
3 Prognosis.
    a. Remission of intrinsic asthma is variable.
    b. Control may be difficult.

Mixed Asthma

Immediate type appears to combine allergic reaction and infection.

Aspirin-induced Asthma (ASA Sensitive)

A type of intrinsic asthma induced by ingestion of aspirin and related compounds.

1 Clinical manifestations spread over a period of time have been described as a 'triad':
    a. Bronchial asthma.
    b. Nasal polyposis.
    c. Severe reactions to aspirin.
2 Onset of symptoms after aspirin ingestion (20 min to 2 hours).
    a. Watery rhinorrhoea, followed by marked flushing of upper part of body.
    b. Nausea, vomiting.
    c. Wheezing, dyspnoea and cyanosis.

Precipitating Factors

Any one of these may trigger an asthmatic attack in person with intrinsic bronchial asthma.

1 Strong odours (fumes): turpentine, paints, chemicals, sprays, heavily scented flowers, perfumes, tobacco smoke.
2 Cold air; sudden barometric changes.
3 Air pollutants.
4 Emotion-triggering situations.

Popular Misconceptions in Asthma

1 That there are exclusive causes of asthma.
2 That most people grow out of asthma.
3 Longstanding asthma leads to permanent damage to the lungs or heart.
4 The dangers of aerosols.
5 Asthma is never fatal.

Medical and Nursing Therapeutic Management

Objective

To achieve sufficient control of symptoms to prevent physical and psychological incapacitation.

1 Treatment must be individualized.
2 Therapy includes concern not only for the physical condition of the person but also for his psychosocial situation and his environment.
3 There is no cure for asthma, but present-day treatment regimes can improve and control the disease.
4 See also Management of the Patient with an Allergy.

Prevention

1 Avoid causative allergens when possible.
2 Immunotherapy (hyposensitization) when applicable—in practice very seldom.
3 Avoid any medications that may aggravate asthma.

Treatment

Environmental Control

1 Control the environment as much as possible to reduce exposure to relevant allergens.
   a. In bedroom carry out regular vacuum cleaning and damp dusting, remove feather pillows and dust collecting articles.
   b. Exclude house pets, to eliminate dander.
   c. Exclude plants, to eliminate mould spores.

Acute Severe Asthma (Status Asthmaticus)

Acute severe asthma is severe bronchial asthma in which the patient has failed to respond to his usual medication. This is a medical emergency and requires rapid therapeutic measures.

Contributing Factors

1 Infection.
2 Dehydration.
3 Overuse of sedation.

Clinical Manifestations

1 Severe dyspnoea with wheeze, but in the late stage no wheeze may be audible.
2 Hypoxia causes changes in the central nervous system: Fatigue, headache, irritability, dizziness, impaired mental functioning.
3 With continued carbon dioxide retention: Muscle twitching, somnolence, flapping tremour.
4 Tachycardia, elevated blood pressure.
5 At very low oxygen levels and high carbon dioxide levels, sudden hypotension may occur.
6 Heart failure.

Table 9.1.   Drugs Used in the Treatment of Asthma, Rhinitis and Allergic Conjunctivitis

Drug	Action	Side-effects
1 Bronchodilators a. Selective β_2 adrenergic drugs, e.g., salbutamol (Ventolin), terbutaline (Bricanyl)	Bronchodilation. Given by aerosol and side-effects are few Orally because blood levels have to be adequate to be effective, may cause side-effects May be given intravenously, as an infusion, or as a wet aerosol	Tremor, tachycardia
b. Atropine-like, e.g., orciprenaline (Alupent), ipratropiumbromide (Atrovent)	Blocks cholinergic receptor sites Bronchodilation is of slow onset, but lasts longer than adrenaline or isoprenaline	Dryness of mouth Urinary retention Contraindiction: in narrow angle glaucoma
2 Catecholamines, e.g., adrenaline	Stimulates alpha- and beta-adrenergic receptors of autonomic nervous system It has short duration of action Given as subcutaneous injection. A 1:1000 (1 mg/ml) solution is used and 0·3 ml injected at $\frac{1}{2}$-hourly intervals	Anxiety, tremor, palpitation, tachycardia and arrhythmia
3 Xanthines, e.g., theophylline (Ronaphyllin, Nuelin), aminophylline (Phyllocontin)	Broncho and vasodilator Given orally, the measurement of drug concentration levels in the serum is necessary to ensure that it is within 'therapeutic range'	May cause severe gastric irritation, nausea, vomiting, cardiac arrythmias, epilepsy
4 Sodium cromoglycate bronchial inhalation (Intal), for nasal inhalation (Lomusol) and for the eyes (Opticrom)	Sodium cromoglycate inhibits the release from sensitized cells of mediators of the allergic reaction	Occasional irritation of the throat and trachea may occur when taking Intal in powder form
5 Antihistamines Ethanolamines (e.g., Dramamine) Alkylamines (e.g., Piriton) Phenothiazines (e.g., Phenergan, Vallergan)	Antagonizes the main actions of histamine in the body, probably by occupying the receptor sites in the effector cells to the exclusion of histamine; they do not prevent the production of histamine	Sedation with the inability to concentrate, lassitude, hypotension, muscular weakness. Sedative effects when they occur may diminish after a few days Other side-effects include gastrointestinal disturbances, headaches, blurred vision, tinnitus, elation or

(continued)

Table 9.1 (*cont.*)

Drug	Action	Side-effects
		depression, dryness of the mouth, difficulty in micturition
6 Corticosteroids a. Systemic, e.g., prednisone, prednisoline, hydro-cortisone	No clear idea how these drugs benefit asthmatics. Thought to influence the responsiveness of bronchial β-adrenoreceptors and thus modifying broncho-motor tone May also inhibit prosta-glandin biosynthesis	High doses given for long periods cause weight gain, fluid retention, diabetes mellitus, hypertension, osteoporosis, proximal myopathy, hypokalaemia, easy bruising of skin, adrenal suppression, growth retardation in children, may mask some signs of infection Abrupt withdrawal of oral corticosteroids may pre-cipitate acute adrenal insufficiency
b. Topical, e.g., beclomethasone dipropionate (Beconase, Becotide)	As above Beclomethasone dipropion-ate is rapidly destroyed in the gut and therefore causes no side-effects due to lack of systemic absorption	Inhaled steroids have been known to cause oro-pharyngeal thrush and hoarseness of the voice Beconase may cause epistaxis

Treatment

Requires team effort—chest doctor, anaesthetist, physiotherapist and intensive care nursing.

1 Careful monitoring of pH, P_{CO_2}, P_{O_2}, repeatedly, in order to evaluate serially the changes in gas exchange and the patient's response to therapy.

NOTE: In early acute severe asthma, a low P_{O_2} is followed by increased respiratory effort; this leads to low P_{CO_2} (hyperventilation). Then follow fatigue, reduced ventilation and increasing P_{CO_2}.

Nursing Alert: In acute severe asthma the return to a normal or increasing P_{CO_2} does not necessarily mean the asthmatic patient is improving—it may mean a fatigue state which develops just before the patient slips into respiratory failure.

2   Correction of derangement of blood gases (hypoxaemia) and haemoconcentration.
3   Rapid mobilization and removal of bronchial and bronchiolar secretions.
   a. Provide adequate hydration orally and intravenously and use humidified oxygen.
   b. Remove secretions by coughing, suctioning or bronchoscopy.

NOTE: These patients must never be sedated.

MANAGEMENT OF THE PERSON WITH AN ALLERGY

Objectives

1   To assist the patient in recognizing the importance of avoiding offending antigens whenever possible.
2   To make sure that the patient understands how the medication he/she is taking acts, and therefore why it is important that they be taken strictly as instructed.

Measures to Control the Environment

Respiratory Allergies

Encourage the patient to modify his environment as much as he can to avoid causative allergens.

Dietary Allergies

Advise the patient as follows:

1   Recognize the difficulties in trying to determine which foods cause allergic reactions.
2   Develop a pattern of eliminating a certain food for a period of time.
   a. Keep a diary, indicating when food was eliminated from the diet.
   b. Record any allergic reactions or the fact that none occurred.
3   Begin with those foods commonly found to cause reactions—nuts, chocolate, milk, strawberries, eggs, etc.
4   Remember to note contents of prepared foods, canned foods, etc., for the specific ingredients one may wish to avoid.
5   In a restaurant, order those foods which are certain not to include the offending ingredients.

NOTE: Foods are considered a rare cause of respiratory allergic symptoms.

Contact Allergies

Instruct patient as follows:

1   Exert extra effort to avoid household items likely to bring on allergic reactions.
   a. Use gloves to avoid skin contact with detergents, fabric dyes, strong soap powders, etc.

b. Use liquid soaps rather than granules that might permeate the air breathed.
2 Avoid cosmetics unless they are known to be hypoallergenic.
3 Do not rub or scratch itchy skin. (Mild doses of tranquillizers may be necessary if this will assist the patient in such control.)
4 Eliminate items of clothing that irritate the skin, such as those made of wool or nylon. Note that permanent press cottons may be a cause of dermatitis.
5 Avoid overexertion, which causes perspiration and itchiness.

Administration of Medications

1 Warn patients that it is dangerous to drive or use machinery during the first few days of antihistamine therapy since these medications often cause drowsiness. If drowsiness persists either the dosage or type of drug used will need to be changed.
2 Nasal decongestants should not be used repeatedly. They have an unpleasant rebound effect which means that addiction for the sake of relief is a common feature.
3 Inhaled Intal (either in powder form for asthma, liquid form for nose (Lomusol), liquid form for eyes (Opticrom)) or inhaled steroids (Becotide), because they are thought to stabilize mast cells, must be taken prophylactically. For that reason, if treatment is prescribed to be taken four times a day this must be adhered to even if the patient is feeling unwell.
4 Inhaled bronchodilators (Ventolin, Bricanyl) have a recommended dose which should not be exceeded. Patients should be advised that if they do need to take more than the prescribed dose they either need more treatment or current treatment is not being effective, in which case they need to consult their doctor.
5 If taking oral corticosteroids, it is important that the patient carries a steroid card detailing current dosage and that if there is a need to increase the dosage due to infection or at time of an operation, this be done under medical supervision. Similarly if the dosage is being reduced it must be done under supervision.

As with all drugs these must be kept out of the reach of children.

FURTHER READING

Books

Clark, T J H and Godfrey, S (Eds) (1979) Asthma, Chapman & Hall
Collins, J V (1979) Clinical Lung Function Tests, A Synopsis of Chest Disease, J Wright & Sons Ltd
Herbert, W J and Wilkinson, P G (Eds) (1971) A Dictionary of Immunology, Blackwell Scientific Publications
Kusemko, J A (Ed) (1976) Asthma in Children, Pitman Medical
Lane, D J and Storr, A (1979) Asthma. The Facts, Oxford Medical Publications
Mygind, N (1978) Nasal Allergy, Oxford Medical Publications
Rogers, H J, Spector, R G and Trounce, J R (1981) Respiratory System, A Textbook of Clinical Pharmacology, Hodder & Stoughton
Roitt, I (1977) Hypersensitivity, Essential Immunology, Blackwell Scientific Publications
Taussig, M J (1979) Hypersensitivity, Processes in Pathology, Blackwell Scientific Publications

Articles

Brostoff, J (1978) Hay fever, The Practitioner, 220: 532–538

Easty, D L (1978) Allergic disorders of the eye, The Practitioner, 220: 581–590

Morris-Owen, R M (1978) Asthma, The Practitioner, 220: 575–579

Pepys, J (1978) Hypersensitivity diseases of the lung due to extrensic agents, The Practitioner, 220: 541–550

Renwick Vickers, H (1975) Skin diseases: Dermatitis, Medicine, 33 (2): 1949–1957

Verrier Jones, R (1978) Allergic rhinitis in childhood, The Practitioner, 220: 553–558

Walker-Smith J A (1978) Gastroentistinal allergy, The Practitioner, 220: 562–573

INDEX

The Index covers all three volumes of *The Lippincott Manual of Medical-Surgical Nursing*. The figures printed in **bold** type before each entry or group of entries indicate the volume in which that page number or numbers will be found. The page numbers in italic indicate a figure, and page numbers followed by 't' indicate a table.